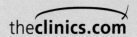

RADIOLOGIC CLINICS

OF NORTH AMERICA

Emergency Cross-Sectional Imaging

Guest Editors

VIKRAM S. DOGRA, MD

SHWETA BHATT, MD

May 2007 • Volume 45 • Number 3

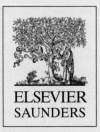

ELSEVIER
SAUNDERS

An imprint of Elsevier, Inc
PHILADELPHIA LONDON TORONTO MONTREAL SYDNEY TOKYO

W.B. SAUNDERS COMPANY

A Division of Elsevier Inc.

1600 John F. Kennedy Boulevard • Suite 1800 • Philadelphia, Pennsylvania 19103-2899

http://www.theclinics.com

RADIOLOGIC CLINICS OF NORTH AMERICA Volume 45, Number 3
May 2007 ISSN 0033-8389, ISBN-13: 978-1-4160-4364-5; ISBN-10: 1-4160-4364-0

Editor: Barton Dudlick

Reprints: For copies of 100 or more, of articles in this publication, please contact the Commercial Reprints Department, Elsevier Inc., 360 Park Avenue South, New York, New York 10010-1710. Tel.: (+1) 212-633-3813; Fax: (+1) 212-462-1935; E-mail: reprints@elsevier.com.

The ideas and opinions expressed in *Radiologic Clinics of North America* do not necessarily reflect those of the Publisher does not assume any responsibility for any injury and/or damage to persons or property arising out of or related to any use of the material contained in this periodical. The reader is advised to check the appropriate medical literature and the product information currently provided by the manufacturer of each drug to be administered to verify the dosage, the method and duration of administration, or contraindications, It is the responsibility of the treating physician or other health care professional, relying on independent experience and knowledge of the patient, to determine drug dosages and the best treatment for the patient. Mention of any product in this issue should not be construed as endorsement by the contributiors, editors, or the Publisher of the productor manufacturers' claims.

Radiologic Clinics of North America (ISSN 0033-8389) is published bimonthly in January, March, May, July, September, and November by Elsevier Inc., 360 Park Avenue South, New York, NY 10010-1710. Business and editorial offices: 1600 John F. Kenedy Boulevard, Suite 1800, Philadelphia, Pennsylvania 19103-2899. Customer Service Office: 6277 Sea Harbor Drive, Orlando, FL 32887-4800. Periodicals postage paid at New York, NY, and additional mailing offices. Subscription prices are USD 259 per year for US individuals, USD 385 per year for US institutions, USD 127 per year for US students and residents, USD 303 per year for Canadian individuals, USD 473 per year of Canadian institutions, USD 352 per year for international individuals, USD 473 per year for international institutions, and USD 171 per year for Canadian and foreign students/residents. To receive student and resident rate, orders must be accompanied by name of affiliated institution, date of term, and the signature of program/residency coordinatior on institution letterhead. Orders will be billed at individual rate until proof of status is received. Foreign air speed delivery is included in all Clinics subscriptionprices. All prices are subject to change without notice. **POSTMASTER:** Send address changes to *Radiologic Clinics of North America,* Elsevier Periodicals Customer Service, 6277 Sea Harbor Drive, Orlando, FL 32887-4800. **Customer Service: 1-800-654-2452 (US). From outside of the US, call (+1) 407-345-4000.**

Radiologic Clinics of North America also published in Greek Paschalidis Medical Publications, Athens, Greece.

Radiologic Clinics of North America is covered in *Index Medicus, EMBASE/Excerpta Medica, Current Contents/Life Sciences, Current Contents/Clinical Medicine, RSNA Index to Imaging Literature, BIOSIS, Science Citation Index,* and *ISI/BIOMED.*

Printed in the United States of America.

EMERGENCY CROSS-SECTIONAL IMAGING

GUEST EDITORS

VIKRAM S. DOGRA, MD
Professor of Radiology, Urology, and Biomedical
Engineering; Associate Chair of Education and
Research; Director of Ultrasound; Director of
Radiology Residency, Department of Imaging
Sciences, University of Rochester Medical Center,
University of Rochester School of Medicine,
Rochester, New York

SHWETA BHATT, MD
Instructor in Radiology, Department of Imaging
Sciences, University of Rochester Medical Center,
University of Rochester School of Medicine,
Rochester, New York

CONTRIBUTORS

JOONG MO AHN, MD
Associate Professor of Radiology, Department of
Radiology, Carver College of Medicine, University
of Iowa Hospitals and Clinics, Iowa City, Iowa

SHWETA BHATT, MD
Instructor in Radiology, Department of Imaging
Sciences, University of Rochester Medical Center,
University of Rochester School of Medicine,
Rochester, New York

JAE YOUNG BYUN, MD, PhD
Professor of Diagnostic Radiology, Department
of Diagnostic Radiology, Division of Abdominal
Radiology, Kangnam St. Mary's Hospital, The
Catholic University of Korea, Seoul, Republic
of Korea

ABRAHAM H. DACHMAN, MD
Professor, Department of Radiology, The
University of Chicago, Chicago, Illinois

M. ROBERT DEJONG, RDMS, RVT, RCDS
Ultrasound Technical Manager, Russell H. Morgan
Department of Radiology and Radiological
Science, Johns Hopkins University, School
of Medicine, Baltimore, Maryland

VIKRAM S. DOGRA, MD
Professor of Radiology, Urology, and Biomedical
Engineering; Associate Chair of Education and
Research; Director of Ultrasound; Director of
Radiology Residency, Department of Imaging
Sciences, University of Rochester Medical Center,
University of Rochester School of Medicine,
Rochester, New York

GEORGES Y. EL-KHOURY, MD
Professor of Radiology and Orthopedic Surgery,
and Director of Musculoskeletal Radiology,
Department of Radiology, Carver College of
Medicine, University of Iowa Hospitals and
Clinics, Iowa City, Iowa

HAMAD GHAZALE, MS, RDMS
Associate Professor and Director, Diagnostic
Medical Sonography Program, Rochester Institute
of Technology, Rochester, New York

ULRIKE M. HAMPER, MD, MBA
Professor of Radiology, Urology and Pathology,
and Director of Ultrasound, Russell H. Morgan
Department of Radiology and Radiological
Science, Johns Hopkins University, School
of Medicine, Baltimore, Maryland

GAURAV JINDAL, MD
Resident in Radiology, Department of Radiology,
University of Pennsylvania Medical Center,
Philadelphia, Pennsylvania

YOUNG JOON LEE, MD
Instructor of Diagnostic Radiology, Department
of Diagnostic Radiology, Division of Abdominal
Radiology, Kangnam St. Mary's Hospital, The
Catholic University of Korea, Seoul, Republic
of Korea

ANGELA D. LEVY, MD, COL, MC, USA
Associate Professor of Radiology and Chief,
Abdominal Imaging, Department of Radiology
and Radiologic Sciences, Uniformed Services
University of Health Sciences, Bethesda, Maryland

MARK E. LOCKHART, MD, MPH
Associate Professor, Department of Radiology,
University of Alabama at Birmingham,
Birmingham, Alabama

SOON NAM OH, MD, PhD
Instructor of Diagnostic Radiology, Department
of Diagnostic Radiology, Division of Abdominal
Radiology, Kangnam St. Mary's Hospital, The
Catholic University of Korea, Seoul, Republic
of Korea

DAVID PAUSHTER, MD
Professor, Department of Radiology, The
University of Chicago, Chicago, Illinois

ADNAN QALBANI, MD
Abdominal and Cross Sectional Imaging Fellow,
The University of Chicago, Chicago, Illinois

CHAD B. RABINOWITZ, MD
Department of Abdominal Imaging and
Interventional Radiology, Massachusetts General
Hospital, Boston, Massachusetts

PARVATI RAMCHANDANI, MD
Professor of Radiology and Chief, Section of
Genitourinary Radiology, Department of
Radiology, University of Pennsylvania Medical
Center, Philadelphia, Pennsylvania

SUNG EUN RHA, MD, PhD
Assistant Professor of Diagnostic Radiology,
Department of Diagnostic Radiology, Division
of Abdominal Radiology, Kangnam St. Mary's
Hospital, The Catholic University of Korea,
Seoul, Republic of Korea

MICHELLE L. ROBBIN, MD
Professor, Department of Radiology, University of
Alabama at Birmingham, Birmingham, Alabama

ALEXANDER V. RYBKIN, MD
Assistant Clinical Professor of Radiology,
Department of Radiology, University of California
San Francisco School of Medicine, San Francisco
General Hospital, San Francisco, California

NAEL SAAD, MBChB
Department of Imaging Sciences, University of
Rochester Medical Center, Rochester, New York

WAEL E.A. SAAD, MBBCh
Department of Imaging Sciences, University of
Rochester Medical Center, Rochester, New York

DUSHYANT V. SAHANI, MD
Director of CT and Assistant Professor of
Radiology, Department of Abdominal Imaging
and Interventional Radiology, Massachusetts
General Hospital, Boston, Massachusetts

ICHIRO SAKAMOTO, MD
Assistant Professor, Department of Radiology
and Radiation Biology, Nagasaki University
Graduate School of Biomedical Sciences,
Nagasaki, Japan

ANURADHA SAOKAR, MD
Department of Abdominal Imaging and
Interventional Radiology, Massachusetts General
Hospital, Boston, Massachusetts

LESLIE M. SCOUTT, MD
Professor of Radiology and Chief, Ultrasound
Section, Yale University, School of Medicine,
New Haven, Connecticut

EIJUN SUEYOSHI, MD
Research Assistant, Department of Radiology and
Radiation Biology, Nagasaki University
Graduate School of Biomedical Sciences,
Nagasaki, Japan

LIJUN TANG, MD
Associate Chief Physician (Radiologist),
Radiological Department of the First Affiliated
Hospital of Nanjing Medical University,
Nanjing, Japan

RUEDI F. THOENI, MD
Professor of Radiology, Department of Radiology,
University of California San Francisco School of
Medicine, San Francisco General Hospital,
San Francisco, California

MASATAKA UETANI, MD
Professor and Chairman, Department of
Radiology and Radiation Biology, Nagasaki
University Graduate School of Biomedical
Sciences, Nagasaki, Japan

DEHANG WANG, MD
Chief Physician (Radiologist), Radiological
Department of the First Affiliated Hospital of
Nanjing Medical University, Nanjing, Japan

THERESE M. WEBER, MD
Professor, Department of Radiology, University
of Alabama at Birmingham, Birmingham,
Alabama

TONGFU YU, MD
Associated Chief Physician (Radiologist),
Radiological Department of the First Affiliated
Hospital of Nanjing Medical University,
Nanjing, Japan

XIAOMEI ZHU, MD
Resident, Radiological Department of the First
Affiliated Hospital of Nanjing Medical University,
Nanjing, Japan

EMERGENCY CROSS-SECTIONAL IMAGING

Volume 45 • Number 3 • May 2007

Contents

Acute pancreatitis is a common disease with potentially serious outcomes. Multiple imaging modalities can be used to evaluate the disease process and its associated complications. Familiarity with the pathogenesis of this disease, indications for imaging, imaging protocols, staging systems, and the strengths and weaknesses of various modalities will help the radiologist optimize patient care.

The most common imaging modality used for diagnosis of aortic disease is CT, followed by transesophageal echocardiography, MRI, and aortography. If multiple imaging is performed, the initial imaging technique most frequently employed is computerized tomography. During the past decade, computed tomographic angiography (CTA) has become a standard non-invasive imaging modality for the depiction of vascular anatomy and pathology. The quality and speed of CTA examinations have increased dramatically as CT technology has evolved from-channel spiral CT systems to multichannel (4-, 8-, 10- and 16-slice) spiral CT system. The quality and speed of CTA is superior to other imaging modalities, and it is also cheaper and less invasive. CTA of the aorta has proven to be superior in diagnostic accuracy to conventional arteriography in several applications.

Recent advances in noninvasive imaging methods, such as CT and MR imaging, have replaced most of invasive angiographic procedures in the diagnosis of acquired aortic disease, decreasing the cost and morbidity of diagnosis. This article reviews and illustrates present MR imaging methods for evaluation of the aorta. Common diseases of the aorta also are discussed with a focus on their unique morphologic and functional features and characteristic MR imaging findings. Knowledge of pathologic conditions of common aortic diseases and proper MR imaging techniques enables accurate and time-efficient aortic evaluation.

State-of-the-art multidetector row CT (MDCT) technology has revolutionized abdominal imaging. The ability of CT to determine if bowel obstruction is present, to localize the obstructive site, to determine degree of obstruction, to diagnose the presence of closed-loop obstruction, and to identify ischemia or perforation of the involved bowel is well established. This article illustrates the usefulness of MDCT in the evaluation of small bowel obstruction and related conditions in adults and emphasizes the benefits of advanced CT applications.

Ultrasound is the initial imaging modality of choice when evaluating the upper extremity venous system. When sonographic findings are equivocal or nondiagnostic, particularly in evaluating the central deep veins, MR venography or catheter venography correlation may be helpful. Ultrasound provides an accurate, rapid, low-cost, portable, noninvasive method for screening, mapping, and surveillance of the upper extremity venous system.

Over the past 2 decades venous ultrasonography has become the standard primary imaging technique for the initial evaluation of patients for whom there is clinical suspicion of deep venous thrombosis (DVT) of the lower extremity veins. This article addresses the role of duplex ultrasonography and color Doppler ultrasonography in today's clinical practice for the evaluation of patients suspected of harboring a thrombus in their lower extremity veins. It reviews the clinical presentation and differential diagnoses, technique, and diagnostic criteria for acute and chronic DVT. In addition, it addresses the sonographic evaluation of venous insufficiency.

Ectopic pregnancy is a high-risk condition that occurs in 1.9% of reported pregnancies. Although the clinical triad of pain, bleeding, and amenorrhea is considered very specific for an ectopic pregnancy, ultrasound plays important role in detecting the exact location of the ectopic pregnancy and also in providing guidance for minimally invasive treatment. This article discusses the main sonographic features of ectopic pregnancy at various common and unusual locations. In addition, it provides insight into the role of hormonal markers in the diagnosis and management of ectopic pregnancy.

Recent advances in cross-sectional imaging, particularly in CT and MR imaging, have given these modalities a prominent role in the diagnosis of fractures of the extremities. This article describes the clinical application and imaging features of cross-sectional imaging (CT and MR imaging) in the evaluation of patients who have occult fractures of the extremities. Although CT or MR imaging is not typically required for evaluation of acute fractures, these modalities could be helpful in the evaluation of the occult osseous injuries in which radiographic findings are equivocal or inconclusive.

Urinary tract injury occurs in 10% of all abdominal trauma patients, and the kidney is the most commonly injured organ in the urinary tract. CT with contrast enhancement is the modality of choice for cross-sectional imaging of renal trauma because it quickly and accurately can demonstrate injury to the renal parenchyma, renal pedicles, and associated abdominal or retroperitoneal organs. This article reviews the mechanism, clinical features, imaging modalities, and CT imaging findings according to the classification of the renal trauma. Trauma to underlying abnormal kidneys, iatrogenic renal injuries, and complications of renal trauma are reviewed also.

Mesenteric ischemia is a difficult clinical diagnosis that requires a high index of clinical suspicion because the clinical and imaging features of intestinal ischemia and infarction overlap with many other intestinal disorders, and patients who have mesenteric ischemia often have coexisting diseases. Multidetecctor CT (MDCT) evaluation of the abdomen is the examination of choice when mesenteric ischemia is suspected because of its ability to provide two-dimensional multiplanar and three-dimensional display of the mesenteric vasculature and small intestine. This article reviews the clinical features, pathophysiology, and MDCT features of mesenteric ischemia.

THE CLINICS ARE NOW AVAILABLE ONLINE!

Access your subscription at:
www.theclinics.com

GOAL STATEMENT
The goal of the *Radiologic Clinics of North America* is to keep practicing radiologists and radiology residents up to date with current clinical practice in radiology by providing timely articles reviewing the state of the art in patient care.

ACCREDITATION
The *Radiologic Clinics of North America* is planned and implemented in accordance with the Essential Areas and Policies of the Accreditation Council for Continuing Medical Education (ACCME) through the joint sponsorship of the University of Virginia School of Medicine and Elsevier. The University of Virginia School of Medicine is accredited by the ACCME to provide continuing medical education for physicians.

The University of Virginia School of Medicine designates this educational activity for a maximum of 15 *AMA PRA Category 1 Credits*™. Physicians should only claim credit commensurate with the extent of their participation in the activity.

The American Medical Association has determined that physicians not licensed in the US who participate in this CME activity are eligible for 15 *AMA PRA Category 1 Credits*™.

Credit can be earned by reading the text material, taking the CME examination online at http://www.theclinics.com/home/cme, and completing the evaluation. After taking the test, you will be required to review any and all incorrect answers. Following completion of the test and evaluation, your credit will be awarded and you may print your certificate.

FACULTY DISCLOSURE/CONFLICT OF INTEREST
The University of Virginia School of Medicine, as an ACCME accredited provider, endorses and strives to comply with the Accreditation Council for Continuing Medical Education (ACCME) Standards of Commercial Support, Commonwealth of Virginia statutes, University of Virginia policies and procedures, and associated federal and private regulations and guidelines on the need for disclosure and monitoring of proprietary and financial interests that may affect the scientific integrity and balance of content delivered in continuing medical education activities under our auspices.

The University of Virginia School of Medicine requires that all CME activities accredited through this institution be developed independently and be scientifically rigorous, balanced and objective in the presentation/discussion of its content, theories and practices.

All authors/editors participating in an accredited CME activity are expected to disclose to the readers relevant financial relationships with commercial entities occurring within the past 12 months (such as grants or research support, employee, consultant, stock holder, member of speakers bureau, etc.). The University of Virginia School of Medicine will employ appropriate mechanisms to resolve potential conflicts of interest to maintain the standards of fair and balanced education to the reader. Questions about specific strategies can be directed to the Office of Continuing Medical Education, University of Virginia School of Medicine, Charlottesville, Virginia.

The authors/editors listed below have identified no financial or professional relationships for themselves or their spouse/partner:
Joong Mo Ahn, MD; Shweta Bhatt, MD (Guest Editor); Jae Young Byun, MD, PhD; M. Robert DeJong, RDMS, RVT, RCDS; Vikram S. Dogra, MD (Guest Editor); Barton Dudlick (Acquisitions Editor); Georges Y. El-Khoury, MD; Hamad Ghazale, MS, RDMS; Ulrike M. Hamper, MD, MBA; Young Joon Lee, MD; Angela D. Levy, MD, COL, MC, USA; Mark E. Lockhart, MD, MPH; Soon Nam Oh, MD, PhD; David Paushter, MD; Adnan Qalbani, MD; Chad B. Rabinowitz, MD; Parvati Ramchandani, MD; Sung Eun Rha, MD, PhD; Michelle L. Robbin, MD; Alexander V. Rybkin, MD; Nael Saad, MBBCh; Wael E.A. Saad, MBBCh; Ichiro Sakamoto, MD; Anuradha Saokar, MD; Leslie M. Scoutt, MD; Elijun Sueyoshi, MD; Lijun Tang, MD; Ruedi F. Thoeni, MD; Tongfu Yu, MD; Masataka Uetani, MD; Dehang Wang, MD; Therese M. Weber, MD; and Xiaomei Zhu, MD.

The authors/editors listed below have identified the following financial or professional relationships for themselves or their spouse/partner:
Abraham H. Dachman, MD is a consultant for EZEM, Inc., iCAD, Inc., and GE Healthcare.
Gaurav Jindal, MD is employed by the University of Pennsylvania as a Radiology resident.
Dushyant V. Sahani, MD is an independent contractor for GE Healthcare and is a consultant for Bracco Diagnostics.

Disclosure of Discussion of Non-FDA Approved Uses for Pharmaceutical and/or Medical Devices.
The University of Virginia School of Medicine, as an ACCME provider, requires that all authors identify and disclose any "off label" uses for pharmaceutical and medical device products. The University of Virginia School of Medicine recommends that each physician fully review all the available data on new products or procedures prior to clinical use.

TO ENROLL
To enroll in the *Radiologic Clinics of North America* Continuing Medical Education program, call customer service at 1-800-654-2452 or sign up online at http://www.theclinics.com/home/cme. The CME program is available to subscribers for an additional annual fee USD 205.

RADIOLOGIC
CLINICS
OF NORTH AMERICA

Radiol Clin N Am 45 (2007) xiii

Preface

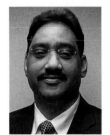 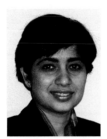

Vikram S. Dogra, MD   Shweta Bhatt, MD
Guest Editors

Vikram S. Dogra, MD
University of Rochester School of Medicine
Department of Imaging Sciences
601 Elmwood Ave., Box 648
Rochester, NY 14642, USA

E-mail address:
vikram_dogra@urmc.rochester.edu

Shweta Bhatt, MD
University of Rochester School of Medicine
Department of Imaging Sciences
601 Elmwood Ave., Box 648
Rochester, NY 14642, USA

E-mail address:
shweta_bhatt@urmc.rochester.edu

Emergency radiology involves examinations for patients of all ages who are acutely ill or injured. The nature of emergency radiology requires practitioners to make prompt and timely decisions about the type of imaging modality to use and then provide quick interpretations of the examinations for an appropriate and timely management.

An area of emergency radiology that does not receive enough focus is the special circumstances surrounding examinations that are given after normal business hours—5:00 PM and beyond. This issue of *Radiologic Clinics of North America* takes a closer look at that aspect of emergency radiology.

A multimodality approach focuses on the three types of cross-sectional imaging most often used in the emergency room: ultrasound, CT, and MR imaging. Relevant topics have been included that will provide up-to-date information for general practitioners as well as radiology residents in an academic setting.

We wish to thank Barton Dudlick and our outstanding contributors for their amazing work and their cooperation. It was a privilege to be guest editors for the 2004 Emergency Radiology issue (Vol. 42, Issue 2) and an honor to have the opportunity to delve deeper into the topic with this issue.

doi:10.1016/j.rcl.2007.04.014

RADIOLOGIC
CLINICS
OF NORTH AMERICA

Radiol Clin N Am 45 (2007) 395–410

ELSEVIER
SAUNDERS

Acute Flank Pain Secondary to Urolithiasis: Radiologic Evaluation and Alternate Diagnoses

Gaurav Jindal, MD, Parvati Ramchandani, MD*

- Imaging
    Abdominal radiography
    Intravenous urography
    Unenhanced CT scanning
    Ultrasonography
- *MR imaging*
- Evaluating the pregnant woman who has acute flank pain
- Alternative diagnoses in patients who have acute renal colic
- References

This article discusses the radiologic management of the patient who has acute flank pain. It describes the evolution of radiologic imaging in patients who present with acute symptoms caused by suspected urolithiasis, the advantages of unenhanced helical CT and the limitations of abdominal radiography, intravenous urography, and ultrasonography in this setting, and the alternative diagnoses encountered within the urinary tract, abdomen, and pelvis.

Acute flank pain or acute renal colic, secondary to urolithiasis, is a common problem in patients presenting to an acute care facility. The lifetime incidence of urolithiasis is estimated at 12% [1], and 2.3% of the population will experience renal colic in their lifetimes [2]. Patients who present with urolithiasis usually are young, between 30 and 60 years of age. Men are affected three times more often than women [3,4].

The classic definition of renal colic is a severe pain that is waxing and waning or spasmodic, beginning abruptly in the flank and increasing rapidly. The pain also may be a steady and continuous discomfort that radiates to the lower abdomen and pelvis as the stone moves distally in the urinary tract. Urinalysis, to evaluate for microhematuria, often is the initial laboratory examination performed in patients who present with suspected renal colic. The presence or absence of microhematuria, however, often is not reliable in determining which patients actually have urinary calculus disease as the cause of the clinical symptoms. Hematuria is not detected in approximately 20% of patients who have documented urinary tract stones [5,6]. Time of onset of pain versus time of examination also may undermine the sensitivity of hematuria as a diagnostic indicator. In a retrospective study of more than 450 patients who had acute ureterolithiasis documented on CT, hematuria was present in 95% on day 1 but in only 65% to 68% on days 3 and 4 [6].

Imaging

Radiologic imaging plays a critical role in the evaluation and management of patients who have acute flank pain. Unenhanced helical CT scanning has

Department of Radiology, University of Pennsylvania Medical Center, 3400 Spruce Street, Philadelphia, PA 19104, USA
* Corresponding author.
E-mail address: ramchanp@uphs.upenn.edu (P. Ramchandani).

0033-8389/07/$ – see front matter © 2007 Published by Elsevier Inc.
radiologic.theclinics.com

doi:10.1016/j.rcl.2007.04.001

supplanted conventional radiography and intravenous urography (IVU) in the evaluation of these patients. CT has the advantages of being both sensitive and specific for the diagnosis of urinary stone disease, with reported sensitivity of 97% to 100% and specificity of 94% to 96% (Fig. 1) [7,8]. Additionally, CT can detect causes of flank pain other than urinary stone disease. Although CT urography is used increasingly for the evaluation of patients who have hematuria and suspected urothelial abnormality, its role in evaluating patients who have acute flank pain is primarily for further evaluation of abnormalities seen on unenhanced CT images that justify further imaging work-up.

Abdominal radiography

Abdominal radiography often is used as a first step in the radiologic work-up of patients who have acute flank pain. Although 90% of urinary tract calculi are composed of calcium salts [9], only 59% of urinary stones are visible on abdominal radiographs [10]. Levine and colleagues [10] retrospectively reviewed abdominal radiographs and CT scans of 178 patients who had acute flank pain and found that abdominal radiographs had a sensitivity of 45% to 59% and specificity of 77% in the detection of urinary tract calculi. They concluded that abdominal radiographs need not be obtained before proceeding to CT scanning in this setting.

Small stones may be difficult to identify on abdominal radiographs, particularly in the presence of overlying bowel gas or fecal material. Levine and colleagues [10] found that the mean size of stones seen on an abdominal radiograph was 4.2 mm, and the mean size of stones not visualized was 3.1 mm. Zagoria and colleagues [11] found that 79% of calculi larger than 5 mm and 95% of calculi with CT attenuation greater than 300 Hounsfield units (HU) were detectable on conventional radiography (Fig. 2). In another study 49% of ureteral calculi visible on unenhanced helical CT scans were visible on the routine CT scout radiographs [12]. Stones composed purely of uric acid account for 5% to 10% of urinary calculi and may not be detectable on abdominal radiographs, regardless of size. Phleboliths may be impossible to distinguish from ureteral stones by abdominal radiography alone, although radiographic findings such as a central lucency or anatomic position may allow the differentiation of these structures from true ureteral calculi [13]. Although phleboliths are most common in the pelvis, gonadal vein phleboliths may cause confusion in the abdomen when assessing for calculi in the lumbar ureter.

An abdominal radiograph is a reasonable initial test in patients who have a history of radiopaque calculi and who present with acute flank pain that is similar to that of previous episodes. In the

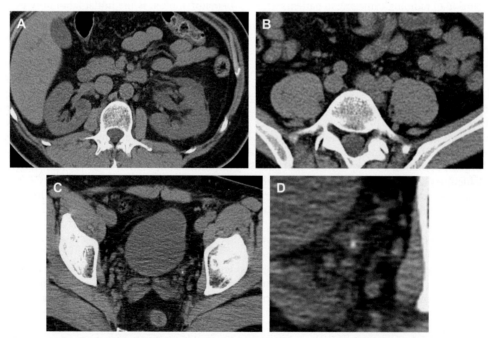

Fig. 1. Noncontrast CT of a 35-year-old man with obstructing calculus in left distal ureter. (*A*) The left kidney is slightly enlarged with anterior perinephric fluid and mild fullness of the left collecting system. (*B*) The left ureter is slightly dilated compared with the right. (*C* and *D*) There is a small calculus in the left distal pelvic ureter. Note the soft tissue thickening around the calculus, the soft tissue rim sign (seen better on the magnified close-up view in panel D).

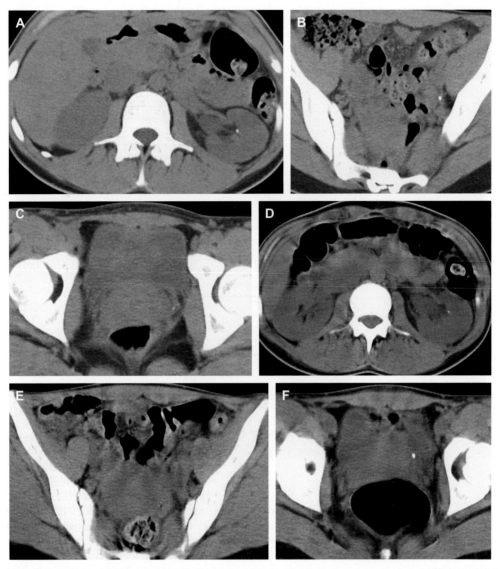

Fig. 2. Noncontrast CT and IVU in a 24-year-old woman who had left flank pain and migrating left ureteral calculus. Panels *A–C* are the images at initial presentation that demonstrate mild left hydronephrosis with (*A*) a small left renal calculus, (*B*) calculus in left sacral ureter and no calculus in the vicinity of the left distal pelvic ureter. (*C*) Note small phlebolith in left pelvis. Panels *D–F* are from a scan done 10 days later when patient presented with worsening left pain. (*A*) There is increased left hydronephrosis. (*B*) No calculus is seen in the left sacral region, but the stone has migrated distally to the left ureterovesical junction. Panels *D–F* are from a scan done 10 days later when the patient presented with worsening left flank pain. (*D*) There is increased left hydronephrosis. (*E, F*) No stone is seen in the left sacral region, but the stone has migrated distally to the left ureterovesical junction. Panels *G–I* are from an IVU done 2 weeks after the second CT when the patient continued to have left flank pain. (*G*) The stone in the left distal ureter is clearly seen on the scout radiograph of the pelvis. (*H*) There is partial obstruction of the left ureter and collecting system to the level of the stone, which is better seen in (*I*) the magnified view of the left distal ureter.

absence of such a history, abdominal radiography may not be of value as an initial examination [10]. If a ureteral calculus is present on CT but is not clearly identifiable on the CT scout view, a conventional abdominal radiograph may be useful for following the progress of the stone for management purposes, especially if the stone is larger than 4 to 5 mm in size and is over 300 HU in density [11].

Intravenous urography

IVU was once the imaging modality of choice in a patient who presented with acute flank pain.

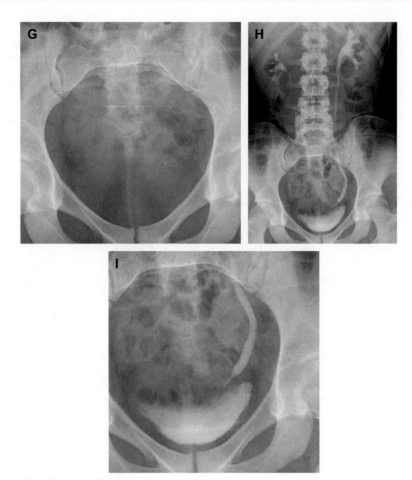

Fig. 2 (continued)

The need to administer intravenous radiographic contrast and the delay in obtaining relevant information about the site of obstruction make IVU a less desirable study than unenhanced CT in an acute pain setting.

The purported advantages of an IVU compared with CT initially were believed to be its ability to display physiologic information regarding the severity of obstruction. Findings on CT, however, can help direct management of the detected stones [14]. Management decisions with a symptomatic stone are based largely on the size and location of the calculus rather than on the degree of obstruction. CT is an excellent technique for determining stone size and location. The radiation exposure to a patient receiving an IVU versus a CT scan depends on the technique used for the two studies but generally is believed to be higher for a CT than for a three-film IVU. This issue is discussed further later in this article.

IVU has a higher sensitivity and specificity than an abdominal radiograph in diagnosing urinary calculus disease as the cause of acute flank pain (64% versus 97, and 92% versus 94%, respectively) [15–17]. Even if a stone is not visible on the scout films, a retrospective effort to look for a stone at the site of obstruction often may allow identification of a small stone. As stated previously, however, IVU is regarded largely as a historical examination in evaluating acute flank pain if CT is readily available.

IVU may have a role in the evaluation of pregnant patients who have acute flank pain when the results of an ultrasonographic examination are negative or equivocal. This issue is addressed further later in this article. Butler and colleagues [18] described the usefulness of single-shot intravenous urography 30 minutes after intravenous contrast injection in this setting. Boridy and colleagues [19] advocate obtaining a scout radiograph, a radiograph collimated to include only the kidneys at 1 and 15 minutes and delayed images as deemed necessary. Even in these patients, CT may be the technique of choice, because it provides a definitive and rapid diagnosis. These advantages outweigh the slightly greater radiation exposure [14,20].

Unenhanced CT scanning

Unenhanced CT scanning is currently the imaging modality of choice for the diagnosis of urolithiasis, particularly in the setting of acute flank pain. The technique has many advantages for patients. It can be performed rapidly without intravenous contrast, can identify and directly measure size of calculi, and can determine the degree of a possible associated urinary tract obstruction. Use of CT scanning in the acute setting has increased dramatically during the past 10 years, raising concerns of overuse and misuse (see Fig. 2). Reports indicate, however, that there has been no decrease in the rate of positive diagnosis of obstructing urinary stones on CT, validating the increased frequency with which CT scans are obtained in the setting of acute flank pain [21]. The overall rate of stone positivity on CT scanning in patients suspected of having renal colic is reported to be 60% to 66% in several studies (Table 1) [21,22]. Additionally, because CT is the diagnostic test of choice to evaluate many acute abdominal problems, a decrease in the stone positivity rate may not necessarily reflect overuse of CT [14].

The accuracy of CT in the diagnosis of obstructive urinary stone disease in patients presenting with acute abdominal and flank pain has been established. The accuracy of CT in stone detection reportedly varies from 96% to 98%, and the sensitivity and specificity of CT for detection of urinary stones are estimated to be 96% and 98%, respectively [7,15,22–27]. Because of its high acquisition speeds, the advent of multidetector CT has improved further the detection of urinary tract calculi [28].

False-negative CT results for stone detection range from 2% to 7% [7,27] and are attributed largely to volume averaging and small stone size. Smaller section widths result in a higher rate of urinary stone detection but add to the dose burden of the patient. Using 147 patients suspected of having renal colic, Memarsadeghi and colleagues [29] recently determined that CT section widths of 1.5 mm and 3.0 mm showed no significant difference in the detection of urinary tract calculi; however, 5.0-mm sections revealed significantly fewer urinary tract stones. They noted that the few missed stones on the 5.0-mm sections were less than 3 mm in diameter. Radiolucent stones, including those secondary to concreted crystals of HIV protease inhibitors, primarily indinavir, are not visible on CT [30]. If a patient who has a history of using these drugs has acute symptoms and secondary signs of obstruction, a presumed diagnosis of a drug-induced stone can be made, even though none is seen.

Accurate determination of stone size is relevant to clinical management, because spontaneous passage of ureteral stones is highly dependent on stone size. In a study of 64 patients, the mean diameter of stones that passed spontaneously was approximately 2.9 ± 2.0 mm, whereas the mean diameter of stones for which conservative therapy failed was 7.9 ± 3.3 mm [31]. CT scans provide more accurate estimates than abdominal radiographs in both the longitudinal and transverse axes [32,33], although these differences did not attain significance for stones between 2 and 13 mm in size. Coronal reconstruction of axial CT scans may be more accurate in predicting the craniocaudal size of a calculus, although the width of the stone is a more important factor in stone passage [34].

Secondary signs of urinary tract obstruction can also be detected on noncontrast helical CT scanning, and the likelihood of these signs increases with increasing duration of pain [35]. Katz and colleagues [36] described the frequency of secondary findings in 54 patients who had CT evidence of ureteral calculi (see Figs. 1 and 2; Fig. 3). Hydronephrosis, perinephric edema, or periureteral edema was seen in 69%, 65%, and 31.4% of patients, respectively. These findings were absent in only 3.7% of patients who had ureteral calculi [36]. The amount of perinephric stranding is related to the time after onset of pain and usually is not seen in the first 2 hours after the onset of pain; maximal stranding may take up to 8 hours after the onset of pain [35]. Absence of hydroureteronephrosis has the strongest negative predictive value for obstruction [27]. When hydroureteronephrosis is present, but no urinary tract calculus can be identified, the differential diagnosis includes a recently passed stone, pyelonephritis, or a stone that is radiolucent or too small to detect. Extensive perinephric edema has

Table 1: CT findings in acute renal colic			
	Hoppe et al [64]	Katz et al [60]	Ahmad et al [65]
Number in study	1500	1000	233
Urinary stone	69%	62%	68%
Additional or alternative diagnosis	71%	10%	12%
Alternate diagnosis only	24%	7.50%	–
Normal	7%	28%	–
Pyelonephritis	3%	1%	1%
Renal cell carcinoma/ renal mass	2%	0.40%	1%
Cholecystitis	0.30%	0.30%	0.40%
Adnexal mass	–	2%	2%

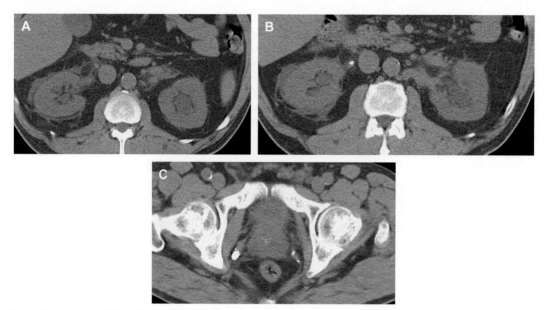

Fig. 3. Noncontrast CT in a 60-year-old man who had right flank pain caused by right proximal ureteral calculus and pelvic phleboliths. (*A*) There is mild bilateral hydronephrosis and perinephric fluid and stranding around the right kidney. Left hydronephrosis is a residual from previous episodes of obstruction caused by stones, illustrating the chronic and recurring nature of urinary calculus disease. (*B*) There is a small calculus in the right proximal lumbar ureter. (*C*) Phleboliths in the pelvis with a "comet-tail" appearance.

been associated with high-grade obstruction as determined by an IVU, whereas mild or no perinephric edema has been associated with no obstruction or low-grade obstruction on IVU (see Figs. 1–3). Boridy and colleagues [37] compared CT with IVU in 47 patients who had acute ureterolithiasis and found that assessing the degree of perinephric edema on CT helped predict the degree of ureteral obstruction on IVU in 94% of patients and correlated inversely with the likelihood of stone passage, thus adding prognostic information. This finding has been disputed in other reports, however [23]. Unilateral perinephric stranding and renal enlargement can be seen in cases of pyelonephritis without associated obstruction. It thus is important to correlate CT findings with clinical history (Fig. 4).

A common dilemma when interpreting a CT scan in a patient who has acute flank pain is the differentiation of phleboliths from ureteral calculi. A soft tissue rim sign may be seen on CT in 50% to 77% of ureteral calculi but is seen in only 0% to 8% of phleboliths (see Fig. 1C, D) [38,39]; reportedly, the specificity of the sign is 92% [39]. The sign is demonstrated as an area of soft tissue attenuation that surrounds a suspected calcified ureteral calculus and seems to depend on the size of the calculus: it tends to be present with 90% of stones smaller than 4 mm or less and absent with stones larger than 5 mm [39]. The absence of a soft tissue rim sign does not exclude the diagnosis of ureteral

stone. The sign also is seen more often with distal stones than with proximal stones (see Fig. 1C, D).

Phleboliths have an associated "tail" of soft-tissue attenuation (the so-called "comet-tail sign") 65% of the time (see Fig. 3C) [40]. A radiolucent center may be useful for identifying phleboliths on an abdominal radiograph; however, in a CT study of 120 phleboliths, 99% did not have a radiolucent center [41]. A combination of these signs probably is the best aid in distinguishing phleboliths from ureteral calculi. On occasion, in a symptomatic patient, there is no choice but to perform a contrast-enhanced CT scan in the excretory phase to distinguish a phlebolith from a ureteral calculus [27]. Rarely, vas deferens calcifications can mimic the appearance of ureteral calculi. Other less common entities that can mimic a ureteral calcification include retained oral contrast material in the bowel and pelvic pathologic conditions containing calcifications. If interpretation of the study is performed electronically on soft copy, the ureter can be traced in most patients, making it easier to determine if a calcification lies within the ureter [14].

The strongest criticism of the use of CT in evaluating patients who have acute abdominal pain has been directed at the increased radiation burden as compared with abdominal radiography. In one study in which 122 patients were assigned randomly to unenhanced CT or to IVU, the mean applied radiation doses were 3.3 mSv for IVU and

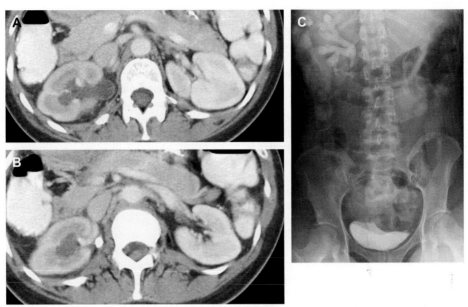

Fig. 4. A 40-year-old woman who had no prior history of stone disease presented with abdominal pain . CT scan was ordered with oral and intravenous contrast because the pain was not typical for renal colic. (*A*) There is a delayed nephrogram in the right kidney caused by high-grade obstruction. (*B*) A dense stone is seen in the proximal right ureter. (*C*) Abdominal radiograph 12 hours later demonstrates continuing high-grade obstruction by the stone, which is obscured by the excreted contrast.

6.5 mSv for unenhanced CT [42]. Other studies indicated a radiation dose for CT of 2.8 to 13.1 mSv for men and 4.5 to 18.0 mSv for women, as compared with 1.5 mSv for an IVU [43,44]. Lack of diagnostic accuracy, however, has led many diagnosticians to consider IVU a less optimal choice for the initial imaging in acute abdominal or flank pain [45]. Moreover, an IVU series containing 10 to 20 images can expose a patient to the same entry skin radiation dose as one nonenhanced abdominal CT examination. The entry skin dose for a typical nonenhanced CT examination is approximately 3 to 5 rad, whereas the entry skin dose for each IVU radiograph is 0.25 to 0.30 rad [7].

There are reports of attempts to reduce radiation dose in this clinical setting. Separate studies by Tack [44] and Rogers [46] support the concept of substantially reducing dose by decreasing milliamps per second (mA/s), resulting in decreased image quality but not necessarily decreased diagnostic capabilities. Heneghan and colleagues [43] compared conventional and reduced-dose CT techniques in acute flank pain with mean mA/s of 160 and 76, respectively, and reported that, compared with the high-dose scan, the low-dose scan had accuracy rates of 91% for nephrolithiasis, 94% for ureterolithiasis, 91% for obstruction, and 92% for normal findings. Increase in pitch also lowers dose in a CT examination. Diel and colleagues [47] examined the use of 5-mm collimation with pitch of 1.5 to 3.0 for a helical CT scanner. Entrance doses were 461 and 553 mR for pitches of 3.0 and 2.5, respectively. That study noted no change in diagnostic accuracy for detection of ureteral calculi when using a pitch of 3.0 or 2.5; image quality decreased at a pitch of 3.0 when compared with a pitch of 2.5, however, and this decrease may limit detection of subtle extraurinary pathologic conditions [47]. Although CT techniques that use reduced mA/s can allow detection of most calculi with less radiation dose, they may not be useful in obese patients. Other techniques such as tube-current modulation may allow the use of low-radiation techniques, even in obese patients [48].

Financial burden also remains a consideration when determining the judicious use of available imaging modalities. One report found that helical CT was faster and only slightly more expensive ($600) than IVU ($400) [8]. Pfister and colleagues [42] showed that direct costs of unenhanced CT and IVU are nearly identical at their institution. Because of its higher rate and more rapid detection of urolithiasis, CT is considered more cost effective overall than IVU in the management of the patient who has acute flank pain [42].

Ultrasonography

Ultrasonography, alone or combined with conventional radiography, has been compared with unenhanced CT. Ultrasonography has a much lower sensitivity (24%–77%) than CT (92%–96%) [49–52]. In Sheafor's [52] study comparing CT and ultrasound, CT depicted 22 of 23 ureteral calculi (sensitivity, 96%). Ultrasound depicted 14 of 23 ureteral calculi (sensitivity, 61%). Differences in sensitivity were statistically significant ($P = .02$). Specificity for each technique was 100%. CT can give a rapid and definitive diagnosis of urinary calculus disease, as well as other abdominal disorders with the same presentation. Ultrasonography often is used as the first imaging procedure in patients who should avoid radiation, such as pregnant women and children. Calculi as small as 0.5 mm may be detectable in optimal conditions. When stones are larger than 5 mm, ultrasound has been shown to have a sensitivity of 96% and specificity of nearly 100% [53].

Identification of ureteral jets within the urinary bladder lumen is helpful for assessing the presence of obstruction. One study showed an absent ureteral jet in 11 of 12 patients who had high-grade obstruction and in 3 of 11 patients who had low-grade obstruction (Fig. 5) [54].

MR imaging

The lack of ionizing radiation makes MR imaging attractive as an imaging alternative to CT. Scanning techniques use either heavily T2-weighted imaging to demonstrate static fluid or gadolinium-enhanced T1-weighted imaging. Although reports indicate that calculi may be detected, small calculi (which are the majority of symptomatic stones) are difficult to detect on MR imaging, Urothelial lesions, blood clots, and debris also can mimic calculi [55,56].

Evaluating the pregnant woman who has acute flank pain

Urinary calculus disease is common in pregnant women, with most women presenting in the second or third trimesters. More than 80% of women pass the calculi spontaneously [20,57,58]; thus, conservative management is prudent at first presentation of symptomatic renal or ureteral stone disease. Imaging should be considered if symptoms are persistent or are associated with signs of infection (see Fig. 5). Transabdominal ultrasound often is the study of first choice [19] and demonstrates renal calculi. The presence of hydronephrosis caused by pregnancy can make the definitive diagnosis of an associated obstructing ureteral calculus difficult, however, unless the calculus is lodged at the ureterovesicular junction; detection may require an endovaginal examination in addition to a transabdominal scan. Evaluation for ureteral jets may provide information regarding the presence of an obstructing calculus. Thus, a complete ultrasound protocol in such patients involves assessment for dilation of the collecting system and ureter, Doppler examination of the segmental intrarenal arteries, imaging for ureteral jets, and transvaginal examination to detect distal ureteral and ureterovesicular stones [59].

As mentioned previously, Butler and colleagues [18] recommended limited IVUs in patients in whom sonographic examination was negative, because in their study of 57 pregnant patients, 40% of calculi were not detected by ultrasound. There is, however, considerable controversy in the literature about the technique, timing, and number of radiographs to be performed in pregnant patients who have renal colic and undergo a limited IVU [19]. Because most patients are in late stages of pregnancy at presentation, identifying a symptomatic ureteral calculus can be difficult on radiographs. Additionally, the exposures required to image the enlarged maternal abdomen with conventional radiography can increase the radiation dose to that of CT [20]. Thus, unenhanced CT may be the best technique to evaluate the symptomatic pregnant woman, as it is in the nonpregnant population. Kenney and colleagues [14] perform a single test slice at the thickest part of the patient's abdomen with reduced dose (80–100 mA, at 140 kV), assess the quality of the image, and perform the examination with the lowest dose that provides adequate quality.

The usefulness of MR imaging in this clinical situation remains a subject of study.

Alternative diagnoses in patients who have acute renal colic

An obstructing ureteral calculus can be mimicked by a host of abdominal and pelvic conditions. It follows, therefore, that imaging evaluations in patients suspected of having a urinary tract stone often reveal an alternate significant diagnosis, and it is important for radiologists not to limit the examination solely to the detection of calculi (Figs. 6–10). The alternative diagnoses span the spectrum of urinary tract pathology unrelated to stone disease, as well extraurinary pathology [7,21,60–63]. It is not possible to discuss all these pathologies in this article. There is concern that the attempts at imaging with reduced radiation dose protocols may decrease the identification of alternative diagnoses because of the noisier images produced by low-dose techniques. Tack and colleagues [44], in a small series, reported that all alternative diagnoses were diagnosed at a very low dose unenhanced CT protocol with imaging at 30 mAs. The detection of alternative pathologies is particularly difficult in patients who have a paucity of fat within the abdomen and pelvis. The alternative

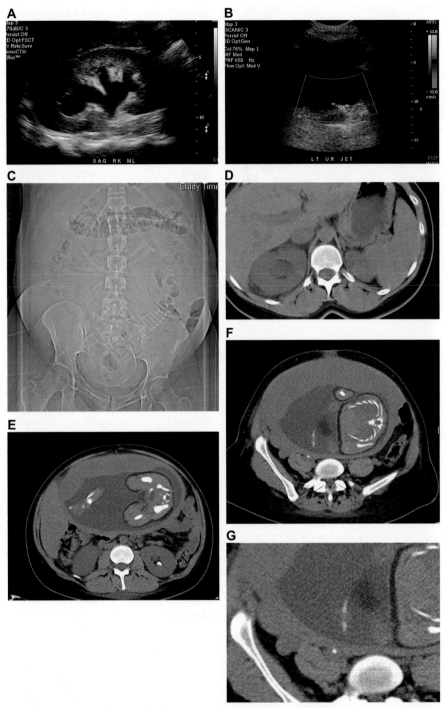

Fig. 5. A woman in the thirty-third week of pregnancy who had a past history of stone disease presented with right flank pain and obstructing right ureteral calculus. (*A*) Renal ultrasound demonstrates right hydronephrosis. No hydronephrosis was seen on the left, but there was a renal calculus (not shown). (*B*) No ureteral jet is visualized on the right side. Panels *C–G* show an unenhanced CT scan done 3 days after the ultrasound because of continuing severe right flank pain. (*C*) The CT scout film demonstrates the fetal skeleton. (*D, E*) There is mild right hydronephrosis and a nonobstructing left renal stone. (*F, G*) A small obstructing right ureteral stone is seen better on the magnified view of the right ureter in panel G. The patient underwent ureteral stent placement.

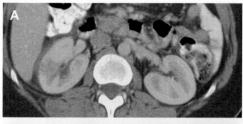

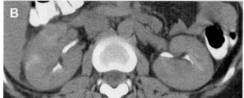

Fig. 6. A 35-year-old woman who had right flank pain and pyelonephritis. The unenhanced CT scan was normal. (*A*) The right nephrogram is focally abnormal, consistent with acute pyelonephritis. (*B*) Delayed image demonstrates persistent enhancement in the same region.

diagnoses that are seen most often are genitourinary disease not related to stones, such as pyelonephritis, renal mass, and adnexal pathology, and gastrointestinal disease, such as appendicitis and diverticulitis [61].

The incidence of extraurinary pathology in patients presenting with renal colic varies in different reports, with most recent studies showing that the incidence of urolithiasis on unenhanced CT examinations done on patients who have acute flank pain is approximately 62% to 69%, whereas the rate of alternate diagnoses is between 10% and 45% [26,64–66]. Hoppe and colleagues [64] found that of the 1500 patients who underwent unenhanced CT because of acute flank pain, 69% had urinary tract calculi (22% had only a urinary tract stone, and 47% had a urinary stone along with an additional diagnosis), whereas 24% had only an

alternate diagnosis. Katz and colleagues [60] retrospectively reviewed 1000 CT examinations done on patients suspected of having renal colic. The incidence of urolithiasis, including recently passed urinary stones, was approximately 62%. There was a 10% incidence of alternate diagnoses, 62% of which were genitourinary in origin. Ahmad and colleagues [65] reviewed 233 consecutive unenhanced CT examinations and identified urinary stones or evidence of recently passed stones in 68% of patients. Overall incidental findings were found in 12% of patients. In another report [26] on patients with their first episode of a suspected kidney stone, 33% had an alternate diagnosis not suspected on clinical grounds, one half of whom had significant disease. Chen and Zagoria [25] studied 100 consecutive patients who had urinary colic. Urinary tract calculi were present in 66% of patients, and extraurinary lesions were present in 16%. A follow up study by Chen and colleagues included an expanded role of nonenhanced CT beyond the evaluation of renal colic. They demonstrated ureteral calculi in only 28% of patients and identified extraurinary lesions in 45%. The incidence of alternate diagnoses is summarized in Table 1. A few of the many alternate diagnoses, including both renal and nonrenal origins, encountered on unenhanced CT examination in the setting of acute flank pain are discussed later.

The diagnosis of alternative pathologies may require the administration of intravenous contrast; Kenney and colleagues [14] found the use of contrast to be necessary in 12% of their patients, either to document that a density was located within the ureter or to evaluate further another abnormality such as pyelonephritis or mass. The decision to extend the unenhanced examination is facilitated if a radiologist assesses the images before the patient is removed from the scanning area; the decision usually is made in concert with the referring physician.

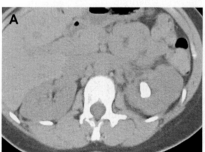

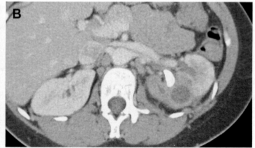

Fig. 7. A 32-year-old woman had left flank pain, left renal calculus complicated by acute pyelonephritis, and a small abscess. (*A*) Noncontrast CT demonstrates a large left renal stone. There is minimal inhomogeneity of the left kidney, which was seen better by adjusting the windows on soft copy viewing (not shown). (*B*) Contrast-enhanced scan demonstrates inhomogeneity of the left nephrogram and a small abscess.

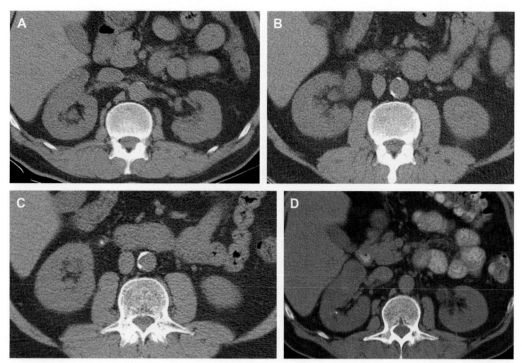

Fig. 8. A 55-year-old man who had history of stone disease and incidental small right renal cell carcinoma that was overlooked on initial CT. Panels *A–C* are the initial CT performed when the patient presented with an obstructing right proximal ureteral calculus. (*A*) A contour abnormality in the anterior aspect of the interpolar region of the right kidney was overlooked. (*B*) There is mild right hydronephrosis and (*C*) a small right ureteral stone. (*D*) A CT done 18 months later for recurrent abdominal pain demonstrates a small new stone in the right kidney and enlargement of the right renal mass.

When unenhanced CT demonstrates unilateral perinephric stranding (bilateral stranding is seen in many older patients and usually denotes no particular clinical significance) and renal enlargement, administration of intravenous contrast should be considered to diagnose pyelonephritis and renal vascular conditions involving the artery or vein [61]. The diagnosis of acute pyelonephritis can be made accurately in most cases with a directed history and physical examination, and imaging studies generally are not necessary. The diagnosis can be suggested by unenhanced CT if the clinical history is appropriate and if findings such as asymmetric perinephric stranding, mild renal enlargement, and/or hydronephrosis are seen. Mild disease, however, may demonstrate no abnormality on unenhanced CT examination. After contrast enhancement, CT findings include those mentioned previously as well as a focal wedge-shaped area of low attenuation or striated enhancement of the kidney (see Figs. 6 and 7). Intra- or extrarenal fluid collections or abscess may be present.

The expanded use of CT scanning over the past 2 decades has made the incidental detection of renal tumors commonplace (see Figs. 8–10). On unenhanced examinations, renal parenchymal neoplasms may be seen as subtle renal contour abnormalities (see Fig. 8), complex masses, or spontaneous subcapsular or perinephric bleeds (which can cause flank pain), whereas urothelial neoplasms are seen as focal soft tissue thickening in the renal sinus, ureter, or bladder (see Figs. 9 and 10).

Rucker [61] and Katz [66] caution that radiologists should be familiar with the appearance of acute appendicitis on unenhanced CT examinations, because the clinical presentation can mimic renal colic. Unenhanced CT demonstrates a normal appendix in 80% of patients who do not have appendicitis [67]. Thus, in all patients suspected of having renal colic in whom the unenhanced CT is not consistent with urinary stone disease, the appendix should be examined carefully, and oral and intravenous contrast should be given as indicated.

Patients who have acute renal vein thrombosis may, infrequently, present with flank pain that can simulate colic caused by a urinary calculus. Most patients are asymptomatic or have no symptoms referable to the kidney, and a pulmonary embolus typically is the only clinical clue to the presence of renal vein thrombosis or deep vein thrombosis.

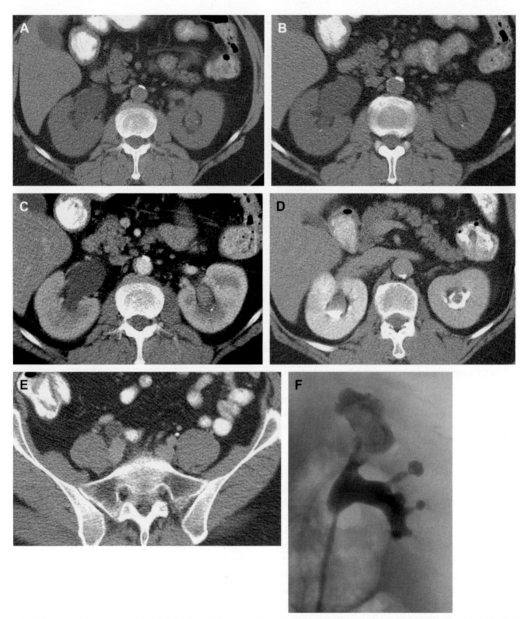

Fig. 9. A 60-year-old woman who had a long history of stone disease presented with right flank pain. (*A, B*) Unenhanced CT scan demonstrates right hydronephrosis, soft tissue mass in left renal sinus, and small bilateral renal calculi. The left renal abnormality was noted, and the patient was given intravenous contrast for additional imaging. Panels *C–E* show contrast-enhanced CT. (*C*) There is enhancement of the left renal sinus mass. Note the small nonobstructing stone in the left kidney in this patient who has a long history of stone disease. Images in excretory phase demonstrate (*D*) right hydronephrosis and a mass in the left collecting system. (*E*) The right ureter is dilated by a small stone at the right ureterovesical junction (not shown), which was the cause of the patient's flank pain. (*F*) Left retrograde pyelogram demonstrates the irregular mass in the left upper pole that proved to be a transitional cell carcinoma.

Patients with the nephrotic syndrome have an increased incidence (10%–40%) of arterial and venous thrombosis, particularly deep vein and renal vein thrombosis. The underlying cause of the observed hypercoagulable state in patients who have nephrotic syndrome is not well understood [68,69]. Renal vein thrombosis is rare in patients who are not nephrotic.

On unenhanced CT, nonspecific signs such as ipsilateral renal enlargement with perinephric edema may be seen. Contrast-enhanced CT scanning or MR imaging will help in establishing the diagnosis

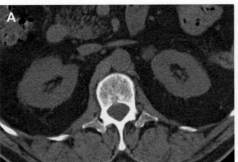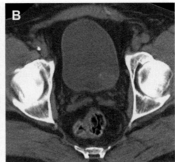

Fig. 10. A 60-year-old man who had left flank pain and incidental bladder carcinoma. (*A*) Unenhanced CT scan demonstrates mild left ureteral dilation. No stone was found. (*B*) Images through the urinary bladder demonstrate an unsuspected small bladder carcinoma.

when suspected in the setting of flank pain in a nephrotic patient.

Acute renal infarction secondary to renal arterial occlusion or thromboembolism may appear unremarkable during the very early stages on nonenhanced CT images. When infarction involves large regions of an involved kidney, the kidney may become enlarged, with preservation of its reniform shape. Contrast enhancement may reveal an absent nephrogram or a cortical rim of enhancement caused by relatively increased blood flow within capsular collateral vessels [70–77]. Clinical presentation varies from the asymptomatic presentation often seen with thromboemboli, to acute flank pain, fever, and other generalized complaints that mimic those of renal colic and acute pyelonephritis that occur with complete occlusion leading to segmental or total renal infarction.

Gynecologic conditions may mimic renal colic clinically. Hemorrhagic ovarian cysts, pelvic inflammatory disease, endometriomas, ovarian torsion, and ovarian neoplasms may present as acute flank pain. Ultrasound plays a critical role in evaluating female pelvic pathology with higher sensitivity and specificity in the detection of gynecologic conditions than either unenhanced or enhanced CT scanning [77–80].

Other gynecologic conditions may be encountered in the setting of acute flank pain. Corpus luteal cysts are prone to hemorrhage during the luteal phase. CT may reveal hemoperitoneum and an adnexal cyst with a ring of peripheral contrast enhancement [80]. The CT appearance of endometriomas is nonspecific, including simple cystic to complex cystic masses. A high-attenuation component may be seen but is nonspecific. Multiplicity of lesions increases the specificity of the diagnosis. CT may be helpful in staging and identifying uncommon sites of implants [81].

CT can be used to diagnose pelvic inflammatory disease when clinical and ultrasound evaluations are inconclusive, in staging, when patients do not

respond to antibiotic therapy, and to detect complications such as abscess and thrombophlebitis. Findings are often bilateral, but one side may be affected more than the other. Salpingitis may appear as a thickened, dilated fallopian tube. The inflamed appendix occasionally may be located in the region of the adnexa and should be identified separately if possible. The tubular appearance helps identify tubo-ovarian abscess. Multiplanar reconstructions often are useful in this setting. Other associated findings include thickening of the pelvic ligaments, loss of definition of the uterine border, infiltration of the pelvic fat, and reactive lymphadenopathy. Sometimes, spread of inflammation to the perihepatic tissues may be visualized, a perihepatitis known as "Fitz-Hugh-Curtis syndrome" [82,83].

In summary, multiple radiologic techniques are available for the evaluation of the patient who has acute renal colic. Unenhanced CT is the modality of choice in the evaluation of patients who have renal colic. It is a fast examination, does not require intravenous contrast administration, and allows accurate determination of stone size and location and assessment of overall stone burden. Several alternate diagnoses may be encountered in the workup of presumed urolithiasis in the setting of acute flank pain and include both renal and nonrenal abdominopelvic pathology. Vigilance is essential to avoid overlooking significant abdominal and pelvic pathology that clinically can mimic acute flank pain caused by urolithiasis.

References

[1] Clark JY, Thompson IM, Optenberg SA. Economic impact of urolithiasis in the United States. J Urol 1995;154(6):2020–4.

[2] Brenner BM, editor. The kidney. Philadelphia: Saunders; 1996. p. 1190–1, 1893–95.

[3] Hiatt RA, Dales LG, Friedman GD, et al. Frequency of urolithiasis in a prepaid medical care program. Am J Epidemiol 1982;115(2):255–65.

[4] Pearle MS, Calhoun EA, Curhan GC. Urologic diseases in America project: urolithiasis. J Urol 2005;173:848–57.

[5] Press SM, Smith AD. Incidence of negative hematuria in patients with acute urinary lithiasis presenting to the emergency room with flank pain. Urology 1995;45:753–7.

[6] Kobayashi T, Nishizawa K, Mitsumori K, et al. Impact of date of onset on the absence of hematuria in patients with acute renal colic. J Urol 2003;170:1093–6.

[7] Smith RC, Verga M, McCarthy S, et al. Diagnosis of acute flank pain: value of unenhanced helical CT. AJR Am J Roentgenol 1996;166:97–101.

[8] Chen MY, Zagoria RJ. Can noncontrast helical computed tomography replace intravenous urography for evaluation of patients with acute urinary tract colic? J Emerg Med 1999;17:299–303.

[9] Herring LC. Observations on the analysis of ten thousand urinary calculi. J Urol 1962;88:545–62.

[10] Levine JA, Neitlich J, Verga M, et al. Ureteral calculi in patients with flank pain: correlation of plain radiography with unenhanced helical CT. Radiology 1997;204(1):27–31.

[11] Zagoria RJ, Khatod EG, Chen MYM. Abdominal radiography after CT reveals urinary calculi: a method to predict usefulness of abdominal radiography on the basis of size and CT attenuation of calculi. AJR Am J Roentgenol 2001;176:1117–22.

[12] Chu G, Rosenfield AT, Anderson K, et al. Sensitivity and value of digital CT scout radiography for detecting ureteral stones in patients with ureterolithiasis diagnosed on unenhanced CT. AJR Am J Roentgenol 1999;173:417–23.

[13] Dunnick RN, Sandler CM, Newhouse JH, et al. Nephrocalcinosis and nephrolithiasis. In: Textbook of uroradiology. 3rd edition. Philadelphia: Lippincott Williams & Wilkins; 2001. p. 178–94.

[14] Kenney PJ. CT evaluation of urinary lithiasis. Radiol Clin North Am 2003;41:979–99.

[15] Miller OF, Rineer SK, Reichard SR, et al. Prospective comparison of unenhanced spiral computed tomography and intravenous urogram in the evaluation of acute flank pain. Urology 1998;52:982–7.

[16] Niall O, Russell J, MacGregor R, et al. A comparison of noncontrast computerized tomography with excretory urography in the assessment of acute flank pain. J Urol 1999;161:534–7.

[17] Yilmaz S, Sindel T, Arslan G, et al. Renal colic: comparison of spiral CT, US and IVU in the detection of ureteral calculi. Eur Radiol 1998;8:212–7.

[18] Bulter EL, Cox SM, Eberts EG, et al. Symptomatic nephrolithiasis complicating pregnancy. Obstet Gynecol 2000;96:753–6.

[19] Boridy IC, Maklad N, Sandler CM. Suspected urolithiasis in pregnant women: imaging algorithm and literature review. AJR Am J Roentgenol 1996;167:869–75.

[20] LeRoy AJ. Imaging of acute maternal diseases in pregnancy. Categorical course in diagnostic radiology at the 92nd Scientific Assembly and Annual Meeting. In: Ramchandani P, editor. Genitourinary radiology syllabus. Chicago: Radiological Society of North America; 2006. p. 271–9.

[21] Kirpalani A, Khalili K, Lee S, et al. Renal colic: comparison of use and outcomes of unenhanced helical CT for emergency investigation in 1998 and 2002. Radiology 2005;236(2):554–8.

[22] Ha M, MacDonald RD. Impact of CT scan in patients with first episode of suspected nephrolithiasis. J Emerg Med 2004;27:225–31.

[23] Boulay I, Holtz P, Foley WD, et al. Ureteral calculi: diagnostic efficacy of helical CT and implications for treatment of patients. AJR Am J Roentgenol 1999;172:1485–90.

[24] Dorio PJ, Pozniak MA, Lee FT Jr, et al. Non-contrast-enhanced helical computed tomography for the evaluation of patients with acute flank pain. Wis Med J 1999;98:30–4.

[25] Chen MY, Zagoria RJ, Saunders HS, et al. Trends in the use of unenhanced helical CT for acute urinary colic. AJR Am J Roentgenol 1999;173:1447–50.

[26] Vieweg J, The C, Freed K, et al. Unenhanced helical computerized tomography for the evaluation of patients with acute flank pain. J Urol 1998;160:679–84.

[27] Fielding JR, Fox LA, Heller H, et al. Spiral CT in the evaluation of flank pain: overall accuracy and feature analysis. J Comput Assist Tomogr 1997;21:635–8.

[28] Ketelslegers E, VanBeers BE. Urinary calculi: improved detection and characterization with thin-slice multidetector CT. Eur Radiol 2006;16(1):161–5; [Epub 2005 Jun 16].

[29] Memarsadeghi M, Heinz-Peer G, Helbich TH, et al. Unenhanced multi-detector row CT in patients suspected of having urinary stone disease: effect of section width on diagnosis. Radiology 2005;235:530–6.

[30] Kopp JB, Miller KD, Mican JA, et al. Crystalluria and urinary tract abnormalities associated with indinavir. Ann Intern Med 1997;127:119–25.

[31] Takahashi N, Kawashima A, Ernst RD, et al. Ureterolithiasis: can clinical outcome be predicted with unenhanced helical CT? Radiology 1998;208:97–102.

[32] Olcott EW, SOmmers FG, Napel S. Accuracy of detection and measurement of renal calculi: in vitro comparison of three-dimensional spiral CT, radiography, and nephrotomography. Radiology 1997;204:19–25.

[33] Parsons JK, Lancini V, Shetye K, et al. Urinary stone size: comparison of abdominal plain radiography and noncontrast CT measurements. J Endourol 2003;17:725–8.

[34] Nadler RB, Stern JA, Kim S, et al. Coronal imaging to assess urinary tract stone size. J Urol 2004;172:962–4.

[35] Varanelli MJ, Coll DM, Levine JA, et al. Relationship between duration of pain and secondary signs of obstruction of the urinary tract on unenhanced helical CT. AJR Am J Roentgenol 2001; 177:325–30.

[36] Katz DS, Lane MJ, Sommer FG. Unenhanced helical CT of ureteral stones: incidence of associated urinary tract findings. AJR Am J Roentgenol 1996;166:1319–22.

[37] Boridy IC, Kawashima A, Goldman SM, et al. Acute ureterolithiasis: nonenhanced helical CT findings of perinephric edema for prediction of degree of ureteral obstruction. Radiology 1999; 213:663–7.

[38] Kawashima A, Sandler CM, Boridy IC, et al. Unenhanced helical CT of ureterolithiasis: value of the tissue rim sign. AJR Am J Roentgenol 1997; 168:997–1000.

[39] Heneghan JP, Dalrymple NC, Verga M, et al. Soft-tissue "rim" sign in the diagnosis of ureteral calculi with use of unenhanced helical CT. Radiology 1997;202:709–11.

[40] Boridy IC, Nikolaidis P, Kawashima A, et al. Ureterolithiasis: value of the tail sign in differentiating phleboliths from ureteral calculi at nonenhanced helical CT. Radiology 1999;211: 619–21.

[41] Traubici J, Neitlich JD, Smith RC. Distinguishing pelvic phleboliths from distal ureteral stones on routine unenhanced helical CT: is there a radiolucent center? AJR Am J Roentgenol 1999; 172:13–7.

[42] Pfister SA, Deckart A, Laschke S, et al. Unenhanced helical computed tomography vs intravenous urography in patients with acute flank pain: accuracy and economic impact in a randomized prospective trial. Eur Radiol 2003;13: 2513–20.

[43] Heneghan JP, Mcguire KA, Leder RA, et al. Helical CT for nephrolithiasis and ureterolithiasis: comparison of conventional and reduced radiation dose techniques. Radiology 2003;229:575–80.

[44] Tack D, Sourtzis S, Delpierre I, et al. Low dose unenhanced MDCT of patients with suspected renal colic. AJR Am J Roentgenol 2003;180: 305–11.

[45] MacKersie AB, Lane MJ, Gerhardt RT, et al. Nontraumatic acute abdominal pain: unenhanced helical CT compared with three-view acute abdominal series. Radiology 2005;237(1):114–22.

[46] Rogers LF. Dose reduction in CT: how low can we go? AJR Am J Roentgenol 2002;179:299.

[47] Diel J, Perlmutter S, Venkataramanan N, et al. Unenhanced helical CT using increased pitch for suspected renal colic: an effective technique for radiation dose reduction? J Comput Assist Tomogr 2000;24:795–801.

[48] Mulkens TM, Daineffe S, De Wijngaert R, et al. Urinary stone disease: comparison of standard dose and low dose with 4D MDCT tube current modulation. AJR Am J Roentgenol 2007;188:553–62.

[49] Catalano O, Nunziata A, Alei F, et al. Suspected ureteral colic: primary helical CT versus selective helical CT alter unenhanced radiography and sonography. AJR Am J Roentgenol 2002;178: 379–87.

[50] Fowler KAB, Locken JA, Duchesne JH, et al. US for detecting renal calculi with nonenhanced CT as a reference standard. Radiology 2002; 222:109–13.

[51] Tublin ME, Dodd GD, Verdile VP. Acute renal colic: diagnosis with duplex Doppler US. Radiology 1994;193:697–701.

[52] Sheafor DH, Hertzberg BS, Freed KS, et al. Nonenhanced helical CT and US in the emergency evaluation of patients with renal colic: prospective comparison. Radiology 2000;217:792–97.

[53] Middleton WD, Dodds WJ, Lawson TL, et al. Renal calculi: sensitivity for detection with US. Radiology 1988;167:239–44.

[54] Burge HJ, Middleton WD, McClennan BL, et al. Ureteral jets in healthy subjects and in patients with unilateral ureteral calculi: comparison with color Doppler US. Radiology 1991;180: 437–42.

[55] Blandino A, Gaeta M, Minutoli F, et al. MR pyelography in 115 patients with a dilated renal collecting system. Acta Radiol 2001;42:532–6.

[56] Sudah M, Vanninen R, Partanen K, et al. MR urography in evaluation of acute flank pain: T2-weighted sequences and gadolinium-enhanced three-dimensional FLASH compared with urography—fast low-angle shot. AJR Am J Roentgenol 2001;176:105–12.

[57] Lewis DF, Robichaux AG III, Jaekle RK, et al. Urolithiasis in pregnancy: diagnosis, management and pregnancy outcome. J Reprod Med 2003; 48:28–32.

[58] Stothers L, Lee LM. Renal colic in pregnancy. J Urol 1992;148:1383–7.

[59] Grenier N, Pariente JL, Trillaud H, et al. Dilatation of the collecting system during pregnancy: physiologic vs. obstructive dilatation. Eur Radiol 2000;10:271–9.

[60] Katz DS, Scheer M, Lumerman JH, et al. Alternative or additional diagnoses on unenhanced helical computed tomography for suspected renal colic: experience with 1000 consecutive examinations. Urology 2000;56:53–7.

[61] Rucker CM, Menias CO, Bhalla S. Mimics of renal colic: alternative diagnoses at unenhanced helical CT. Radiographics 2004;24:S11–28.

[62] Chen MY, Scharling ES, Zagoria RJ, et al. CT diagnosis of acute flank pain from urolithiasis. Semin Ultrasound CT MR 2000;21:2–19.

[63] Smith RC, Levine J, Dalrymple NC, et al. Acute flank pain: a modern approach to diagnosis and management. Semin Ultrasound CT MR 1999;20:108–35.

[64] Hoppe H, Studer R, Kessler TM, et al. Alternate or additional findings to stone disease on unenhanced computerized tomography for acute

flank pain can impact management. J Urol 2006; 175(5):1725–30; [discussion: 1730].

[65] Ahmad NA, Ather MH, Rees J. Incidental diagnosis of diseases on un-enhanced helical computed tomography performed for ureteric colic. BMC Urol 2003;17(3):2.

[66] Katz DS, Jain M. Invited commentary. Radiographics 2004;24:S28–33.

[67] Benjaminov O, Atri M, Hamilton P. Frequency of visualization and thickness of normal appendix at nonenhanced helical CT. Radiology 2002; 225:400–6.

[68] Llach F. Hypercoagulability, renal vein thrombosis, and other thrombotic complications of nephrotic syndrome. Kidney Int 1985;28:429.

[69] Glassock RJ. Diagnosis and natural course of membranous nephropathy. Semin Nephrol 2003; 23:324–32.

[70] Lupetin AR, Mainwaring BL, Daffner RH. CT diagnosis of renal artery injury caused by blunt abdominal trauma. AJR Am J Roentgenol 1989; 153(5):1065–8.

[71] Domanovits H, Paulis M, Nikfardjam M, et al. Acute renal infarction. Clinical characteristics of 17 patients. Medicine 1999;78:386–94.

[72] Carey HB, Boltax R, Dickey KW, et al. Bilateral renal infarction secondary to paradoxical embolism. Am J Kidney Dis 1999;34:752–5.

[73] Cosby RL, Miller PD, Schrier RW. Traumatic renal artery thrombosis. Am J Med 1986;81:890–4.

[74] Ivanovic V, McKusick MA, Johnson CM, et al. Renal artery stent placement: complications at a single tertiary care center. J Vasc Interv Radiol 2003;14:217–25.

[75] Krishnan P, Anandh U, Fernandes DK, et al. Renal failure in a patient with primary antiphospholipid syndrome. J Assoc Physicians India 2002;50:964–6.

[76] Lumerman JH, Hom D, Eiley D, et al. Heightened suspicion and rapid evaluation with CT for early diagnosis of partial renal infarction. J Endourol 1999;13:209–14.

[77] Thompson SK, Goldman SM, Shah KB, et al. Acute non-traumatic maternal illnesses in pregnancy: imaging approaches. Emerg Radiol 2005;11(4):199–212.

[78] Webb EM, Green GE, Scoutt LM. Adnexal mass with pelvic pain. Radiol Clin North Am 2004; 42(2):329–48.

[79] Houry D, Abbott JT. Ovarian torsion: a fifteen year review. Ann Emerg Med 2001;38:156–9.

[80] Hertzberg BS, Kliewer MA, Paulson EK. Ovarian cyst rupture causing hemoperitoneum: imaging features and the potential for misdiagnosis. Abdom Imaging 1999;24:304–8.

[81] Umaria N, Offliff JF. Imaging features of pelvic endometriosis. Br J Radiol 2001;74:556–62.

[82] Wilbur AC, Aizenstein RI, Napp TE. CT findings in tuboovarian abscess. AJR Am J Roentgenol 1992;158:575–9.

[83] Langer JE, Dinsmore BJ. Computed tomographic evaluation of benign and inflammatory disorders of the female pelvis. Radiol Clin North Am 1992;30:831–42.

ELSEVIER
SAUNDERS

RADIOLOGIC
CLINICS
OF NORTH AMERICA

Radiol Clin N Am 45 (2007) 411–422

Current Concepts in Imaging of Appendicitis

Alexander V. Rybkin, MD, Ruedi F. Thoeni, MD

- Anatomy and pathogenesis of appendicitis
- Clinical features of appendicitis
- Selection of imaging modality for diagnosing appendicitis

CT of appendicitis
Ultrasound diagnosis of appendicitis
MR imaging of appendicitis
- Summary
- Acknowledgments
- References

There are more than 250,000 new cases of acute appendicitis in the United States every year [1], and appendicitis is the most common cause of acute abdominal pain requiring surgery. Early diagnosis is crucial to the success of therapy, which consists of surgical removal of the inflamed appendix before it perforates. It has long been recognized that rapid and accurate diagnosis of appendicitis improves patient outcome [2]. CT and ultrasound are widely recognized as very useful in the timely diagnosis of appendicitis. MR imaging is emerging as an alternative to CT in pregnant patients and in patients who have an allergy to iodinated contrast material. This articles reviews the current imaging methods and diagnostic features of appendicitis.

Anatomy and pathogenesis of appendicitis

Vermiform appendix is a blind-ended loop of bowel that arises from the cecum 3 to 4 cm below the ileocecal valve. Although the base of the appendix is relatively fixed, its tip usually is freely mobile. Therefore, location of the appendix is highly variable. In an anatomic study of 10,000 patients [3], the most common location was paracolic/retrocolic, with the appendix extending superiorly

(65% of cases). Other locations for the appendix were the iliac fossa (31%), retrocecal (2.5%), and paricecal/peri-ileal regions (1.5%). A more recent imaging-based study showed that in only 4% is the appendix located at the classic McBurney point (the junction of the lateral and middle third of the line between the anterior superior iliac spine and the umbilicus) [4].

Appendicitis occurs when a fecalith, fecal matter, or lymphoid hyperplasia obstructs the appendix. Obstruction leads to inflammation, rising intraluminal pressures, and ultimately ischemia. Subsequently, the appendix enlarges and incites inflammatory changes in the surrounding tissues, such as in the pericecal fat and peritoneum. If untreated, the inflamed appendix eventually perforates.

Appendicitis occurs most often in the second decade of life (at a median age of 22 years) [5], with a lifetime risk of 8.6% for males and 6.7% for females [1]. The overall rate of perforation is about 26% and is believed to result largely from the delay in initial presentation, although the in-hospital delay in diagnosis may play a role [6]. When the appendix perforates, surgical morbidity and mortality increase sharply. Mortality increases from

Department of Radiology, University of California San Francisco School of Medicine, San Francisco General Hospital, 1001 Potrero Ave., 1x57E, San Francisco, CA 94110, USA
E-mail address: manxray@yahoo.com (R.F. Thoeni).

doi:10.1016/j.rcl.2007.04.003

0.0002% to 3%, and morbidity increases from 3% to 47% [5]. These numbers underscore the importance of speed and high accuracy in diagnosing appendicitis.

Clinical features of appendicitis

Patients who have appendicitis typically present with diffuse abdominal pain, anorexia, nausea, vomiting, and subsequent migration of pain to the right lower quadrant. This pattern, although suggestive, is present in only 50% to 60% of patients who have appendicitis [7]. Atypical symptoms can result from variability in the location of the appendix [8]. The characteristic clinical picture frequently is absent in young children (before the age of 5 years), who cannot provide adequate history, and in the elderly, whose peritoneal symptoms may be blunted. The elevated rates of appendiceal perforation in these groups (45% and 51%, respectively, compared with 25.8% in the general population) reflect the difficulty in making the clinical diagnosis [5,7]. Laboratory abnormalities may include leukocytosis and elevated C-reactive protein, which are observed frequently but also can occur in many other conditions.

The differential diagnosis of appendicitis includes a long list of common gastrointestinal and genitourinary disorders (Box 1). Before the widespread use of imaging, the accuracy of clinical diagnosis of appendicitis was around 80% [2], which led to the traditional teaching that a rate of up to 20% for pathologically normal appendices at appendectomy ("negative appendectomy") was acceptable. It also was noted that the rate of negative appendectomy was inversely proportional to the rate of perforation. If the diagnostic criteria

---

Box 1: Differential diagnosis of appendicitis
Acute mesenteric adenitis
Acute gastroenteritis
Pelvic inflammatory disease
Urinary tract infection
Ureteral stone
Ruptured Graafian follicle
Epiploic appendagitis
Endometriosis
Ovarian torsion
Ruptured ectopic pregnancy
Meckel's diverticulum
Intussusception
Crohn's disease
yersiniosis
Perforated peptic ulcer
Henoch-Schönlein purpura

were more stringent, fewer patients would receive early appendectomy, putting those who had equivocal symptoms at a greater risk of perforation. Since the introduction of routine cross-sectional imaging for appendicitis, some institutions have experienced a drop in the negative appendectomy rate to 3% without increase in the rate of perforation; this experience demonstrates the significant impact of modern imaging upon diagnosis and management of these patients [9].

Selection of imaging modality for diagnosing appendicitis

Ultrasound and abdominal CT have a distinct advantage over clinical assessment alone in diagnosing appendicitis [10,11]. Doria and colleagues [12] performed a meta-analysis of the studies published between 1986 and 2004 to assess the accuracy of CT and ultrasound. CT had a pooled sensitivity and specificity of 94% and 95%, respectively, in children and 94% and 94%, respectively, in adults. Ultrasound had a pooled sensitivity and specificity of 88% and 94%, respectively, in children, and 83% and 93%, respectively, in adults. Studies that compared CT and ultrasound directly confirmed that CT was more sensitive than ultrasound [13,14]. Another disadvantage of ultrasound is that its success depends strongly on the knowledge, skill, and patience of the sonologist. In a landmark article published in *The New England Journal of Medicine*, Rao and colleagues [10] advocated the routine use of CT in all patients who met admission criteria for suspected appendicitis. This study showed that routine CT improved patient outcome and reduced hospital costs for managing appendicitis. This study helped make CT the preferred modality for diagnosing appendicitis.

Since then the usefulness of routine use of CT imaging has come under increasing scrutiny, primarily in the surgical and pediatric literature. Specifically, the beneficial effects of routine CT imaging on patient outcome as manifested by decreased rates of negative appendectomy and perforation have been challenged [15,16]. Surgical research also suggested that routine CT offers no advantage in patients who have a classic clinical presentation of appendicitis [17,18]. Unnecessary CT imaging may even lead to delay in diagnosis and treatment of appendicitis. A more targeted approach, which uses imaging only in clinically equivocal cases, is emerging.

The use of CT imaging in adult men suspected of having appendicitis often is not indicated, because there usually is less clinical uncertainty [18]. Women of childbearing age, however, benefit greatly from preoperative imaging, whether by CT or ultrasound [19]. A number of gynecologic conditions (eg, pelvic inflammatory disease, ruptured Graafian follicles, endometriosis, ovarian torsion) may simulate the clinical presentation of appendicitis, reducing the accuracy of clinical work-up to 65% in this group, compared with 82% in the rest of the population [5]. Both CT and ultrasound can be helpful, but CT seems to have an advantage over ultrasound in sensitivity (95% versus 61%) [12].

Children are another subgroup that merits special consideration. Although CT seems to have an advantage over ultrasound and clinical evaluation alone in preventing negative appendectomy and perforation [20], concerns over radiation exposure limit the use of this modality. Children are more susceptible than adults to the effects of ionizing radiation. The best available theoretical models suggest that a single abdominal CT may raise the lifetime risk of fatal cancer in a child. This elevation of lifetime risk is greater for a child than for an adult by a full order of magnitude [21]. Even so, an abdominal CT examination, if done in the first year of life, would contribute only 0.35% to the background lifetime cancer mortality. Although this contribution is small, it is preventable. Therefore, many institutions use ultrasound as the initial step, followed by CT only if sonographic diagnosis is uncertain. This approach seems to have excellent accuracy, with reported sensitivity of 94% to 99% and specificity of 94% to 95% [11,22–24].

Radiation exposure also is an important factor in managing pregnant patients. Fetal exposure from abdominal multidetector CT performed in the first trimester may double the likelihood of childhood cancer (from 1 to 2 in 600) [25]. Consequently, ultrasound is usually the first study attempted. Although high accuracy of ultrasound in pregnancy has been reported [26], several factors limit its usefulness. The appendix may be displaced from its expected location by the gravid uterus. The enlarged uterus also may make graded compression difficult. MR imaging has emerged recently as a useful second-line technique and seems to have a high accuracy and low failure rate [27,28]. The use of MR imaging eliminates radiation exposure of the fetus, avoids the operator dependency of ultrasound, and facilitates rendering alternative diagnoses, such as ovarian torsion or renal obstruction.

CT of appendicitis

CT techniques

There are several valid approaches to CT of appendicitis. Most of the validated protocols use helical CT. These protocols differ in the use of intravenous (IV), oral, or rectal contrast and in the extent of anatomic coverage. The use of thin sections (at least 5 mm) through the region of the appendix seems to be a common feature. The most common approach uses IV and oral contrast and covers the entire abdomen and pelvis [29,30]. The high accuracy of this technique for the diagnosis of appendicitis has long been established (sensitivity 96%; specificity 89%; accuracy 94%) [13]. The main advantage of this technique is its ability to establish alternative or concurrent diagnoses. This ability is particularly important in patients whose clinical presentations are equivocal, because these patients have a greater chance of having alternative conditions, such as pelvic inflammatory disease. Scanning the entire abdomen allows easy visualization of appendices in nonstandard positions, including the right upper quadrant. The best results are achieved when the cecum is opacified by contrast, allowing detection of secondary colonic pathology. To take advantage of oral contrast in this way, one must wait 1 hour or more after administration of oral contrast to image the patient. This delay is the main disadvantage of this protocol, although it is unclear if it is long enough to adversely effect outcomes.

An alternative, more focused method, advocated by Rao and colleagues, involves administration of rectal contrast and scanning only the lower abdomen (below the lower pole of the right kidney) and upper pelvis [9,10,31]. The reported sensitivity, specificity, and accuracy of this technique are 98%. When used for all patients who met criteria for admission for appendicitis, this approach reduced the negative appendectomy rate from 20% to 3%; however, it yielded an alternative explanation of the patient's symptoms in only 39% of the cases that were negative for appendicitis [31]. Wise and colleagues [32] compared this focused technique with an unfocused abdominopelvic CT with IV contrast. Although the accuracy was not significantly different, the interpreting radiologists reported more confidence in positive cases when the focused technique was used. The nonfocused technique yielded more confidence in a negative result. This experience is not surprising, because enteric contrast is very helpful in establishing the diagnosis of appendicitis. Jacobs and colleagues [33] compared a similar focused technique (the only difference being oral administration of enteric contrast) with a nonfocused technique with IV and oral contrast and demonstrated that a nonfocused approach had higher sensitivity. In one case, the focused technique missed an inflamed appendix that was out of the limited field view of the study. Another study compared the usefulness of focused and nonfocused techniques in cases that were negative for appendicitis [34]. The unfocused protocol established alternative diagnoses in significantly more cases (56%) than the focused technique. The focused protocol missed several diagnoses that needed immediate surgery. Clearly, the nonfocused technique allows a more complete examination than the targeted protocol.

Another well-studied technique is unenhanced CT of the abdomen and pelvis [35–38]. The advantages of this approach are speed and lack of patient preparation. This technique also avoids the inherent risks of exposure to IV contrast medium, which may include allergic reactions and nephrotoxicity. In a patient population, in which appendicitis was clinically suspected, this protocol yielded sensitivity of 96%, specificity of 99%, and accuracy of 97% [37,38]. Although the accuracy of unenhanced CT is excellent for the diagnosis of appendicitis, its overall usefulness is less clear. In patients who did not have appendicitis, alternative diagnoses were achieved only 35% of the time [35]. Detection of abnormalities by unenhanced CT is considerably easier when there is ample intra-abdominal fat. Thin patients, such as children and young women, may be particularly difficult to examine without intravenous contrast material.

At the University of California, San Francisco, the authors and colleagues use a reconstructed slice thickness of 3 to 5 mm for the helical scanner and of 2.5 to 5 mm or thinner as needed for the multidetector scanner. The patients initially are imaged supine, but in difficult cases the author finds it helpful to obtain additional images with the patient in left or right lateral decubitus position. The author and colleagues routinely administer IV, oral, and rectal contrast in their CT protocol for appendicitis, which yields excellent accuracy for appendicitis and alternative diagnoses. They traditionally have used positive enteric contrast. More recently they have had excellent results with neutral contrast material or plain water. This approach which has the advantage of optimal small bowel distention. The use of rectal contrast shortens the delay of diagnosis, because it is not necessary to wait for oral contrast to reach the cecum. Rectal contrast helps identify the appendix in difficult cases [31]. It allows exquisite imaging of the colon, which is helpful because large bowel pathology can resemble appendicitis [37]. Opacification of the rectum and sigmoid also can help distinguish pelvic organs, such as ovaries, from adjacent bowel loops. The patient discomfort associated with administration of rectal contrast and the risks of IV contrast are the disadvantages of this approach. A recent survey found that 21% of academic institutions use CT with IV, oral, and rectal contrast for diagnosis of appendicitis [29].

CT findings of appendicitis

On CT The inflamed appendix appears as an enlarged blind-ending tubular structure, frequently associated with inflammatory stranding in the surrounding fat (Fig. 1). Identification of the appendix is possible with most of the modern CT protocols. The entire appendix should be examined, from cecal insertion to the tip, and the largest transverse diameter should be reported. Traditionally, the threshold diameter of 6 mm was used for diagnosis of appendicitis. Among patients who were prescreened by physical examination and

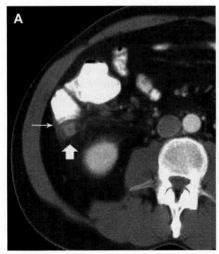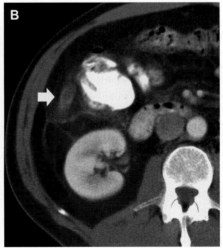

Fig. 1. Axial CT images demonstrate uncomplicated appendicitis. (*A*) An enhancing enlarged appendix is seen near the cecal tip (*thick arrow*) surrounded by inflammatory fat stranding. The adjacent cecal wall is thickened (*thin arrow*). (*B*) A slightly higher image demonstrates the inflamed appendix (*thick arrow*) as it courses superiorly along the ascending colon.

ultrasound, enlargement of the fluid-filled appendix above 6 mm had independent sensitivity of 93% and specificity of 92% [39]. In a general population, however, the threshold of 6 mm may be too low. Studies of healthy adults revealed that the normal range of appendiceal size in an adult patient is 3 to 10 mm [40]. In 42% of normal adults the appendiceal diameter was greater than 6 mm. It has been suggested that appendices in the range of 6 to 10 mm should be considered indeterminate [40,41]. When the appendix is within this range, secondary signs, such as fat stranding or cecal changes, are needed for a definitive diagnosis of appendicitis on CT. When such secondary signs are absent, Daly and colleagues [41] advocate using an appendiceal threshold size of 9 mm.

Thickening of the appendiceal wall of over 1 mm (sensitivity 66%, specificity 96%) and abnormal enhancement (sensitivity 75%, specificity 85%) have been proposed as additional signs of appendicitis [39]. The thickness of the wall can be difficult to measure precisely even with electronic calipers, however.

The inflamed appendix usually does not fill with rectal contrast or gas, but if the point of obstruction is not at the base, a small amount of fluid or contrast can leak into the proximal portion of the appendix. Gas also may be present within the inflamed appendix because of the presence of gas-forming microorganisms [31]. Therefore the presence of contrast or gas within the appendix should not be used to exclude appendicitis. Appendicoliths are visualized in 20% to 40% of cases of appendicitis and may confer a greater risk of perforation. Visualization of an appendicolith in the presence of secondary inflammatory findings strongly suggests appendicitis, even if the appendix itself is not visualized [30].

Signs of inflammation in the structures adjacent to the appendix are useful, because appendiceal size alone does not allow a confident diagnosis. Periappendiceal fat stranding has sensitivity of 87% and specificity of 74% in a prescreened population [39]. Fat stranding (and thickening of lateroconal fascia) lacks specificity for appendicitis because it can occur in such mimickers of appendicitis as Crohn's disease, infectious colitis, and diverticulitis. Focal inflammatory thickening of the cecum is common at the cecal apex (sensitivity of 69%) (Fig. 2). Cecal wall thickening also may create the appearance of funneling of the cecal wall toward the origin of the appendix (Fig. 3). This appearance is termed "cecal arrowhead" sign (sensitivity of 23%). The rare "cecal bar" sign is seen when the inflamed cecal wall is interposed between cecal contents and a proximal obstructing appendicolith (Fig. 4) [42]. Both the arrowhead sign and the cecal bar sign can be diagnosed only if positive contrast is present in the cecum. When the cecal wall thickening is circumferential, the thickening is more likely to be caused by intrinsic bowel pathology, such as colitis, than by appendicitis [37]. If the appendix is not visualized, the absence of inflammatory findings makes appendicitis unlikely [43].

The signs of perforated appendicitis include phlegmon, abscess, extraluminal gas, extraluminal appendicolith, and focal defect in the enhancement of the appendiceal wall (Fig. 5). In patients who are known to have appendicitis, identification of any one of these five findings has a reported sensitivity of 95% and specificity of 100% for perforation [44]. The presence of a phlegmon is the least specific sign.

Ultrasound diagnosis of appendicitis

Sonographic technique

Puylaert [45] proposed the sonographic graded compression technique for diagnosis of appendicitis in 1986. With the patient supine, a linear-array high-frequency transducer is used to compress the right lower quadrant while imaging. The use of harmonic imaging may facilitate visualization of the appendix and the relevant surrounding structures [46]. The examiner slowly applies gentle pressure with the transducer to displace the air-filled bowel loops, which commonly obscure the sonographic evaluation of the peritoneal cavity. The inflamed appendix is relatively fixed and can be imaged by this technique in most cases. Transverse images usually are the most helpful for identification of the cecum and the appendix. Longitudinal images of the appendix subsequently are obtained for complete demonstration of its morphology. It is helpful to ascertain that the visualized structure is blind-ending, to differentiate it from the adjacent terminal ileum. One also should strive to image the tip, because inflammation can be limited to the distal appendix. Color Doppler images of the appendiceal wall can be obtained; these images may be helpful in equivocal cases [47].

Compression usually is started at the point of maximal tenderness, which helps identify the site of the inflamed appendix. When a patient can self-localize the site of maximal pain, there is a significant sonographic finding at this site 94% of the time [48]. Interaction of the sonologist with the patient therefore is crucial to the success of the examination. The proper examination should not be hurried. Compressing the abdomen slowly, in a graded fashion, allows the bowel time to move out of the right lower quadrant. Fast compression usually is ineffective and can be very painful to a patient who has peritonitis. Jerky compression

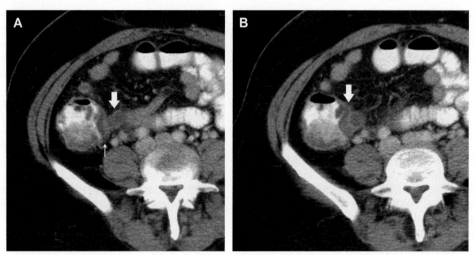

Fig. 2. Focal cecal wall thickening in a patient who has appendicitis. (A) Axial CT image demonstrates the relationship between the origin of the enlarged appendix (*thick arrow*) and the focal edema in the wall of the cecum (*thin arrow*). (B) A slightly lower cut demonstrates the focal wall thickening of the cecum (*thick arrow*). The majority of the cecal wall is normal. Care should be taken not to confuse focal cecal wall thickening with an ileocecal valve, which normally contains fat.

also may rupture an appendix on the verge of perforation.

Several additional maneuvers have be been shown to facilitate visualization of the appendix [49,50]. Applying pressure posteriorly with the left hand directed toward the transducer helps improve the degree of compression and is reported to increase the rate of visualization of the appendix to 95% [49]. Lee and colleagues [50] have advocated another intriguing technique called "upward graded compression." This technique consists of forceful

upward sweeps with the transducer to displace the cecum and appendix upward. This technique may be particularly useful when the appendix is low lying or pelvic. Putting the patient in left lateral decubitus position may be helpful in visualizing a retrocecal appendix [51].

Sonographic findings

The appendix appears on ultrasound as a lamellated, elongated, blind-ending structure (Fig. 6). Unlike normal bowel, the inflamed appendix is

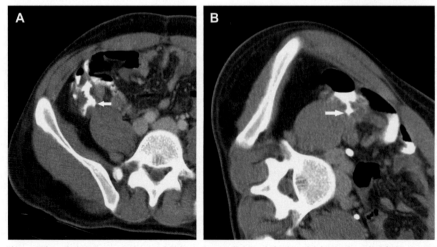

Fig. 3. Cecal arrowhead sign in a patient who has appendicitis. (A) The thickened wall of the cecum seems to "funnel" contrast material toward the origin of the appendix (*arrow*). This appearance is termed the "*cecal arrowhead*" sign. (B) The patient was scanned in left lateral decubitus position. The image demonstrates another example of the cecal arrowhead sign (*arrow*).

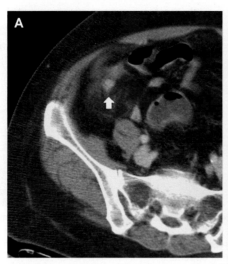
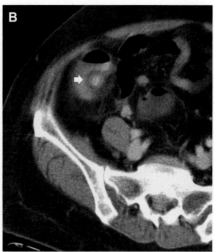

Fig. 4. Appendicolith and the cecal bar sign in appendicitis. (*A*) An appendicolith is identified at the origin of the inflamed appendix (*arrow*). (*B*) This cut is slightly superior to the cut in panel A. The appendicolith is seen again and is separated from the contrast material by the thickened wall of the cecum (*arrow*). This appearance is termed the "cecal bar sign." Note the difference between the density of the appendicolith and the density of the contrast within the cecum.

fixed, noncompressible, and appears round on transverse images. Measurements of appendix are performed with full compression. Traditionally, the diagnosis of appendicitis is made when the diameter of the compressed appendix exceeds 6 mm [52]. The size criterion remains the most important sonographic sign of appendicitis, with reported sensitivity of 98% [53]; however the threshold of 6 mm has been called into question. Just as with CT,

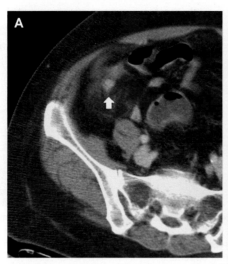

Fig. 5. Perforated appendicitis. This image demonstrates a focal defect in the enhancement of the wall of the appendix (*arrow*). Adjacent to this defect is a small focus of free gas and extensive fat stranding/early phlegmon.

sonographic studies of normal individuals show that up to 23% of normal patients have appendiceal sizes greater than 6 mm [54]. The ultrasound department at the San Francisco General Hospital uses a threshold of 7 mm to improve the specificity of their sonographic evaluation (Fig. 7).

Inflammatory changes in the fat surrounding the appendix sometimes are detectable by ultrasound and can be used in the diagnosis of appendicitis. The inflamed fat appears brightly echogenic and noncompressible. Appendiceal perforation can be diagnosed when the appendix demonstrates irregular contour or when periappendiceal fluid collections are identified (Fig. 8). Appendicoliths are seen in 30% of appendicitis cases and may confer a higher risk of perforation [47].

Doppler examination usually reveals increased vascularity in and around the acutely inflamed appendix. Doppler examination is useful as an adjunct sign of appendicitis when the appendiceal measurement is equivocal (Fig. 9) [55]. When increased flow is seen, it is a sensitive sign of appendicitis (reported sensitivity of 87%) [56], but blood flow decreases in advanced inflammation, when intraluminal pressures exceed perfusion pressures. Doppler signal is diminished when the appendix is gangrenous or close to necrosis. Therefore, Doppler examination cannot reliably distinguish between normal and abnormal appendix.

Multiple studies revealed that the appendix is visualized more easily when it is inflamed. Whether the appendix is visualized also depends on the skill of the operator; for an experienced sonologist,

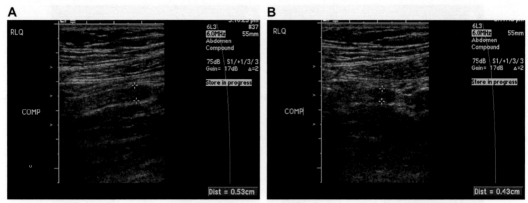

Fig. 6. Sonographic appearance of a normal appendix. (*A*) Longitudinal image of the appendix its normal lamellated appearance. Measurement was performed under compression. Diameter of less than 6 mm has an excellent negative predictive value for appendicitis. (*B*) Transverse image of the appendix, taken under compression, demonstrates compressibility (deformation) of the normal appendix.

armed with modern equipment, nonvisualization has a negative predictive value of 90% [53]. Cases of perforated appendicitis can be particularly easy to miss, because the appendix usually is decompressed. Therefore, nonvisualization should be interpreted with caution. When appendix is visualized, its shape can be used to exclude appendicitis [57]. The most significant finding is an ovoid shape on transverse section of the appendix throughout its length. (Inflamed appendices usually are round in transverse section.) This finding is particularly useful when compressibility of the appendix cannot be assessed, for example when the appendix is located in the pelvis.

MR imaging of appendicitis

MR imaging technique

MR imaging has a limited role in the work-up of suspected appendicitis. Although the use of MR imaging avoids ionizing radiation, it has several disadvantages, including high cost, long duration of studies, and limited availability on an emergent basis. At the UCSF School of Medicine the use of MR imaging is limited to pregnant patients in whom ultrasound is inconclusive.

There are no known adverse effects of MR imaging in human pregnancy, but the safety of MR imaging has not been proven unequivocally [58]. Although tissue heating from radiofrequency pulses

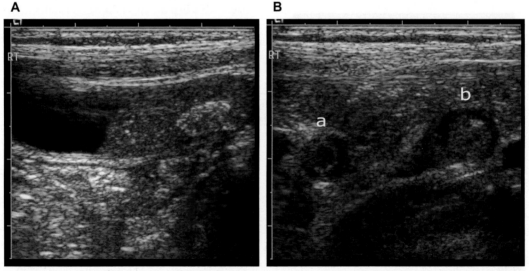

Fig. 7. Sonographic appearance of appendicitis. (*A*) Longitudinal image demonstrates an enlarged appendix with an appendicolith at its tip. Notice sonographic shadowing from the appendicolith. The diameter of the appendix was 11 mm. (*B*) Transverse image demonstrates two cross sections of the appendix (*a* and *b*), as it curves in and out of the plane of the probe. Inflammation seems to be limited to the distal appendix (*b*).

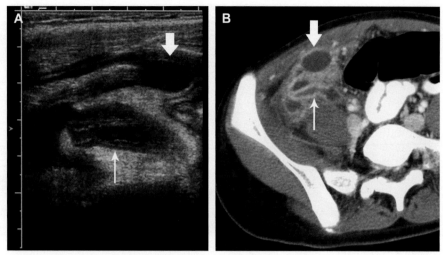

Fig. 8. Perforated appendicitis. (*A*) Transverse gray-scale ultrasound image demonstrates a relatively decompressed appendix (*thin arrow*) surrounded by fluid and hyperechoic inflamed fat. An abscess is identified superficial to the appendix (*thick arrow*). (*B*) Axial CT image in the same patient demonstrates the appendix (*thin arrow*) and the abscess (*thick arrow*). Note the appearance of the inflammatory fat on ultrasound and CT.

and acoustic stimulation potentially could harm the fetus, these concerns remain theoretical [59,60]. Gadolinium easily crosses the placenta and enters fetal circulation. It remains there for an indefinite amount of time, excreted by the fetal kidneys and subsequently swallowed by the fetus with amniotic fluid [61]. Although there is no evidence of mutagenic or teratogenic effects of gadolinium in humans, mutagenic effects were seen in animal studies [62]. Therefore the author and colleagues take a conservative approach and avoid using gadolinium when possible. It should be avoided at all costs in the first trimester.

Incesu and colleagues [28] suggested the use of fat-suppressed fast spin echo T2 and gadolinium-enhanced T1 sequences for the diagnosis of appendicitis. This technique was found to be superior to sonography in sensitivity and equal to it in specificity. The UCSF School of Medicine uses a protocol that includes fast spin echo T2 sequences in axial and coronal planes performed on a 1.5-Tesla MR imaging scanner. If needed, gadolinium is administered, but only in patients beyond the first trimester. Using a similar noncontrast technique, Cobben and colleagues [63] showed that MR imaging is far superior to ultrasound in pregnant patients. Ultrasound failed to identify the appendix in 11 of 12 patients. MR imaging, on the other hand, correctly diagnosed appendicitis in three patients, without false positives.

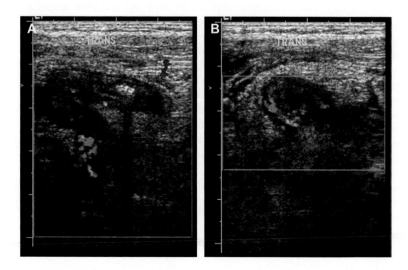

Fig. 9. Color Doppler images of acute appendicitis. (*A*) Longitudinal image of the appendix demonstrates an appendicolith, but the size of the appendix was equivocal. (*B*) Transverse image with color Doppler demonstrates focally increased flow in the wall of the appendix. Note the hyperechoic inflamed fat surrounding the appendix.

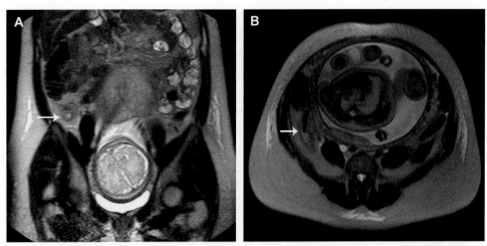

Fig. 10. MR imaging of acute appendicitis in a pregnant woman. (*A*) Coronal single-shot fast spin echo sequence demonstrates an enlarged fluid-filled appendix (*arrow*). (*B*) Axial single-shot fast spin echo sequence again demonstrates the enlarged appendix (*arrow*). The elongated low signal intensity structures seen within the appendix turned out to be appendicoliths.

MR imaging findings of appendicitis

On MR imaging, the appendix is identified as a tubular structure with intraluminal T1 and T2 prolongation. Appendicitis is diagnosed using thresholds of the size used for CT (Fig. 10). Inflammatory changes are visualized as T2 hyperintensity in the periappendiceal fat. In pregnant women, the abdomen must be examined carefully for an unusual location of the appendix because the pregnant uterus displaces the appendix significantly. In one MR imaging study, the kidneys could be evaluated for hydronephrosis, which was detected in four of nine patients who did not have appendicitis [63].

Summary

Today imaging is an important part of the work-up of appendicitis. In the academic setting, CT, ultrasound, and MR imaging are extremely accurate and helpful in preventing unnecessary operations and appendiceal perforation. As multiple studies reported high sensitivity and specificity of these imaging modalities, their use in the community became increasingly commonplace. Sobering evidence subsequently came to light, however. A population-based outcomes study of appendicitis in 86,000 patients in Washington state revealed that misdiagnosis and perforation rates have not decreased after widespread introduction of modern imaging techniques [13]. Several studies suggested that indiscriminate use of imaging does not improve patient outcomes [6,14,16–18,64].

There are several reasons why diagnostic tests may not perform in the community as well as in the academic milieu. Studies may not be performed with optimal protocols. They may not be targeted to the appropriate subgroups of patients. Communication with treating physicians may break down, rendering interpretations ineffectual. The results of the imaging studies may not be integrated correctly with the clinical data.

Solving these problems may involve shifting the focus of study from the imaging modalities in isolation to the health delivery system as a whole. Several institutions have accomplished this shift by integrating diagnostic imaging into standardized clinical guidelines for management of appendicitis. These clinical guidelines define when particular imaging modalities are used and how their results affect management. They permit uniform, targeted approaches for specific patient groups, such as children and women of childbearing age. When imaging is viewed as a part of a larger system, quality control can be applied to imaging and also to the system as a whole. Several recent studies have validated the benefits of such standardized guidelines on patient outcomes [23,65–67]. This integrative approach seems to be the promising new frontier in the diagnosis of appendicitis.

Acknowledgments

The authors are grateful to Dr. Loretta Strachowski for her editorial comments.

References

[1] Addiss DG, Shaffer N, Fowler BS, et al. Epidemiology of appendicitis and appendectomy in the United States. Am J Epidemiol 1990;132(5): 910–25.

[2] Berry J, Malt RA. Appendicitis near its centenary. Ann Surg 1984;200(5):567–75.

[3] Wakeley CPG. Position of the vermiform appendix as ascertained by analysis of 10,000 cases. J Anat 1933;67:277–83.

[4] Oto A, Ernst RD, Mileski WJ, et al. Localization of appendix wit MDCT and influence of findings on choice of appendectomy incision. AJR Am J Roentgenol 2006;187:987–90.

[5] Jaffe BM, Berger DH. The appendix. In: Brunicardi FCB, Andersen DK, Billiar TR, et al, editors. Schwartz's principles of surgery. 8th edition. New York: McGraw-Hill; 2005. p. 1119–37.

[6] York D, Smith A, Phillips JD, et al. The influence of advanced radiographic imaging on the treatment of pediatric appendicitis. J Pediatr Surg 2005;40:1908–11.

[7] Silen W. Acute appendicitis and peritonitis. In: Kasper DL, Braunwald E, Fauci AS, et al, editors. Harrison's principles of internal medicine. 16th edition. New York: McGraw-Hill; 2005. p. 1805–8.

[8] Birnbaum BA, Wilson SR. Appendicitis at the millennium. Radiology 2000;215:337–48.

[9] Rhea JT, Halpern EF, Ptak T, et al. The status of appendiceal CT in an urban medical center 5 years after its introduction: experience with 753 patients. AJR Am J Roentgenol 2005;184:1802–8.

[10] Rao PM, Rhea JT, Novelline RA, et al. Effect of computed tomography of the appendix on treatment of patients and use of hospital resources. N Engl J Med 1998;338:141–6.

[11] Garcia Peña BM, Mandl KD, Kraus SJ, et al. Ultrasonography and limited computed tomography in the diagnosis and management of appendicitis in children. JAMA 1999;282(11):1041–6.

[12] Doria AS, Moineddin R, Kellenberger CJ, et al. US or CT for diagnosis of appendicitis in children and adults? A meta-analysis. Radiology 2006;241:83–94.

[13] Balthazar EJ, Birnbaum BA, Yee J, et al. Acute appendicitis: CT and US correlation in 100 patients. Radiology 1994;190(1):31–5.

[14] Terasawa T, Blackmore CC, Bent S, et al. Systematic review: computed tomography and ultrasonography to detect acute appendicitis in adults and adolescents. Ann Intern Med 2004;141: 537–46.

[15] Flum DR, Morris A, Koepsel T, et al. Has misdiagnosis of appendicitis decreased over time? A population-based analysis. JAMA 2001;286:1748–53.

[16] Vadeboncoeur TF, Heister RR, Behling CA. Impact of helical computed tomography on the rate of negative appendicitis. Am J Emerg Med 2006;24:43–7.

[17] Lee SL, Walsh AJ, Ho HS. Computed tomography and ultrasonography do not improve and may delay the diagnosis and treatment of acute appendicitis. Arch Surg 2001;135:556–62.

[18] Stephen AE, Segev DL, Ryan DP, et al. The diagnosis of acute appendicitis in the pediatric population: to CT or not to CT. J Pediatr Surg 2003; 38(3):367–71.

[19] Bendeck SE, Nino-Murcia M, Berry GJ, et al. Imaging for suspected acute appendicitis: negative appendectomy and perforation rates. Radiology 2002;225:131–6.

[20] Applegate KE, Sivit CJ, Salvador AE, et al. Effect of cross-sectional imaging on negative appendectomy and perforation rates in children. Radiology 2001;220:103–7.

[21] Brenner DJ, Elliston CD, Hall EJ, et al. Estimated risks of radiation-induced fatal cancer from pediatric CT. AJR Am J Roentgenol 2001;176:289–96.

[22] Old JL, Dusing RW, Yap W, et al. Imaging for suspected appendicitis. Am Fam Physician 2005;71: 71–8.

[23] Smink DS, Finkelstein JS, Garcia-Pena BM, et al. Diagnosis of acute appendicitis in children using a clinical practice guideline. J Pediatr Surg 2004; 39(3):458–63.

[24] Hernandez JA, Swischuk LE, Angel CA, et al. Imaging of acute appendicitis: US as the primary imaging modality. Pediatr Radiol 2005;35: 392–5.

[25] Hurwitz LM, Yoshizumi T, Reiman RE, et al. Radiation dose to the fetus from body MDCT during early gestation. AJR Am J Roentgenol 2006; 186:871–6.

[26] Lim HK, Bae SH, Seo GS. Diagnosis of acute appendicitis in pregnant women: value of sonography. AJR Am J Roentgenol 1992;159:539–42.

[27] Oto A, Ernst RD, Shah R, et al. Right-lower-quadrant pain and suspected appendicitis in pregnant women: evaluation with MR imaging–initial experience. Radiology 2005;234:445–51.

[28] Incesu L, Coskun A, Selcuk MB, et al. Acute appendicitis: MR imaging and sonographic correlation. AJR Am J Roentgenol 1997;168:669–74.

[29] O'Malley ME, Halpert E, Mueller PR, et al. Helical CT protocols for the abdomen and pelvis: a survey. AJR Am J Roentgenol 2000;175:109–13.

[30] Macari M, Balthazar EJ. The acute right lower quadrant: CT evaluation. Radiol Clin North Am 2003;41:1117–36.

[31] Rao PM, Rhea JT, Novelline RA, et al. Helical CT combine with contrast material administered only through the colon for imaging of suspected appendicitis. AJR Am J Roentgenol 1997;169: 1275–80.

[32] Wise SW, Labuski MR, Kasales CJ, et al. Comparative assessment of CT and sonographic techniques for appendiceal imaging. AJR Am J Roentgenol 2001;176:933–41.

[33] Jacobs JE, Birnbaum BA, Macari M, et al. Acute appendicitis: comparison of helical CT diagnosis—focused technique with oral contrast material versus nonfocused technique wit oral and

intravenous contrast material. Radiology 2001; 220:683–90.

[34] Kamel IR, Goldberg SN, Keogan MT, et al. Right lower quadrant pain and suspected appendicitis: nonfocused appendiceal CT—review of 100 cases. Radiology 2000;217:159–63.

[35] Malone AJ, Wolf CR, Malmed AS, et al. Diagnosis of acute appendicitis: value of unenhanced CT. AJR Am J Roentgenol 1993;160:763–6.

[36] Malone AJ. Unenhanced CT in the evaluation of the acute abdomen: the community hospital experience. Semin Ultrasound CT MR 1999;20:68–76.

[37] Lane MJ, Liu DM, Huynh MD, et al. Suspected acute appendicitis: nonenhanced helical ct in 300 consecutive patients. Radiology 1999;213:341–6.

[38] Ege G, Akman H, Sahin A, et al. Diagnostic value of unenhanced helical CT in adult patients with suspected acute appendicitis. Br J Radiol 2002; 75:721–5.

[39] Choi D, Park H, Lee YR, et al. The most useful findings for diagnosing acute appendicitis on contrast-enhanced helical CT. Acta Radiol 2003; 44:574–82.

[40] Tamburrini S, Brunetti A, Brown M, et al. CT appearance of normal appendix in adults. Eur Radiol 2005;15:2096–103.

[41] Daly CP, Cohan RH, Francis IR, et al. Incidence of acute appendicitis in patients with equivocal CT findings. AJR Am J Roentgenol 2005;184: 1813–20.

[42] Rao PM, Rhea JT, Novelline RA. Sensitivity and specificity of the individual CT signs of appendicitis: experience with 200 helical appendiceal CT examinations. J Comput Assist Tomogr 1997;21: 686–92.

[43] Nikolaidis P, Hwang CM, Miller FH, et al. Incidence of acute appendicitis when secondary inflammatory changes are absent. AJR Am J Roentgenol 2004;183:889–92.

[44] Horrow MM, White DS, Horrow JC. Differentiation of perforated from nonperforated appendicitis at CT. Radiology 2003;227:46–51.

[45] Puylaert JBCM. Acute appendicitis: US evaluation using graded compression. Radiology 1986;158:355–60.

[46] Rompel O, Huelsse B, Bodenschatz K, et al. Harmonic US imaging of appendicitis in children. Pediatr Radiol 2006;36(12):1257–64.

[47] Puylaert JBCM. Ultrasonography of the acute abdomen: gastrointestinal conditions. Radiol Clin North Am 2003;41:1227–42.

[48] Chesbrough RM, Burkhard TK, Balsara ZN, et al. Self-localization in US of appendicitis: an addition to graded compression. Radiology 1993; 187:349–51.

[49] Lee JH, Jeong YK, Hwang JC, et al. Graded compression sonography with adjuvant use of a posterior manual compression technique in the sonographic diagnosis of acute appendicitis. AJR Am J Roentgenol 2002;178:863–8.

[50] Lee JH, Jeong YK, Park KB, et al. Operator-dependent techniques for graded compression sonography to detect the appendix and diagnose acute appendicitis. AJR Am J Roentgenol 2005; 184:91–7.

[51] Rioux M. Sonographic detection of the normal and abnormal appendix. AJR Am J Roentgenol 1992;158:773–8.

[52] Jeffrey RB, Laing FC, Townsend MD. Acute appendicitis: sonographic criteria based on 250 cases. Radiology 1988;167:327–9.

[53] Kessler N, Cyteval C, Gallix B, et al. Appendicitis: evaluation of sensitivity, specificity, and predictive values of US, Doppler US, and laboratory findings. Radiology 2004;230:472–8.

[54] Rettenbacher T, Hollerweger A, Macheiner P, et al. Outer diameter of the vermiform appendix as a sign of acute appendicitis: evaluation at US. Radiology 2001;218:757–62.

[55] Lim HK, Lee WJ, Kim TH, et al. Appendicitis: usefulness of color Doppler US. Radiology 1996;201:221–5.

[56] Quillin SP, Siegel MJ. Appendicitis: efficacy of color Doppler sonography. Radiology 1994; 191:557–60.

[57] Rettenbacher T, Hollerweger A, Macheiner P, et al. Ovoid shape of the vermiform appendix: a criterion to exclude acute appendicitis—evaluation with US. Radiology 2003;226:95–100.

[58] Pates JA, Twickler DM. The use of radiographic modialities to diagnose infection in pregnancy. Clin Perinatol 2005;32:789–802.

[59] Leyendecker JR, Gorengaut V, Brown JJ. MR imaging of maternal diseases of he abdomen and pelvis during pregnancy and immediate postpartum period. Radiographics 2004;24:1301–16.

[60] De Wilde JP, Rivers AW, Price DL. A review of the current use of magnetic resonance imaging in pregnancy and safety implications for the fetus. Prog Biophys Mol Biol 2005;87:335–53.

[61] Shellock FG, Kanal E. Safety of magnetic resonance imaging contrast agents. J Magn Reson Imaging 1999;10:477–84.

[62] Webb JAW, Thomsen HS, Morcos SK. The use of iodinated and gadolinium contrast media during pregnancy and lactation. Eur Radiol 2005; 15:1234–40.

[63] Cobben LP, Groot I, Haans L, et al. MRI for clinically suspected appendicitis during pregnancy. Am J Roentgenol 2004;183:671–5.

[64] Martin AE, Vollman D, Adler B, et al. CT scans may not reduce the negative appendectomy rate in children. J Pediatr Surg 2004;39:886–90.

[65] Garcia Pena BM, Taylor GA, Fishman SJ, et al. Effect of an imaging protocol on clinical outcomes among pediatric patients with appendicitis. Pediatrics 2002;110:1088–93.

[66] Garcia Pena BM, Cook EF, Mandl KD. Selective imaging strategies for the diagnosis of appendicitis in children. Pediatrics 2004;113:24–8.

[67] Kosloske AM, Love CL, Rohrer JE, et al. The diagnosis of appendicitis in children: outcomes of a strategy based on pediatric surgical evaluation. Pediatrics 2004;113:29–34.

ELSEVIER
SAUNDERS

RADIOLOGIC
CLINICS
OF NORTH AMERICA

Radiol Clin N Am 45 (2007) 423–445

Computer Tomography for Venous Thromboembolic Disease

Wael E.A. Saad, MBBCh*, Nael Saad, MBBCh

- Thromboembolic pulmonary embolism
  Imaging modalities
  Emergence of CT pulmonary angiography as the principle diagnostic modality
  Advances in the technology of CT pulmonary angiography
  Multidetector CT pulmonary angiography technique and protocol
  CT pulmonary angiography findings of pulmonary embolism
  Causes of misdiagnoses of pulmonary embolism (imaging pitfalls)
  Diagnostic performance of CT pulmonary angiography
- Deep venous thrombosis
  Diagnostic modalities
  Technique and protocol of multidetector indirect CT venography
  CT venography findings of deep venous thrombosis
  Diagnostic performance of CT venography
- Nonthromboembolic pulmonary embolism
  Types of nonthromboembolic pulmonary emboli and individual CT findings
- References

Venous thromboembolic disease is composed of two disease entities: pulmonary thromboembolism/pulmonary embolism (PE) and deep venous thrombosis (DVT). Dislodgement of thrombus in the deep veins of the extremities produces emboli that travel to the lung and become entrapped in the pulmonary arteries. Clinical signs and symptoms of venous thromboembolic disease often are nonspecific; as a result, the diagnosis may be difficult. If left untreated, PE can lead to a potentially fatal outcome. Furthermore, anticoagulation therapy may lead to bleeding complications. Therefore accurate imaging diagnosis plays a large role in the management of these patients [1].

When approaching the imaging diagnosis of venous thromboembolic disease, diagnostic imaging modalities can be classified into (1) imaging tests for PE, (2) imaging tests for DVT, and (3) imaging tests for both PE and DVT. Both cross-sectional angiography modalities—CT angiography and MR angiography/MR venography—are in the third category [1].

This article focuses on CT angiography as the diagnostic modality for PE . To begin, the definition, morphologic and pathogenic classifications (types) of PE must be discussed briefly. The general term "pulmonary thromboembolus" refers to a space-occupying intraluminal entity that is foreign to the lumen of the pulmonary artery. Pulmonary arterial embolism can be classified generally as thrombotic or nonthrombotic PE (Box 1) [2]. Almost all space-occupying lesions in the pulmonary arteries are

Department of Imaging Sciences, University of Rochester Medical Center, Rochester, NY, USA
* Corresponding author.
E-mail address: wspikes@yahoo.com (W.E.A. Saad).

0033-8389/07/$ – see front matter © 2007 Elsevier Inc. All rights reserved.
radiologic.theclinics.com

doi:10.1016/j.rcl.2007.04.011

---

truly thromboembolic in nature. The focus of this article is on these lesions. Other types of space-occupying pulmonary artery lesions are discussed briefly in the latter part of this article.

Thromboembolic pulmonary embolism

Pulmonary thromboembolism is the third most common cardiovascular disease after myocardial infarction and stroke (cerebrovascular accidents) [3,4]. The incidence of pulmonary thromboembolism is 69 cases per 100,000 inhabitants in the United States; 175,000 to 250,000 cases in North America annually lead to an estimated 50,000 annual deaths [5–9]. The thousands of deaths are, in part, the result of the process often going undetected. Even when PE is diagnosed, the 3-month mortality, according to the Pulmonary Embolism Registry, is 17.5% [10,11]. Thirty percent of patients who have PE are seen first in the emergency department [12].

Imaging modalities

Traditionally, thromboembolic disease has been screened by lower extremity ultrasound examination for DVT and ventilation-perfusion scintigraphy with or without confirmation with pulmonary arteriography for PE. In recent years, new diagnostic examinations have been introduced including D-dimer assay and CT pulmonary angiography (CTPA). These new examinations have improved physicians' diagnostic ability but have added complexity to diagnostic protocols. Table 1 summarizes the various

diagnostic examinations used to diagnose PE [1,2,13].

Emergence of CT pulmonary angiography as the principle diagnostic modality

For years ventilation-perfusion scintigraphy occupied a central role in the diagnostic triage of potential PE patients. Ventilation-perfusion scintigraphy, however, was nondiagnostic (giving an indeterminate or intermediate probability) for PE in 39% of cases and had a reader confidence level of 54% [12–14]. Furthermore, ventilation-perfusion scintigraphy rarely provided other cardiovascular and/or cardiopulmonary diagnoses other than PE that could explain symptoms in 50% to 60% of patients suspected of having PE [15]. Moreover, a seldom-mentioned disadvantage of ventilation-perfusion scintigraphy is its reliance on the level of clinical suspicion as part of the diagnosis of the probability of the presence of PE [12,16]. That is, ventilation-perfusion scintigraphy is rarely a stand-alone diagnostic examination. In summary, because of the high number of nondiagnostic examinations, the inability to use ventilation-perfusion scintigraphy as a stand-alone diagnostic examination, and its inability to provide diagnoses other than PE, ventilation-perfusion scintigraphy is no longer the modality of choice for the emergent diagnosis of PE.

CTPA, on the other hand, is both highly sensitive and specific. Multidetector CT (MDCT) has sensitivity ranging from 83% to 94%, specificity ranging from 94% to 100%, and a reader confidence of 90% [14,17–20]. The indeterminate examination rate is 6% to 7%. Moreover, CTPA provides a non-PE diagnosis in 70% of patients who were initially suspected of having PE but were found not to have PE (more than 50% of patients initially suspected of having PE) [15,18]. Table 2 demonstrates the conditions that can mimic PE clinically for which CT may help in their diagnosis [21]. A brief comparison between the performance of ventilation-perfusion scintigraphy and CTPA is found in Table 3. In addition, CTPA is a stand-alone diagnostic examination with 24-hour availability in tertiary care centers. (Box 2 provides the advantages of CTPA.) As a result, in many institutions CTPA has supplanted ventilation perfusion scintigraphy, which is reserved for cases in which there is increased patient motion and respiratory motion artifact, poor right-heart function, or contraindications to the use of intravenous radiographic contrast medium [22–26]. Fig. 1 shows the 10-year data (1992–2001) from a single institution collected by Wittram and colleagues [27]. As Fig. 1 shows, a statistically significant decline in the use of ventilation-perfusion scintigraphy (P = .003) and also in the number of diagnostic pulmonary

Table 1: Diagnostic modalities for pulmonary embolism

Modality	Cardinal Findings	Advantages	Disadvantages	Sensitivity	Specificity
Chest radiograph	Atelectasis Westermark sign Pleural effusion Hampton's hump Fleischner sign	Inexpensive No contrast allergies	Inaccurate	Poor	Nonspecific
Ventilation perfusion scintigraphy	Ventilation perfusion mismatch	No contrast allergies	Inaccurate: 39%–57% indeterminate/ intermediate probability	Relatively high	Relatively poor
Pulmonary angiography	Filling defect in pulmonary artery; wedge paucity of affected segment	Reference standard Can measure pulmonary pressures	Invasive Mortality 0.3% Morbidity 1%–3%	High	Highest
Tracheoesophageal echocardiogram	Filling echogenic defects in pulmonary artery; evaluation of right-heart function	No IV contrast load Evaluate cardiac status, especially in pulmonary hypertension or large PE	Not readily available Operator dependent Semi-invasive (intrusive)	Relatively poor	
MR angiography	Filling defect in pulmonary artery; parenchymal infiltrates; pleural effusion	No radiation No iodinated contrast	Sensitive to patient motion and dyspnea Expensive Time-consuming Not readily available	Relatively high: 68%–87%	High: 97%
CT angiography	Filling defect in pulmonary artery; parenchymal infiltrates; pleural effusion	Accurate Available Can be used in the same setting to evaluate for DVT Provides other diagnoses (cardiopulmonary and cardiovascular)	IV contrast load	High MDCT: 83%–94%	High MDCT: 94%–100%

Abbreviations: DVT, deep venous thrombosis; IV, intravenous; MDCT, multidetector CT; PE, pulmonary embolus.
Data from Refs. [1,2,22].

angiograms ($P = .02$) coincided, circa 1997, with the introduction of single-detector spiral CTPA as a new diagnostic modality for the diagnosis of PE. The pattern of the graph represents a classic replacement of an old technology by a new one [27]. The decline in pulmonary angiograms with the advent of CTPA may, in part, represent the replacement of pulmonary angiography by CTPA [21,27,28]. Some authors recently have challenged the sensitivity of pulmonary angiography and have compared it with the sensitivity of multidetector CTPA (MD-CTPA) [28].

Table 2: Conditions that can mimic pulmonary embolism clinically and that can have findings on CT that may help in diagnosis

Thoracic Condition	CT Findings
Pericarditis	Pericardial thickening ± calcifications Pericardial effusion
Myocardial infarction	Filling defect in the coronary artery Lack of enhancement of coronary artery Perfusion defect in myocardium
Aortic dissection	Dissection flap Aortic dilation Aortic dual lumen with varying attenuation
Esophagitis	Wall thickening Periesophageal stranding/ inflammation
Esophageal rupture	Left-sided pleural effusion (hydro-pneumothorax) Hydro-pneumo mediastinum
Pneumonia	Air space disease (infiltrates) Ground-glass opacities Enlarged lymph nodes
Bronchogenic carcinoma	Lung mass Infiltrates Enlarged lymph nodes
Pleural disease	Air (pneumothorax) Pleuritis (pleural effusion, thickening)
Rib abnormalities	Rib fractures Rib tumors/metastasis

Data from Wittram C, Maher MM, Yoo AF, et al. CT angiography of pulmonary embolism: diagnostic criteria and causes misdiagnosis. Radiographics 2004;24:1219–38.

Advances in the technology of CT pulmonary angiography

When reviewing the diagnostic performance of CTPA over the years, one must be aware of numerous variables within the studies. These variables include patient selection, extent of thrombus evaluated/area of pulmonary vasculature evaluated, interpretation criteria, experience of the reader, and the level of technology used [8,21–23]. The use of MDCT probably has had the greatest impact on the improved diagnostic performance of CTPA. The ability to cover larger axial chest slabs at one moment in time (using 8, 16, 32, or 64 slices) considerably abbreviates acquisition time, reducing patient and respiratory motion problems. In addition, reducing collimation to 1 mm has improved spatial resolution [29–31]. With these technologic advances, the sensitivity of CTPA has improved from 37% to 94% to 83% to 96%, and its specificity has improved from 81% to 100% to 94% to 100% [17,18,28–34].

Multidetector CT pulmonary angiography technique and protocol

Intravenous access is obtained or, if already established, is assessed for adequacy. At least an 18- or 20-gauge catheter (cannula) is introduced in an antecubital vein. Certain high-pressure central lines can be used as well as high-pressure peripherally inserted central catheters. The total contrast injection ranges from 120 to 140 mm of 300-mg/mL nonionic iodinated contrast medium at 3 to 4 mL/s [21,35,36]. If higher iodinated contrast concentrations (> 300 mg/mL) are used, the injection rate can be reduced [35]. A bolus-tracking technique with a region of interest centered on the main pulmonary artery and a threshold trigger of 125 Hounsfield units (HU) can be used [35–37]. This technique allows precise timing of the image acquisition whatever the degree of the patient's right-heart failure or pulmonary hypertension, if any [35].

Detection of emboli relies on optimal opacification of the pulmonary arteries at the time of image acquisition. The degree of opacification is influenced by the volume of intravenous contrast medium injected, the contrast injection rate, the patient's cardiac throughput/output in relation to the timing of the scan, and section collimation [24,30,36,38–44]. The lungs are imaged from the top of the aortic arch to the dome of the diaphragm [45]. Imaging is performed during suspended full inspiration, with the patient's arms above the patient's head [36,37]. This position allows spreading of the pulmonary vessels and reduces the crowding of the lung parenchyma and pulmonary vessels. The position also reduces beam-hardening artifact. The direction of the scan is somewhat controversial, however. Washington and colleagues [46] recommended the caudal-cranial direction; whereas Remy-Jardin and colleagues [45] and Hargaden and colleagues [36] showed that the direction of image acquisition does not affect the overall quality of the CT pulmonary angiogram examination. Hargaden and colleagues [36], however, added that scanning in the cranial-caudal direction significantly improves upper-lobe pulmonary artery enhancement.

Most 16-detector (slice) CT scanners can scan the pulmonary arteries within 8 to 20 seconds, making the technique feasible within a single breathhold [35]. (Thirty-two– and 64-detector CT scanners

Table 3: Diagnostic performance characteristics of ventilation-perfusion scintigraphy and CT pulmonary angiography

Characteristic	Ventilation-Perfusion Scintigraphy	Multidetector CT Pulmonary Angiography[b]
Reader confidence	54%	90%
Indeterminate diagnosis	39%	6%–7%
Effect of underlying lung disease and contorted rib-cage anatomy	Significantly affected	Rarely affected
Non–pulmonary embolism diagnosis rate	<5% (not specific)	50%–55% (highly specific)
Sensitivity	Relatively sensitive[a]	83%–94%
Specificity	Poor	94%–100%

[a] Forty-one percent of patients suspected of having PE would be labeled as "high probability" on ventilation-perfusion scintigraphy with a sensitivity of 88%.
[b] Multidetector CT pulmonary angiography is the latest technology; earlier performance numbers are lower for single-detector CT pulmonary angiography.
Data from Refs. [12–15,18,28].

now are commercially available.) Collimation (detector width) has been described as less than 3 mm, but the thinnest possible collimation with current technology is between 0.5 and 1.0 mm [35]. Thinner collimation increases spatial resolution and allows detailed display and evaluation of the segmental and subsegmental pulmonary artery branches [35]. Collimation is increased intentionally to between 1.5 and 2.5 mm when the patient has tachypnea or weighs more than 250 pounds (112 kg) [21,35,44]. Increasing the collimation/detector width for tachypnea reduces the total scan time and thus reduces respiratory motion artifact [35]. Increasing collimation for increased patient body habitus reduces noise and improves scan quality [35]. Increased collimation, however, reduces the spatial resolution and reduces sensitivity in detecting PE, especially at the subsegmental pulmonary artery level [21,44].

To improve image quality in patients who have larger body habitus, it may be necessary to increase the X-ray dose/technique to 120 to 140 kV as well as increasing collimation [21]. Reducing the X-ray dose for patients undergoing CT examinations is important. For slender patients weighing less than 70 kg (< 155 pounds) the CT tube voltage can be reduced to 80 to 100 kV [35]. Furthermore, manufacturers have developed a promising tool (using a tube current modulation system) that allows the tube voltage to adapt to the patients' morphotype. The dose is delivered according to the attenuation of the tissues scanned and, consequently, can reduce the dose by 10% to 30% depending on the scan volume [47].

Multiplanar and three-dimensional reconstructions are generated at a reconstruction interval

that is half that the detector width (collimation value). For example, if the collimation is 1.25 mm in patients weighing less than 250 pounds, the reconstruction interval is 0.625 mm. If the collimation is 2.5 mm in patients weighing more than 250 pounds, the reconstruction interval is 1.25 mm [21]. The reformatted images can help differentiate between true PE and a variety of patient-related,

Box 2: **Advantages and disadvantages of CT pulmonary angiography over other diagnostic modalities**

Advantages
Sensitivity and specificity > 90% (for multidetector CT with 1-mm collimation)
Diagnostic value outside pulmonary arteries (50%–55% of patients initially suspected of having PE)
Widespread availability
Rapid acquisition of examination
Patient- and physician-oriented, with high acceptance
Relatively inexpensive and cost effective compared with ventilation-perfusion scintigraphy and pulmonary angiography
High negative predictive value; is not affected by underlying lung disease

Disadvantages
Increased radiation dose, especially with multidetector CT
Effect of contrast dose/load on renal function (particularly in patients who have diabetes or borderline renal function)
Low risk of contrast reaction (< 0.5%)

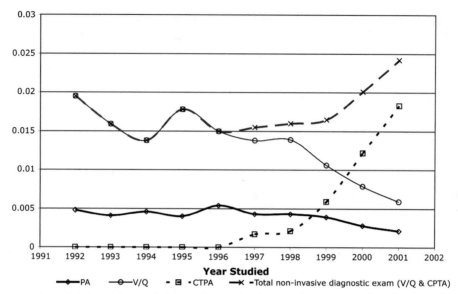

Fig. 1. The number of different types of diagnostic examinations per inpatient used to diagnose clinically suspected pulmonary emboli. PA, pulmonary angiogram per inpatient; V/Q, Ventilation-perfusion scintigram per inpatient; CTPA, CT pulmonary angiogram per inpatient. (*Data from* Wittram C, Maher MM, Yoo AF, et al. CT angiography of pulmonary embolism: diagnostic criteria and causes misdiagnosis. Radiographics 2004;24:1219–38; and Wittram C, Meehan MJ, Halpern EF, et al. Trends in thoracic radiology over a decade at a large academic medical center. J Thorac Imaging 2004;19:164–70.)

technical, anatomic, and pathologic factors that can mimic PE [21].

CT pulmonary angiography findings of pulmonary embolism

PE incidentally noted on noncontrast chest CT can be seen in the central pulmonary arteries as hyperattenuated defects in the relatively dilated pulmonary artery (Fig. 2) [48]. Large acute central PE (discovered by CT with or without contrast enhancement) adds an acute strain on the right heart and puts the patient at risk for circulatory collapse. Early detection of acute right ventricular failure allows implementation of the most appropriate therapeutic strategy [21]. Some morphologic abnormalities that suggest right ventricular failure can be quantified/appreciated by CTPA [21,49,50]:

Right ventricular dilation (short axis of right ventricle > short axis of left ventricle) (Fig. 3)

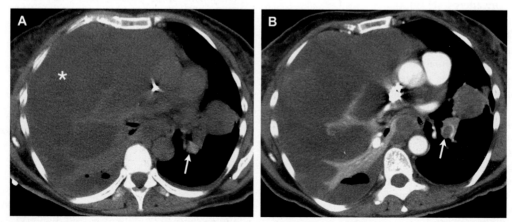

Fig. 2. A 52-year-old woman who has metastatic sarcoma involving the right thoracic cavity (*asterisk* in panel A). (*A*) Non–contrast-enhanced axial CT demonstrating an area of hyperattenuation in the left interlobar pulmonary artery (*arrow*). (*B*) Contrast-enhanced CT confirms the presence of an acute pulmonary embolus (*arrow*).

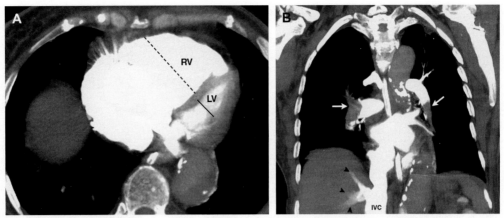

Fig. 3. A 79-year-old woman presenting with chest pain and hypoxia. (*A*) CT scan shows right ventricular dilation. The short axis (*dashed line*) of the right ventricle (*RV*) is larger than the short axis (*solid line*) of the left ventricle (*LV*). (*B*) Coronal reformatted CT image shows bilateral pulmonary artery emboli (*arrows*) with reflux of contrast into the inferior vena cava (*IVC*) and the hepatic veins (*arrowheads*).

Deviation of the intraventricular septum toward the left ventricle

Contrast refluxes into the hepatic veins (see Fig. 3)

Pulmonary embolic index greater than 60%

Findings of acute PE by CTPA (Table 4) include [21–25,51–54]

Complete arterial occlusion; artery may be enlarged (Fig. 4)

Centrally located partial filling defect

"Polo mint sign": if axial image acquired is perpendicular to the long axis of the affected pulmonary artery segment (Fig. 5)

"Railway track sign" or "tram-track sign": if axial image acquired is parallel to the long axis of the affected pulmonary artery segment (Fig. 6)

Peripheral or eccentric intraluminal filling defect forming an acute angle with the pulmonary arterial wall (Fig. 7) [23,46,51]

Other nonspecific/secondary signs

Wedge-shaped area of hyperattenuation in the peripheral lung field that may represent pulmonary infarction (Fig. 8) [52]

Linear lung parenchymal bands (Fig. 9) [52]

Oligemia: distal pulmonary artery is attenuated (smaller caliber) (Fig. 10) [54]

Basal and/or local pleural effusion (> 60% of PE cases) (see Fig. 9)

Signs of right-heart strain [21,49,50]

Table 4: CT pulmonary angiography in acute and chronic pulmonary emboli	
CTPA Findings in Acute Pulmonary Embolus	**CTPA Findings in Chronic Pulmonary Embolus**
Pulmonary arterial occlusion with enlarged pulmonary artery caliber	Pulmonary arterial occlusion with diminished pulmonary artery caliber
Partial filling defect with acute angles with pulmonary artery wall	Partial filling defect with obtuse angles with pulmonary artery wall
Extrapulmonary artery findings:	Extrapulmonary artery findings:
Wedge shaped infiltrate	Mosaic perfusion pattern
Linear parenchymal bands	Prominent bronchial collaterals
Pleural effusion	
Right heart strain:	Pulmonary hypertension:
R dilation (RV > LV)	MPA diameter > 33 mm
Deviation of IVS toward the LV	Pericardial effusion
Reflux of contrast into hepatic veins	Pruning of the pulmonary vasculature

Abbreviations: IVS, Intraventricular septum; LV, left ventricle; MPA, main pulmonary artery; RV, right ventricle.
Data from Refs. [21,23–25,51–54]

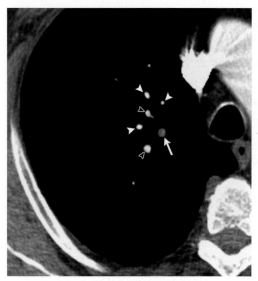

Fig. 4. Acute pulmonary embolus in an 81-year-old man presenting with syncope. The right apical segmental pulmonary artery (*arrow*) is completely occluded and is larger than the adjacent pulmonary arteries (*white arrowheads*). Black arrowheads indicate pulmonary veins.

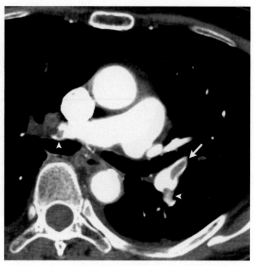

Fig. 6. Acute pulmonary embolus in an 88-year-old woman presenting with syncope and hypoxia. CT shows a central filling defect with contrast on either side, the "railway track sign" (*arrow*). Additional pulmonary emboli (*arrowheads* are seen also).

Findings of chronic PE by CTPA (see Table 4) include [21] Complete occlusion of artery that is smaller in caliber than adjacent patent vessels

Peripheral crescent-shaped intraluminal filling defect forming an obtuse angle with the pulmonary arterial wall [21]

Contrast filling small channels in thickened pulmonary arteries caused by recannulated chronically thrombosed and organized pulmonary arteries [21]

A web or flap within the pulmonary artery (having a morphology similar to a dissection flap) (Fig. 11)

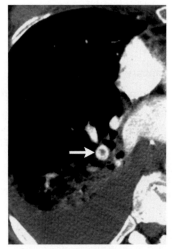

Fig. 5. Partial central filling defect with a ring of contrast circumferentially in the right interlobar artery. This is the classic appearance of the "polo mint sign" (*arrow*) of acute pulmonary embolism.

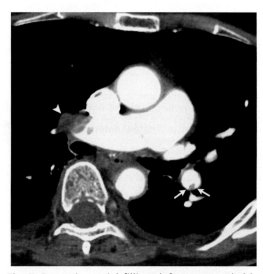

Fig. 7. Eccentric partial filling defect surrounded by contrast that forms acute angles with the arterial wall (*arrows*). The patient also had an acute pulmonary embolus involving the right main pulmonary artery (*arrowhead*).

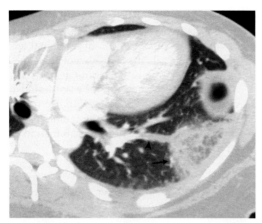

Fig. 8. Acute segmental pulmonary embolus (*arrowhead*) in the lateral basal segment of the left lower lobe with an area of wedge-shaped hyperattenuation (*arrow*) that may represent an infarct.

Formation of collateral arteries from the systemic bronchial arteries (Fig. 12)
Other ancillary signs (signs of pulmonary hypertension) [46,51,55,56]
   Mosaic perfusion pattern
   Main pulmonary artery diameter more than 33 mm
   Pericardial effusion
   Pruning of the pulmonary vasculature

Causes of misdiagnoses of pulmonary embolism (imaging pitfalls)

Diagnostic difficulties that may lead to the misdiagnosis of PE have many causes. These pitfalls can be classified as patient-related factors, technical factors, anatomic factors, and pathologic factors (Box 3) [21].

Diagnostic performance of CT pulmonary angiography

Contrast-enhanced chest CT obtained for reasons other than investigating possible PE (when there is no clinical suspicion for PE) have found PE incidentally in 1.0% to 1.5% of the general inpatient and outpatient population [64,65]. This incidence rises to 4.0% to 5.0% in the inpatient and/or oncology patient population [65,66]. The incidence of PE detected by CT obviously rises further, to 9% to 27%, with dedicated contrast-enhanced CTPA in patients clinically suspected of having PE [67–69]. These incidences based on patient populations are tabulated in Table 5.

Despite the noninvasive nature of CTPA, the modality is not without complications, but almost all of these complications are minor. In a study addressing 1095 consecutive CTPA examinations, all complications were minor (0.6%, n = 7/1095). These minor complications included mild allergic reactions to iodinated contrast (0.4%, n = 4/1095), contrast intravasation (0.2%, n = 2/1095), and transient renal failure in diabetic patients (0.1%, n = 1/1095). The results of MD-CTPA are summarized in Table 6 [28].

The sensitivity and specificity of CTPA are high. They have increased with the advent of MDCT from a sensitivity of 37% to 94% and specificity of 81% to 100% for single-detector spiral CT to an overall sensitivity of 83% to 94% and specificity of 94-100% for 4- to 16-detector MDCT [17,18,28,32–34]. In addition, the negative predictive value of MD-CTPA is 93% to 96% [28,70]. It is believed that with improved technology (the use of

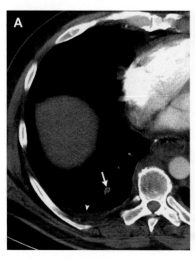
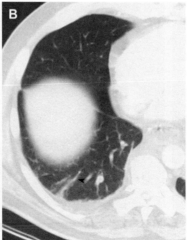

Fig. 9. A 51-year-old woman presenting with shortness of breath and cough. (*A*) Axial CT image in soft tissue widow shows an acute pulmonary embolus (*arrow*) and an ancillary finding of a small pleural effusion (*arrowhead*). (*B*) Lung window settings of the same axial image demonstrate an additional ancillary finding of a linear band of atelectasis (*arrowhead*).

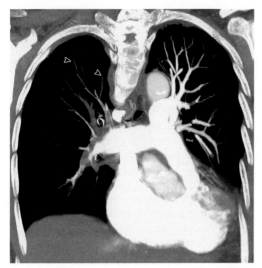

Fig. 10. Coronal CT reformatted image showing oligemia of the right upper lobe in a patient who has acute pulmonary embolism. The pulmonary arterial branches to the right upper lobe (*arrowheads*) are smaller in caliber than those on the left side.

more than 16 detectors and with collimation of 1 mm or less) both the sensitivity and specificity of CTPA would consistently be above 94% [22,29–31]. The percentage of CTPA examinations that are deemed indeterminate is low (6.2%) for a noninvasive test in this clinical setting [18], particularly when compared with the indeterminate examination rate (39%) of ventilation-perfusion scintigraphy [12]. This reduction of more than six-fold in the indeterminate examination rate is the principal reason CTPA has prevailed over ventilation-perfusion scintigraphy (see Table 3) [12]. The reader of the CTPA, however, must evaluate the level at which the CTPA examination is deemed

indeterminate and decide whether the CTPA examination is negative for PE at the lobar and segmental levels and indeterminate at the subsegmental level or indeterminate at the lobar/segmental level. When the examination is indeterminate, the clarity or extent of parenchymal lung disease should be assessed also. Based on the level of indeterminacy and the extent of lung disease, the radiologist can recommend further diagnostic examination as shown in Table 7.

Diagnostic performance of CT pulmonary angiography for subsegmental pulmonary embolism

The incidence of isolated subsegmental PE in patients who are clinically suspected of having PE is not known exactly [71]. Most authors estimate it to be 4% to 6%, but, depending on the population studied and the inclusion criteria, it has been estimated to be as high as 17% of the population suspected of having PE [12,22,71–74]. Nevertheless, the clinical significance of isolated subsegmental PE is unclear, especially in patients who do not have baseline cardiopulmonary dysfunction [22,71]. It has been suggested that isolated peripheral emboli are less important clinically, and hence a lower detection rate can be tolerated [75–77].

PE are more difficult to appreciate by CTPA when evaluating subsegmental pulmonary arteries because the subsegmental pulmonary arteries are small in caliber, have limited contrast enhancement in relation to the finite spatial resolution of CT, and have an orientation that is not ideal for contrast imaging [78]. As a result, isolated subsegmental PE reduce the sensitivity of CTPA by 15% to 23% and its specificity by 3% to 14%. Therefore the sensitivity of CTPA for detecting subsegmental PE is 82% to

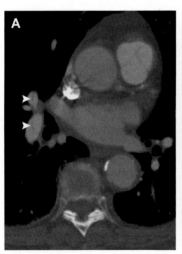

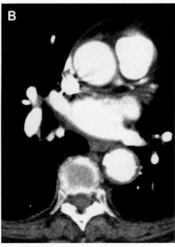

Fig. 11. A 74-year-old woman who had with history of uterine cancer and pulmonary emboli presented with chest pain. (*A*) Weblike filling defects (*arrowheads*) representing chronic pulmonary emboli are seen on the bone window settings. (*B*) These defects are not detected on mediastinal window settings.

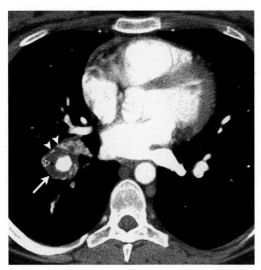

Fig. 12. A 20-year-old woman who had Behcet's disease and a known pulmonary artery aneurysm presented with hemoptysis. The axial CT image demonstrates a pulmonary artery aneurysm with mural thrombus (*arrow*). Gas (*open arrowhead*) is seen within the thrombus because of fistulization with an adjacent bronchus. Dilated bronchial arteries (*white arrowheads*) are seen along the wall of the aneurysm because of chronic pulmonary emboli.

87%, and its specificity is 92% to 94% [62,79–81]. Conventional pulmonary angiography may not be superior to thin-collimation (1 mm) MD-CTPA even at the subsegmental level, however [81]. One study comparing thin-collimation (1 mm) CTPA and conventional pulmonary angiography in a cast porcine model demonstrated no statistical significance in the sensitivity of the two modalities (87% for both) at the subsegmental level [81].

Deep venous thrombosis

DVT of the lower extremities is considered the most likely (> 90% of cases) source of PE. One percent to 8% of patients who have DVT develop fatal PE [82]. In the clinical setting of established PE, the lower extremities are still considered the likely source even when diagnostic examinations are negative for DVT. The pathogenesis in latter scenario is referred to as the "big-bang theory": it is hypothesized that all the DVT in both lower extremities mobilizes to the pulmonary arteries, leaving little evidence behind in the lower extremity veins.

Diagnostic modalities

Ultrasound examination of the lower extremities is used to evaluate for DVT. Other modalities such as D-dimer assay, plethysmography, MR venography,

and CT venography are used also, however [5,82–85]. The sensitivity and specificity of these diagnostic examinations are shown in Table 8 [5,82–85]. CT venography consists of contrast-enhanced axial CT images of the upper thigh and pelvis with an approximate 3-minute delay from the original CTPA examination. As discussed later, this contrast-enhanced CT examination, also known as "indirect CT venography," is performed in conjunction with CTPA and not as a stand-alone or independent CT examination.

ELISA D-dimer assay is an assay for D-dimer, a degradation product of cross-linked fibrin blood clot. Levels of D-dimer typically are elevated in patients who have acute venous thromboembolism as well as a variety of nonthrombotic conditions (eg, recent major surgery, hemorrhage, trauma, pregnancy, or cancer) [82,86]. D-dimer assays generally are sensitive, but their sensitivity varies depending on the quality of the examination and the time spent in obtaining the results: more time and a higher-quality kit give a higher sensitivity [87,88]. Generally, the D-dimer assay is a sensitive test with poor specificity. That is, it is good test for eliminating suspected conditions, and it is used commonly as a pretest for more specific and more anatomic (imaging) investigational examinations (eg, CTPA and indirect CT venography) [82].

Technique and protocol of multidetector indirect CT venography

The images are acquired 3 minutes (180 seconds) after the start of contrast injection for the CTPA examination [5,89,90]. The axial images are obtained from the top of the iliac crest (lower vena cava) down to the knees (popliteal veins) [5,89,90]. Four millimeter × 2.5 collimation at 120kV is used [5,89,90].

CT venography findings of deep venous thrombosis

Findings of DVT by CT venography are reminiscent of the findings of PE by CTPA. The intraluminal pathology and the imaging modality are the same (the location of the potentially affected vessels is different), and therefore the imaging findings are the same. An intravascular filling defect is the cardinal and most specific sign of DVT. This filling defect can occupy the lumen of the vessel either partially or completely [22]. When it occupies the vein completely, the vein diameter is increased in the setting of acute DVT.

Diagnostic performance of CT venography

Indirect CT venography increases the sensitivity of MD-CTPA from 83% to 90%. Indirect CT venography allows "one stop-shopping," that is, two

Box 3:   Imaging pitfalls in the diagnosis of pulmonary embolism

Patient-related factors
Respiratory motion artifact [21]

> This artifact is the most common cause of indeterminate CTPA.
> Respiratory motion artifact makes it difficult to evaluate subsegmental pulmonary arteries.
> This artifact is reduced by increased slice number MDCT and increased collimation thickness to reduce shorter breathholds.

Image noise [21]

> Large patient body habitus can increase quantum mottle.
> Image noise makes it difficult to evaluate segmental and subsegmental pulmonary arteries.
> Image noise can be reduced by increasing collimation thickness to reduce noise.

Flow-related artifact [21,57,58]

> Flow-related artifact causes a relatively low-attenuation segment within the lower lobe pulmonary arteries that has ill-defined margins but still has a moderate enhancement of more than 78 HU
> This artifact Is caused by a poor mixture of blood and contrast material leading to poor contrast enhancement in the lower lobe pulmonary arteries (indeterminate CTPA).
> Flow-related artifact most likely results from inspiration, which draws in unenhanced blood entering the right atrium, right ventricle, and pulmonary arteries from the inferior vena cava just before image acquisition (Fig. 13).

Technical factors
Window setting [21]

> Very bright vessel contrast can obscure small PE (see Fig. 11).
> Ideal window settings (width and level) differ among patients.
> Window width of 700 HU and level of 100 HU usually are appropriate for most segmental and subsegmental studies.

Streak artifact [21]

> Streak artifact is caused by beam-hardening artifact from dense contrast in the superior vena cava.
> Artifact may overlie the right pulmonary artery and/or the right upper lobe pulmonary artery segments (Fig. 14).
> This artifact is reduced by flushing the superior vena cava with normal saline following the initial contrast bolus (saline chase) using a dual injection.

Lung algorithm artifact [59]

> This algorithm is a special frequency reconstruction that creates artifacts that can mimic pulmonary emboli.
> Changing the algorithm to a standard algorithm can eliminate these artifacts.

Partial volume artifact [21]

> Partial volume artifact results from axial imaging of an axially oriented vessel. The apparent filling defect mimics pulmonary emboli.
> The margins usually are not sharp, and the artifact usually is seen on one axial image.
> Partial volume artifact is reduced by decreasing the collimation (detector width).

Stair-step reformatting artifact [21]

> Stair-step reformatting artifact consists of low-attenuation lines seen traversing a vessel on coronal and/or sagittal reformatted images.
> This artifact is accentuated by cardiac and respiratory motion.
> Stair-step reformatting artifact is reduced by reconstructing the raw axial data with a 50% overlap before 3-D image reconstruction.

Anatomic factors
Lymph nodes: partial volume averaging effect [60]

> Knowledge of hilar and pulmonary lymph node anatomy may help, although this anatomy may vary among patients.
> Reducing collimation (detector width) helps reduce this artifact.
> Careful evaluation of coronal and sagittal reconstructions helps with difficult cases.

(continued on next page)

Box 3: (continued)

Vascular bifurcation [46]

Vascular bifurcations on axial images may mimic linear filling defects/PE.
Reducing collimation (detector width) helps reduce this artifact.
Careful evaluation of coronal and sagittal reconstructions helps identify these normal structures.

Misidentification of pulmonary veins for pulmonary arteries [61]

Filling defects in the pulmonary veins caused by admixture flow artifact may be seen. This misidentification is a double fault: mistaking the defect for a true filling defect (an embolus) and mistaking the involved pulmonary vein segment for a pulmonary artery.
Following the pulmonary veins back and forth from the left atrium through contiguous images helps prevent mistaking the pulmonary vein segment for a pulmonary artery.

Pathologic factors
Mucus plug [21]

A mucus plug in the bronchus with enhancement of the wall may mimic a PE (**Fig. 15**).
Misidentification is avoided by viewing the bronchus on contiguous images.

Perivascular edema [21]

Perivascular edema is caused by left-heart failure that produces peri-bronchovascular interstitial thickening.
Perivascular edema appears as chronic PE
Other findings of heart failure can be seen.

Localized increase in vascular resistance [58,62]

Pulmonary consolidation including atelectasis can cause regional vascular crowding (vessels adjacent to one another become closer) and also can increase the vascular resistance, leading to reduced flow in the pulmonary arteries in that region.
Slow flow causes reduced contrast admixture (poor enhancement) that may make the normal vessel look thrombosed (false positive) or may lead the reader to overlook an underlying PE (false negative).
The apparently unenhancing pulmonary artery segment is actually enhancing by more than 78 HU.

Pulmonary artery stump in situ thrombus [63]

Patient has had a recent pneumonectomy or lobe resection.
Thrombus is found only in the blind-ended pulmonary artery stump.

Primary pulmonary artery sarcoma (see later discussion)
Tumor emboli (see later discussion)

---

examinations studying two related entities of the same pathologic process: thromboembolic venous disease [18]. The statistical results of indirect CT venography as an independent examination are tabulated in Table 9 [5,91–95]. The advantages and disadvantages of this examination are tabulated in Box 4 [5,22,91–95].

Nonthromboembolic pulmonary embolism

Nonthrombotic PE and the broader differential, filling defects within the pulmonary artery, can be classified into malignant filling defects/PE, autologous nonmalignant filling defects/PE (iatrogenic or noniatrogenic), and iatrogenic (foreign body) PE.

Types of nonthromboembolic pulmonary emboli and individual CT findings

Primary pulmonary artery sarcoma

Primary pulmonary artery sarcomas are pulmonary artery angiosarcomas and are uncommon. They present as lobulated, heterogeneously enhancing masses/filling defects in the pulmonary arteries [21,96,97]. In addition, they show expansion or distension in the affected segment of the pulmonary artery [21,98] and/or focal breakthrough of the pulmonary artery wall and extravascular spread [21,98]. Because they show enhancement, they may be confused with chronic thromboembolic PE, which also may enhance, but sarcomas usually form acute angles with the pulmonary artery lumen, as do acute thromboembolic PE [21].

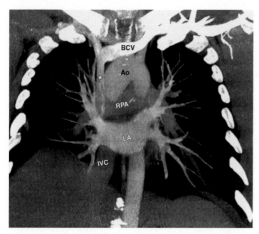

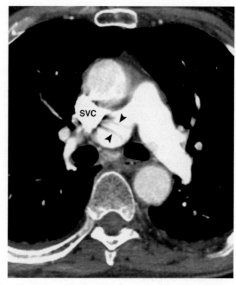

Fig. 13. Deep inspiration during the scan draws unenhanced blood from the inferior vena cava (*IVC*) into the right atrium. The unenhanced blood displaces the contrast-enhanced blood entering the right atrium from the left brachiocephalic vein (*BCV*) and superior vena cava (*asterisk*) from the pulmonary arteries and into the pulmonary veins, left atrium (*LA*) and eventually the aorta (*Ao*). This process is demonstrated by the unenhanced right pulmonary artery (*RPA*) on this coronal slab maximum-intensity projection image.

Fig. 14. Beam hardening from dense contrast in the superior vena cava (*SVC*) causes streak artifact (*arrowheads*) that overlies the right pulmonary artery and may simulate a pulmonary embolus.

Pulmonary artery tumor emboli

Small tumor emboli at the segmental and subsegmental pulmonary artery level are more common than larger, more central, lobar and main pulmonary artery tumor emboli [21]. In fact, tumor emboli are seen in up to 26% of autopsies but are identified infrequently by CT [2,99]. In addition, tumor emboli often are associated with superadded recent and/or organizing thrombi [100,101]; this association may create confusion and lead to misdiagnosis.

Primary tumors that more commonly cause small peripheral tumor emboli include prostate, breast, and hepatocellular carcinomas and adenocarcinomas of the gastrointestinal tract such as stomach and pancreas [100]. Small peripheral tumor emboli produce segmental and subsegmental pulmonary artery vascular dilation and beading that increases in size over time, enhances, and gives

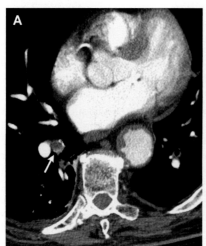

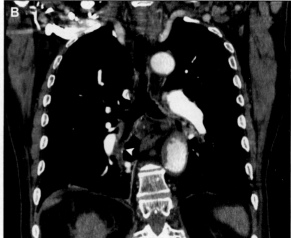

Fig. 15. (*A*) A mucus plug in the bronchus intermedius with enhancement of the bronchial wall (*arrow*) may mimic a pulmonary embolus. (*B*) Coronal reformat image shows that the filling defect is in fact within the bronchus (*arrowhead*) and not a pulmonary artery.

Table 5: Incidence of pulmonary embolism in various patient populations detected by contrast-enhanced chest CT

Patient Population	Incidence (%)	Increase from Baseline
All patients without clinical suspicion of pulmonary embolism	1–1.5	Baseline
Inpatients and/or oncology patients without clinical suspicion of pulmonary embolism	4–5	2.5-fold to fivefold
Patients with clinical suspicion of pulmonary embolism (CT pulmonary angiographic examination)	9–27	Sixfold to 27-fold

The examination was not necessarily performed using dedicated contrast-enhanced chest CT (CT pulmonary angiography).
Data from Refs. [21,64–69,71].

a tree-in-bud appearance [2,21,102,103]. In addition, associated heterogeneous focal or diffuse lung opacities may be seen because of the lymphangitic spread of tumor (lymphangitic carcinomatosis) [104]. The tree-in-bud appearance has two different pathogenic explanations: the filling of the centrilobular arteries with tumor cells and thrombotic microangiopathy [2,103,105–107].

Large tumor emboli are less common and are similar in appearance to primary sarcoma of the pulmonary artery [21]. Primary tumors that more commonly cause larger tumor emboli include renal cell carcinoma, hepatocellular carcinomas, and choriocarcinomas (tumors that commonly invade the inferior vena cava) [101].

Pulmonary septic embolism and septic thromboembolism

Septic emboli to the pulmonary arteries usually are bacterial; parasitic or mycotic infections are less common [108]. Common predisposing factors are tricuspid valve endocarditis, drug addiction, alcoholism, immune deficiencies, infected indwelling central catheters or pacemaker wires, and lymphoma [109,110]. Septic thromboembolism in which the source is an infected deep venous thrombus (septic thrombophlebitis) also may occur. A particular entity that can be diagnosed in its entirety by a contrast-enhanced chest CT, including dedicated CTPA, is Lammier's disease, septic venous thrombosis of the jugular vein with distal pulmonary septic embolization. The jugular vein is distended and thrombosed with enhancing wall and perivascular soft tissue at the base of the neck in the upper cuts of the chest CT. At the same time there may be segmental and subsegmental PE with typical parenchymal lung findings of septic PE.

Typical parenchymal lung findings include bilateral, usually peripheral, lung nodules that are predominantly in the lower lung lobes and often demonstrate cavitary changes [2,46–48]. These nodules vary in size and degree of cavitation reflecting repeated episodes of embolic showers [2]. Other CT parenchymal findings include subpleural wedge-shaped heterogeneous areas of increased density with rimlike enhancement [2,46–48]. In addition septic PE are complicated by empyema [2].

Hydatid pulmonary embolism

Hydatid PE is a rare complication of cardiac or hepatic echinococcosis caused by the infestation of *Echnococcus granulosus* [2]. The sources of hydatid PE are an hepatic or abdominal cystic lesion that has ruptured into the hepatic veins or inferior vena cava or a pulmonary cystic lesion that has

Table 6: Efficacy of multidetector CT pulmonary angiography

Criterion	Value
Sensitivity	83%–94%
Specificity	94%–100%
Negative predictive value	93%–96%
Percentage of indeterminate exams	6%–7%
Reader confidence	≥ 90%
Interobserver agreement	0.63–0.94 (k) (high)
Major complications	< 0.1%
Minor complications	0.6%
Pulmonary embolism rate 3–6 months after an initially negative MD-CTPA	0.9%–3.0%
Fatal pulmonary embolism rate 3–6 months after an initially negative MD-CTPA	0.2%–0.5%

Data from Refs. [17–20,28,67–71].

Table 7: Evaluation and management (diagnostic triage) of an indeterminate CT pulmonary angiography examination depending on the pulmonary artery level of indeterminacy and the degree of lung opacification

Level of Indeterminacy	Clear lungs	Opacified lungs
Lobar/segmental	V/Q[a] Repeat CTPA	Pulmonary angiogram Repeat CTPA
Subsegmental	Pulmonary angiogram Clinical significance?[b]	Lung disease explains clinical picture: No other examinations Lung disease does not explain clinical picture: Pulmonary angiogram Clinical significance?

Abbreviations: CTPA, CT pulmonary angiogram; C/P, Clinical picture (clinical suspicion of pulmonary embolus); V/Q, ventilation-perfusion scintigram.
[a] V/Q scintigraphy following indeterminate CTPA is particularly useful if there is significant motion (respiratory or patient tremor motion) artifact.
[b] The incidence of patients who have isolated subsegmental PE in the setting of the clinical suspicion of PE is probably 4% to 6%. There is a controversy, however, regarding the clinical significance of a false-negative subsegmental CTPA examination (subsegmental PE not appreciated by CTPA) and whether missing the diagnosis and not treating patients is detrimental or not.

ruptured into the superior vena cava or right atrium [2]. CT findings include occlusion of the pulmonary artery branches with cystic lesions, which can be confirmed by MR imaging [2].

Fat pulmonary embolism

Fat PE is an infrequent complication of long-bone fractures. It occurs in 0.5 to 3% of simple, isolated femoral fractures; but its incidence has been reported to be as high as 20% in massive or complicated traumas [2]. Less common causes include hemoglobinopathy, major burns, pancreatitis, overwhelming infection, malignancy, and liposuction procedures [2]. The insult to the pulmonary vascular bed is twofold. The first is the obstructive event of the pulmonary arteries, as in any PE event. The second is the production of free fatty acids that initiates a toxic reaction in the endothelium that is associated with an inflammatory response with accumulation of neutrophils and other inflammatory cells that cause further damage to the vasculature [2].

A combination of pulmonary, cerebral, and cutaneous symptoms occurs within 12 to 24 hours of the traumatic event [2]. These symptoms are referred to as "fat embolism syndrome" and can be fatal in up to 20% of clinically diagnosed cases. The time interval between the instigating traumatic event and the appearance of radiographic findings is 1 to 2 days [2]. The CT findings, which consist of widespread patchy areas of parenchymal opacities (increased permeability edema), resemble acute respiratory distress syndrome [2]. Other findings on early, high-resolution CT may include ill-defined

Table 8: Sensitivity and specificity of various diagnostic examinations evaluating for lower extremity deep venous thrombosis

Examination	Above-Knee DVT		Below-Knee DVT	
	Sensitivity	Specificity	Sensitivity	Specificity
D-dimer assay[a]	85%–99%	50%–68%	85%–99%	50%–68%
Plethysmography	Modest	Poor	Poor	Poor
Ultrasound	94%–97%	94%	64%–73%	94%
CT venography	95% (89%–100%)	97% (92%–100%)	95% (89%–100%)	97% (92%–100%)
MR venography	92%	95%	92%	95%

[a] The D-dimer assay is an ELISA with varying sensitivity and specificity based on the particular expense and time constrains for the examination.
Data from Refs. [5,82–85,87,88].

Table 9: **Efficacy of indirect CT venography**

Criterion	Value
Effect on sensitivity of CT pulmonary angiography	Increases (from 83% to 90%)
Effect on specificity of CT pulmonary angiography	No significant effect
Sensitivity	89%–100%
Specificity	92%–100%
Positive predictive value	67%–100%
Negative predictive value	97%–100%
Major complication rate[a]	< 0.1%
Minor complication rate[a]	0.6%

[a] The complication rates displayed are from a CTPA series. Because all complications related to CTPA were related to contrast injection and contrast reaction, the authors assume that the complication rates are the same for indirect CT venography.
Data from Refs. [5,18,91–95].

centrilobar and subpleural nodules (in 20%–85% of cases), interlobar septal thickening (in 50%–60% of cases) and/or ground-glass opacities (in 75%–80% of cases).

Silicone (polydimethylsiloxane) pulmonary embolism
Silicone PE is caused by the intravasation of silicone into the blood stream, most often from illegal, nonmedical cosmetic injections. The clinical manifestations are similar to those of fat embolism. Radiographically there are bilateral diffuse patchy infiltrates (alveolar hemorrhage).

Amniotic fluid pulmonary embolism
Amniotic fluid PE is a complication of pregnancy and delivery with a maternal mortality reaching

Box 4: **Advantages and disadvantages of indirect CT venography**

Advantages
Offers one combined examination for PE and DVT
High diagnostic accuracy
Ability to detect nonthromboembolic pathology
Availability of examination (24 × 7)
Reproducibility (not operator dependent)

Disadvantages
Radiation exposure
Contrast nephropathy
Not a bedside examination
High cost
Can be significantly affected by streak artifact (eg, from hardware)

80% [2]. This complication occurs when amniotic fluid escapes into the blood stream through small uterine venule tears during natural labor, surgery (including cesarean sections), or trauma during surgery [2]. When amniotic fluid PE is associated with labor, 70% of patients suffer from symptoms during spontaneous labor, and 30% of patients suffer from symptoms after parturition [2]. The diagnosis is primarily clinical and circumstantial. Clinical manifestations include central nervous system irritability such as hyperreflexia and convulsions [2]. The radiographic findings are nonspecific and supportive. The diffuse bilateral heterogeneous areas of increased opacity are indistinguishable from pulmonary edema [2].

Air pulmonary embolism
Pulmonary air embolus almost always results from iatrogenic causes and/or conditions such as transthoracic needle sampling, barotrauma from positive-pressure ventilation, supradiaphragmatic central venous catheter placement, or intravenous drug or contrast injection. It occurs in 23% of patients undergoing intravenous contrast injection for CT examinations [2]. In addition, this complication can occur in decompression sickness, when nitrogen gas is formed and embolizes in the pulmonary arteries [2]. The risk of death is associated the volume of air/gas and with the rate of air/gas accumulation within the circulation (right-heart and/

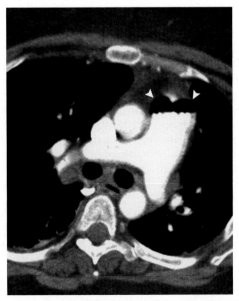

Fig. 16. Axial CT image shows air (*arrowheads*) in the nondependent portion of the main pulmonary artery caused by air in the connecting tubing from the power injector.

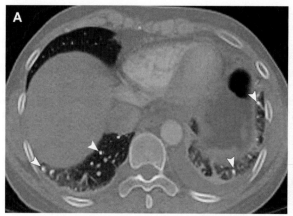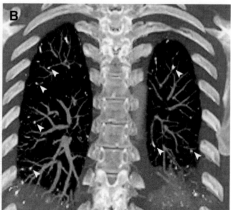

Fig. 17. A patient presented with dyspnea after undergoing transcatheter sclerosis of a cerebral arterio-venous malformation using glue. (*A*) Axial and (*B*) coronal reformatted images demonstrate numerous, peripherally located high-density pulmonary emboli (*arrowheads*).

or pulmonary circulation) [2]. The minimal lethal volume is reported to be 300 to 500 mL of air, and the minimal lethal injection rate is reported to be 100 mL/s [2]. Death occurs when a segment of blood is displaced almost entirely by a compressible column of gas within the right-heart/pulmonary circulation. Because this column of gas is compressible and does not move, it interrupts the circulation.

Air is seen by CT as nonattentuating pockets in any location, from the systemic veins such as the subclavian vein and superior vena cava, to the right atrium, and to the central (Fig. 16) and/or peripheral pulmonary arteries [2].

Talc pulmonary embolism

Talc and cellulose are common fillers added drugs intended for oral consumption or for inhalation. Such drugs include amphetamines, methylphenidate, hydromorphone, or dextropropoxyphene [2]. When drugs intended to be taken orally are injected, the insoluble materials of microcrystalline cellulose and/or talc embolize to the pulmonary arteries and create a nidus for a chronic granulomatous (Giant cell) inflammatory reaction [2].

On CT the condition appears as multiple nodules that may expand to involve larger opacities. In addition, there is fibrosis and later scaring as well as a tree-in-bud appearance on thin CT slices [2].

Cotton fiber pulmonary embolism

Cotton fiber PE is caused by cotton fibers that enter the blood stream when narcotics or intravenous medication is injected through cotton swabs or when fibers become detached from guidewires during angiography [2].

Iodinated oil pulmonary embolism

Iodinated oil embolism occurs from diagnostic and therapeutic interventional radiology procedures such as lymphangiography, hepatic artery chemoembolization for hepatocellular carcinoma, and systemic vascular malformation glue embolization/sclerosis [2]. Lymphangiography probably is the most common historical cause [2], but the authors of this article believe that, with the declining use of lymphangiography and the increasing use of interventional procedures in managing hepatocellular carcinoma and vascular malformations, the latter two are or will become the major causes of iodinated oil embolization and particularly chemoembolization.

Iodinated oil embolism from lymphangiography usually is seen as diffuse, fine nodules of increased opacity, and the patients usually are asymptomatic [2]. Iodinated oil embolism from hepatocellular carcinoma chemoembolization appears as parenchymal pulmonary infiltrates 2 to 5 days after the embolization and is accompanied by symptoms such as hemoptysis, cough, and dyspnea [2]. Hepatocellular carcinoma in livers demonstrating hepatic arterial to hepatic venous shunting and the use of small particles in the chemoembolization iodinated oil–particulate embolism concoction may increase the incidence of pulmonary artery embolization after chemoembolization. By CT, the embolus is seen as a high-density (high-attenuation) intravascular lesion, possibly with an associated wedge-shaped parenchymal lesion, if any (Fig. 17). Symptoms from glue PE depend on the

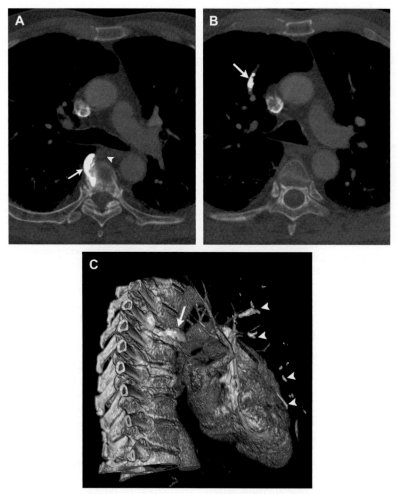

Fig. 18. A 70-year-old woman underwent vertebroplasty for multilevel thoracic vertebral insufficiency compression fractures secondary to advanced osteopenia. (*A*) Axial CT image demonstrates extravasation of cement from the vertebral body (*arrow*) with the azygous vein (*arrowhead*) in close proximity. (*B*) High-density cement is seen in a pulmonary artery (*arrow*) caused by the intravasation of the cement into the systemic venous circulation and subsequent embolization to the lungs. (*C*) Three-dimensional volume-rendered image demonstrating extravasated cement from a thoracic vertebral body (*arrow*) and several cement emboli in peripheral pulmonary arteries (*arrowheads*).

size of the PE and the patient's cardiopulmonary reserve.

Metallic mercury pulmonary embolism
Intravenous injection of liquid mercury, whether accidental or intentional, is rare [2]. Most patients who suffer from mercury pulmonary embolization experience little or no toxic effects [2]. Most short-term symptoms are caused by the embolic (pulmonary artery obstructive) process itself along with the resultant, if any, pulmonary infarction [2]. CT findings include diffusely scattered high-density foci in the pulmonary arteries. Findings may be permanent or may resolve gradually [2].

Cement (polymethylmethacrylate) pulmonary embolism
Cement PE occurs form intravasation of radiopaque cement from vertebroplasty procedures from the vertebral body into the perivertebral venous plexus and into the systemic veins. CT findings include high-density tubular embolus in the pulmonary arteries. In the lower cuts of the CT, paravertebral contrast leaks may be depicted (Fig. 18) [2].

Iatrogenic pulmonary embolism caused by a plastic or metal alloy foreign body
Objects used in the medical field include that have been reported as causing PE include catheter

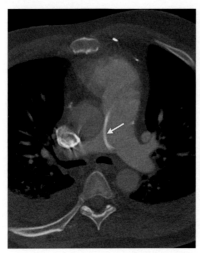

Fig. 19. Axial CT image demonstrates a catheter fragment (*arrow*) that embolized into the main pulmonary artery.

fragments (Fig. 19), metal stents, angioplasty balloon fragments, wires, metal coils, and, rarely, vena caval filter fragments [2]. All these foreign bodies can be seen and identified on CT scouts and axial images.

References

[1] Meltem G, Goodman LR, Washington L. Venous thromboembolic disease: where does multidetector computed tomography fit? Cardiol Clin 2003;21:631–8.

[2] Han D, Lee KS, Franquet T, et al. Thrombotic and nonthrombotic pulmonary arterial embolism: spectrum of imaging findings. Radiographics 2003;23:1521–39.

[3] Anderson FA Jr, Wheeler B, Goldberg RJ, et al. A population-based perspective of the hospital incidence and case fatality rates of deep vein thrombosis and pulmonary embolism: the Worcester DVT study. Arch Intern Med 1991; 151:933–8.

[4] Giuntini C, Ricco GD, Marini C, et al. Pulmonary embolism: epidemiology. Chest 1995; 107(Suppl):3S–9S.

[5] Begemann PGC, Bonacker M, Kemper J, et al. Evaluation of deep venous system in patients with suspected pulmonary embolism with multi-detector CT: a prospective study in comparison to Doppler sonography. J Comput Assist Tomogr 2003;27:399–409.

[6] Silverstein MD, Helt JA, Mohr DN, et al. Trends in the incidence of deep vein thrombosis and pulmonary embolism: a 25-year population-based study. Arch Intern Med 1998;158: 585–93.

[7] Goodman LR. 1999 Plenary session: Friday imaging symposium: CT diagnosis of pulmonary embolism and deep venous thrombosis. Radiographics 2000;20:1201–5.

[8] Rathbun SW, Raskob GE, Whitsett TL. Sensitivity and specificity of helical computed tomography in the diagnosis of pulmonary embolism: a systematic review. Ann Intern Med 2000; 132:227–32.

[9] Stauffer JL. Pulmonary thromboembolism. In: Tierney LM, McPhee SJ, Papdakis MA, editors. Current medical diagnosis and management. 36th edition. Stamford (CT): Appleton & Lange; 1997. p. 290–7.

[10] Goldhaber SZ. Pulmonary embolism. N Engl J Med 1998;339:93–104.

[11] Goldhaber SZ, Visani L, De Rosa M. Acute pulmonary embolism: clinical outcomes in the International Cooperative Pulmonary Embolism Registry (ICOPER). Lancet 1999;353:1386–9.

[12] The PIOPED investigators. Value of the ventilation/perfusion scan in acute pulmonary embolism: results of the Prospective Investigation of Pulmonary Embolism Diagnosis (PIOPED). JAMA 1990;263:2753–9.

[13] van Rossum AB, Treurniet FE, kieft GJ, et al. Role of spiral volumetry computed tomographic scanning in the assessment of patients with clinical suspicion of pulmonary embolism and an abnormal ventilation/perfusion lung scan. Thorax 1996;51:23–8.

[14] Cross JJ, Kemp PM, Walsh CG, et al. A randomized trial of spiral CT and ventilation perfusion sscintigraphy for the diagnosis of pulmonary embolism. Clin Radiol 1998;53:177–82.

[15] MacDonald SLS, Mayo JR. Computed tomography of acute pulmonary embolism. Semin Ultrasound CT MR 2003;24:217–31.

[16] Holbert JM, Costello P, Federle MP. Role of spiral computed tomography in the diagnosis of pulmonary embolism in the emergency department. Ann Emerg Med 1999;33:520–8.

[17] Russo V, Piva T, Lovato L, et al. A new gold standard in the diagnosis of pulmonary embolism? State of the art diagnostic algorithms. Radiol Med 2005;109:49–61.

[18] Stein PD, Fowler SE, Goodman LR, et al. for the PIOPED Investigators. Multidetector computed tomography for acute pulmonary embolism. N Engl J Med 2006;354(22):2317–27.

[19] Raptopoulos V, Boiselle PM. Multidetector row spiral CT pulmonary angiography: comparison with single-detector row spiral CT. Radiology 2001;221:606–13.

[20] Patel S, Kazerooni EA, Cascade PN. Pulmonary embolism: optimization of small pulmonary artery visualization at multidetector row spiral CT. Radiology 2003;227:445–60.

[21] Wittram C, Maher MM, Yoo AF, et al. CT angiography of pulmonary embolism: diagnostic criteria and causes misdiagnosis. Radiographics 2004;24:1219–38.

[22] Kanne JP, Lalani TA. Role of computed tomography and magnetic resonance imaging for

deep venous thrombosis and pulmonary embolism. Circulation 2004;109(Suppl I):I15–21.

[23] Ghaye B, Remy J, Remy-Jardin M. Non-traumatic thoracic emergencies: CT diagnosis of acute pulmonary embolism: The first 10 years. Eur Radiol 2002;12:1886–905.

[24] Remy-Jardin M, Mastora I, Remy J. Pulmonary embolus imaging with multislice CT. Radiol Clin North Am 2003;41:507–19.

[25] Powell T, Muller NL. Imaging of acute pulmonary thromboembolism: should spiral computed tomography replace the ventilation-perfusion scan? Clin Chest Med 2003;24:29–38.

[26] Johnson MS. Current strategies for the diagnosis of pulmonary embolus. J Vasc Interv Radiol 2002;13:12–23.

[27] Wittram C, Meehan MJ, Halpern EF, et al. Trends in thoracic radiology over a decade at a large academic medical center. J Thorac Imaging 2004;19:164–70.

[28] Paterson ID, Schwartzman K. Strategies incorporating spiral CT for the diagnosis of acute pulmonary embolism: a cost-effectiveness analysis. Chest 2001;119:1791–800.

[29] Blachere H, Latrabe V, Montaudon M, et al. Pulmonary embolism revealed on helical CT angiography: comparison with ventilation-perfusion radionuclide lung scanning. Am J Roentgenol 2000;174:1041–7.

[30] Remy-Jardin M, Remy J, Baghaie F, et al. Clinical value of thin collimation in the diagnostic workup of pulmonary embolism. Am J Roentgenol 2000;175:407–11.

[31] Herold CJ. Spiral computed tomography of pulmonary embolism. Eur Respir J 2002;35(Suppl):13S–21S.

[32] Drucker EA, Rivitz SM, Shepard JA, et al. Acute pulmonary embolism: assessment of helical CT for diagnosis. Radiology 1998;209:235–41.

[33] Pruszcyk P, Torbicki A, Pacho R, et al. Noninvasive diagnosis of suspected severe pulmonary embolism: transesophageal vs. spiral CT. Chest 1997;112:722–8.

[34] Otmani A, Tribouilloy C, Leborgne L, et al. Valeur diagnostique de l'echographie cardiaque et de l'angioscanner thoracique helicoidal pour le diagnostic de l'embolie pulmonaire aigue. Ann Cardiol Angeiol (Paris) 1998;47:707–15.

[35] Napoli A, Fleischmann D, Chan FP, et al. Computed tomography angiography: state-of-the-art imaging using multidetector-row technology. J Comput Assist Tomogr 2004;28(Suppl 1):S32–45.

[36] Hargaden GC, Kavanagh EC, Fitzpatrick P, et al. Diagnosis of pulmonary emboli and image quality at CT pulmonary angiography: influence of imaging direction with multidetector CT. Clin Radiol 2006;61:600–3.

[37] Kirchner J, Kickuth R, Laufer U, et al. Optimized enhancement in helical CT: experiences with a real-time bolus tracking system in 628 patients. Clin Radiol 2000;55:368–73.

[38] Remy-Jardin M, Remy J, Wattinne L, et al. Central pulmonary thromboembolism: diagnosis with spiral volumetric CT with the single-breath-hold technique: comparison with pulmonary angiography. Radiology 1992;185:381–7.

[39] Ghaye B, Szapiro D, Mastoora I, et al. Peripheral pulmonary arteries: how far in the lung does multi-detector row spiral CT allow analysis? Radiology 2001;219:629–36.

[40] Remy-Jardin M, Remy J, Artaud D, et al. Peripheral pulmonary arteries: optimization of the spiral CT acquisition protocol. Radiology 1997;204:157–63.

[41] Hu H, He HD, Foley WD, et al. Four multidetector-row helical CT: image quality and volume coverage speed. Radiology 2000;215:55–62.

[42] Remy-Jardin M, Baghale F, Bonnel F, et al. Thoracic helical CT: influence of subsecond scan time and thin collimation on evaluation of peripheral pulmonary arteries. Eur Radiol 2000;10:1297–303.

[43] Schoepf UJ, Kessler MA, Reiger CT, et al. Multislice CT imaging of pulmonary embolism. Eur Radiol 2001;11:2278–86.

[44] Schoepf UJ, Holznecht N, Helmberger TK, et al. Subsegmental pulmonary emboli: improved detection with thin-collimation multidetector row spiral CT. Radiology 2002;222:483–90.

[45] Remy-Jardin M, Remy J, Spiral CT. Angiography of the pulmonary circulation. Radiology 1999;212:615–36.

[46] Washington L, Goodman LR, Gonyo MB. CT for thromboembolic disease. Radiol Clin North Am 2002;46:751–71.

[47] Schoepf UJ, Becker CR, Hofmann LK, et al. Multislice CT angiography. Eur Radiol 2003;13:1946–61.

[48] Kanne JP, Gotway MB, Thoongsuwan N, et al. Six cases of acute central pulmonary embolism revealed on unenhanced multidetector CT of the chest. AJR Am J Roentgenol 2003;180:1661–4.

[49] Contractor S, Maldjian PD, Sharma VK, et al. Role of helical CT in detecting right ventricular dysfunction secondary to acute pulmonary embolism. J Comput Assist Tomogr 2002;26:587–91.

[50] Wu AS, Pezzullo JA, Cornan JJ, et al. CT pulmonary angiography: quantification of pulmonary embolus as a predictor of patient outcome-initial experience. Radiology 2004;230:831–5.

[51] Gottschalk A, Stein PD, Goodman LR, et al. Overview of prospective investigation of pulmonary embolism diagnosis II. Semin Nucl Med 2002;32:173–82.

[52] Coche EE, Muller NL, Kim K, et al. Acute pulmonary embolism: ancillary findings at spiral CT. Radiology 1998;207:753–8.

[53] Reissig A, Heyne JP, Kroegel C. Sonography of lung and pleura in pulmonary embolism: sono-morphologic characterization and comparison with spiral CT scanning. Chest 2001;120: 1977–83.

[54] Woodard PK, Roger Y. Diagnosis of pulmonary embolism with spiral computed tomography and magnetic resonance angiography. Curr Opin Cardiol 1999;14(5):442–52.

[55] Edwards PD, Bull RK, Coulden R. CT measurement of main pulmonary artery diameter. Br J Radiol 1998;71:1018–20.

[56] Baque-Juston MC, Wells AU, Hansell DM. Pericardial thickening or effusion in patients with pulmonary artery hypertension: a CT study. AJR Am J Roentgenol 1999;172:361–4.

[57] Gosselin MV, Rassner UA, Thieszen SL, et al. Contrast dynamics during CT pulmonary angiogram: analysis of an inspiration associated artifact. J Thorac Imaging 2004;19:1–7.

[58] Wittram C, Maher MM, Halpern E, et al. The Hounsfield unit values of acute and chronic pulmonary emboli [abstract]. In: Radiological Society of North America Scientific Assembly and Annual Meeting Program. Oak Brook (IL): Radiological Society of North America; 2003. p. 678.

[59] Swensen SJ, Morin RL, Aughenbaugh GL, et al. CT reconstruction algorithm selection in the evaluation of solitary pulmonary nodules. J Comput Assist Tomogr 1995;19:932–5.

[60] Remy-Jardin M, Remy J, Artaud D, et al. Spiral CT of pulmonary embolism: technical considerations and interpretative pitfalls. J Thorac Imaging 1997;12:103–17.

[61] Beigelman C, Chartrand-Lefebvre C, Howarth NO, et al. Pitfalls in diagnosis of pulmonary embolism with helical CT angiography. AJR Am J Roentgenol 1998;171:579–85.

[62] Goodman LR, Curtin JJ, Mewissen MW, et al. Detection of pulmonary embolism in patients with unresolved clinical and scintigraphic diagnosis: helical CT versus angiography. AJR Am J Roentegenol 1995;164:1369–74.

[63] Wechsler RJ, Salazar AM, Gessner AJ, et al. CT of in situ vascular stump thrombosis after pulmonary resection for cancer. AJR Am J Roentgenol 2001;176:1423–5.

[64] Winston CB, Wechsler RJ, Salazar AM, et al. Incidental pulmonary emboli detected at helical CT: Effect on patient care. Radiology 1996; 201:23–7.

[65] Gosselin MV, Rubin GD, Leung AN, et al. Unsuspected pulmonary embolism: prospective detection on routine helical CT scans. Radiology 1998;208:209–15.

[66] Storto ML, Di Credico A, Guido F, et al. Incidental detection of pulmonary emboli on routine MDCT of the chest. AJR Am J Roentgenol 2005;184:264–7.

[67] Kuroki M, Nishino M, Takahashi M, et al. Incidence of pulmonary embolism in younger versus older patients using CT. J Thorac Imaging 2006;21:167–71.

[68] Nilsson T, Olausson A, Johnsson H, et al. Negative spiral CT in pulmonary embolism. Acta Radiol 2002;43:486–91.

[69] SBU. Report no. 158. Venous thromboembolism: prevention, diagnosis and treatment. A systematic review. Stockholm (Sweden): The Swedish State Health Technology Board; 2002.

[70] Ost D, Rozenshtein A, Saffran L, et al. The negative predictive value of spiral computed tomography for the diagnosis of pulmonary embolism in patients with nondiagnostic ventilation-perfusion scans. Am J Med 2001;110: 16–21.

[71] Gladish GW, Choe DH, Marom EM, et al. Incidental pulmonary emboli in oncology patients: prevalence, CT evaluation, and natural history. Radiology 2006;240:246–55.

[72] Stein PD, Henry JW, Gottschalk A. Reassessment of pulmonary angiography for the diagnosis of pulmonary embolism: relation of interpreter agreement to the order of the involved pulmonary arterial branch. Radiology 1999;210:689–91.

[73] Diffin DC, Leyendecker JR, Johnson SP, et al. Effect of anatomic distribution of pulmonary emboli on interobserver agreement in the interpretation of pulmonary angiography. AJR Am J Roentgenol 1998;171:1085–9.

[74] Oser RF, Zuckerman DA, Gutierrez FR, et al. Anatomic distribution of pulmonary emboli at pulmonary angiography: implications for cross-sectional imaging. Radiology 1996;199: 31–5.

[75] Remy-Jardin M, Remy J, Deschildre F, et al. Diagnosis of pulmonary embolism with spiral CT: comparison with pulmonary angiography and scintigraphy. Radiology 1996;200:699–706.

[76] Weinstein MC, Fineberg HV. Clinical decision analysis. Philadelphia: WB Saunders Company; 1980.

[77] van Erkel AR, van Rossum AB, Bloem JL, et al. Spiral CT angiography for suspected pulmonary embolism: a cost effectiveness analysis. Radiology 1996;201:29–36.

[78] Kauczor HU, Heussel CP, Thelen M. Update on diagnostic strategies of pulmonary embolism. Eur Radiol 1999;9:262–75.

[79] van Rossum AB, Pattynama PM, Tijn A Ton ER, et al. Pulmonary embolism: validation of spiral CT angiography. Radiology 1996;201:467–70.

[80] Woodard PK. Pulmonary arteries must be seen before they can be assessed. Radiology 1997; 204:11–2.

[81] Baile EM, King GG, Muller NL, et al. Spiral computed tomography is comparable to angiography for the diagnosis of pulmonary embolism. Am J Respir Crit Care Med 2000;161:1010–5.

[82] Scarvelis D, Wells PS. Diagnosis and treatment of deep-vein thrombosis. CMAJ 2006;175(9): 1087–92.

[83] Andrews EJ Jr, Fleischer AC. Sonography for deep venous thrombosis: current and future applications. Ultrasound Q 2005;21:213–25.

[84] Goodacre S, Sampson F, Stevenson M, et al. Measurement of the clinical and cost-effectiveness of non-invasive diagnostic testing strategies for deep vein thrombosis. Health Technol Assess 2006;10(15):1–168, iii-iv.

[85] Kearon C, Julian JA, Newman TE, et al. Noninvasive diagnosis of deep vein thrombosis. Ann Intern Med 1998;128:663–77.

[86] Kelly J, Rudd A, Lewis RR, et al. Plasma D-dimer in the diagnosis of venous thromboembolism. Arch Intern Med 2002;162:747–56.

[87] de Monye W, Huisman M, Pattynama P. Observer dependency of the SimpliRED D-dimer assay in 81 consecutive patients with suspected pulmonary embolism. Thromb Res 1999;96:293–8.

[88] Ginsberg J, Wells P, Kearon C, et al. Sensitivity and specificity of a rapid whole-blood assay for D-dimer in the diagnosis of pulmonary embolism. Ann Intern Med 1998;129:1006–11.

[89] Loud PA, Grossman ZD, Klippenstein DL, et al. Combined CT venography and pulmonary angiography: a new diagnostic technique for suspected thromboembolic disease. AJR Am J Roentgenol 1998;170:951–4.

[90] Yankelevitz DF, Gamsu G, Shah A, et al. Optimization of combined CT pulmonary angiography with lower extremity CT venography. AJR Am J Roentegenol 2000;174:67–9.

[91] Loud PA, Katz DS, Klippenstein DL, et al. Combined CT venography and pulmonary angiography in suspected thromboembolic disease: diagnostic accuracy for deep venous evaluation. AJR Am J Roentgenol 2000;174:61–5.

[92] Garg K, Kemp JL, Wojcik D, et al. Thromboembolic disease: comparison of combined CT pulmonary angiography and venography with bilateral leg sonography in 70 patients. AJR Am J roentgenol 2000;175:997–1001.

[93] Duwe KM, Shiau M, Budorick NE, et al. Evaluation of the lower extremity veins in patients with suspected pulmonary embolism: a retrospective comparison of helical CT venography and sonography. AJR Am J Roentgenol 2000; 175:1525–31.

[94] Coche EE, Hamoir XL, Hammer FD, et al. Using dual-detector helical CT angiography to detect deep venous thrombosis in patients with suspicion of pulmonary embolism: diagnostic value and additional findings. AJR Am J Roentgenol 2001;176:1035–9.

[95] Wildberger JE, Mahnken AH, Sinha A-M, et al. Abklarung von lungenembolie und venoser thromboembolie mittels mehrschicht-spiral-CT. Fortschr Rntgenstr 2002;174:301–7.

[96] Chow B, Wittram C, Lee VW. Unilateral absence of pulmonary perfusion mimicking pulmonary embolism. AJR Am J Roentgenol 2001;176: 1423–5.

[97] Cox JE, Chiles C, Aquino SL, et al. Pulmonary artery sarcomas: a review of clinical and radiologic features. J Comput Assist Tomogr 1997; 21:750–5.

[98] Yi CA, Lee KS, Choe YH, et al. Computed tomography in pulmonary artery sarcoma: distinguishing features from pulmonary embolic disease. J Comput Assist Tomogr 2004;28:34–9.

[99] Schriner RW, Ryu JH, Edwards WD. Microscopic pulmonary tumor embolism causing subacute cor pulmonale: a difficult ante mortem diagnosis. Mayo Clin Proc 1991;66:143–8.

[100] Kane RD, Hawkins HK, Miller JA, et al. Microscopic pulmonary tumor emboli associated with dyspnea. Cancer 1975;36:1473–82.

[101] Winterbauer RH, Elfenbein IB, Ball WC Jr. Incidence and clinical significance of tumor embolization in lungs. Am J Med 1968;187:797–801.

[102] Shepard JA, Moore EH, Templeton PA, et al. Pulmonary intravascular tumor emboli: dilated and beaded peripheral pulmonary arteries at CT. Radiology 1993;187:797–801.

[103] Tack D, Nollevaux MC, Gevenois PA. Tree-in-bud pattern in neoplastic pulmonary emboli. AJR Am J Roentgenol 2001;176:1421–2.

[104] Rossi SE, Goodman PC, Franquet T. Nonthrombotic pulmonary emboli. AJR Am J Roentgenol 2000;174:1499–508.

[105] Franquet T, Giminez A, Prats R, et al. Thrombotic microangiopathy of pulmonary tumors: a vascular cause of tree-in-bud pattern on CT. AJR Am J Roentgenol 2002;179:897–9.

[106] von herbay A, Illes A, Waldherr R, et al. Pulmonary tumor thrombotic microangiopathy with pulmonary hypertension. Cancer 1990;66: 587–92.

[107] Pinckard JK, Wick MR. Tumor-related thrombotic pulmonary microangiopathy: review of pathologic findings and pathophysiologic mechanisms. Ann Diagn Pathol 2000;4:154–7.

[108] Fred HL, Harle TS. Septic pulmonary embolism. Am Fam Physician GP 1970;1:81–7.

[109] Roberts WC, Buchbinder NA. Right-sided valvular infective endocarditis: a clinicopathologic study of twelve necropsy patients. Am J Med 1972;53:7–19.

[110] Huang RM, Naidich DP, Lubat E, et al. Septic pulmonary emboli: CT radiographic correlation. AJR Am J Roentgenol 1989;153:41–5.

ELSEVIER
SAUNDERS

RADIOLOGIC
CLINICS
OF NORTH AMERICA

Radiol Clin N Am 45 (2007) 447–460

Cross-Sectional Imaging in Acute Pancreatitis

Anuradha Saokar, MD, Chad B. Rabinowitz, MD,
Dushyant V. Sahani, MD*

- Disease classification
- Patient management
- Role of imaging
- CT
  Technique
  Imaging findings
  CT severity index

- MR imaging
- Ultrasound
- Percutaneous cross-sectional
    imaging–guided interventions
- Summary
- References

Acute pancreatitis is responsible for more than 220,000 annual hospital admissions in the United States [1]. Gallstones and alcohol abuse are the most common causes of acute pancreatitis. Biliary pancreatitis is highest among patients who have small gallstones (less than 5 mm in diameter) or microlithiasis [1,2]. Less common causes of acute pancreatitis are hypertriglyceridemia, hypercalcemia, medications, ductal obstruction caused by tumor, trauma, endoscopic retrograde cholangio-pancreaticography, and developmental abnormalities including pancreas divisum and annular pancreas. No matter the underlying cause of acute pancreatitis, inflammation is triggered by premature activation of pancreatic enzymes with resultant autodigestion of the pancreatic parenchyma. The inflammatory process may remain localized to the pancreas, spread to regional tissues, or even involve remote organ systems resulting in multiorgan failure and occasional death. Furthermore, ischemic/reperfusion injury has been recognized increasingly as an important mechanism in the pathogenesis of acute pancreatitis, especially in patients who have severe necrotizing pancreatitis [3].

Clinically, acute pancreatitis generally presents with upper abdominal pain and may be accompanied by vomiting, fever, tachycardia, and leukocytosis. The clinical diagnosis is supported by an elevation of the serum amylase and lipase in excess of three times the upper limit of normal [4].

Disease classification

In 1992, the International Symposium on Acute Pancreatitis held in in Atlanta, Georgia, established a clinically based classification system and defined and standardized certain terminologies commonly associated with acute pancreatitis [5]. Acute pancreatitis is classified as mild or severe, based on the presence of local complications and organ failure [5,6]. Organ failure is assessed best using clinical and laboratory parameters, whereas local complications are evaluated by imaging, the criterion standard being contrast enhanced CT [5,7,8]. This classification helps identify patients who have severe disease and who require close monitoring and ICU care.

Mild acute pancreatitis (also known as "interstitial" or "edematous" pancreatitis) is a more common

Department of Abdominal Imaging and Interventional Radiology, Massachusetts General Hospital - White 270, 55 Fruit Street, Boston, MA 02114, USA
* Corresponding author.
E-mail address: dsahani@partners.org (D.V. Sahani).

0033-8389/07/$ – see front matter © 2007 Published by Elsevier Inc.
radiologic.theclinics.com

doi:10.1016/j.rcl.2007.04.002

and self-limiting disease with minimal organ dysfunction and an uneventful recovery. Pathologically, the mild form of acute pancreatitis is characterized by interstitial edema and, infrequently, by microscopic areas of parenchymal necrosis [5].

Severe acute pancreatitis, also known as "necrotizing pancreatitis," occurs in 20% to 30% of all patients and is associated with organ failure and/or local complications such as necrosis, abscess, or pseudocyst [5]. Overall, the mortality associated with severe acute pancreatitis ranges from 10% to 30% [1,9]. Pathologic findings include macroscopic areas of focal or diffuse pancreatic necrosis, fat necrosis, and hemorrhage in the pancreas and peripancreatic tissues [5]. Pancreatic parenchymal necrosis usually is limited to the periphery of the gland; only rarely does necrosis involve the entire gland [10,11].

Patient management

An important initial step in the management of acute pancreatitis is the assessment of disease severity. Although mild pancreatitis can be managed conservatively, severe acute pancreatitis requires a more aggressive approach including ICU care and possible surgical or percutaneous interventions [1].

The severity of pancreatitis can be assessed by specific laboratory values that measure systemic inflammatory response, such as C-reactive protein, and by using scoring systems that assess inflammation, organ failure, and imaging findings [1,7]. Several scoring systems that combine clinical and laboratory parameters have been devised in an attempt to identify patients who have severe pancreatitis [12–17]. Ranson's scoring system is used commonly and comprises five clinical criteria measured at admission and six measured at 48 hours [12]. Criteria measured at admission reflect the local inflammatory effects of pancreatic enzymes; those measured at 48 hours represent later, systemic effects. The fulfilling of three or more Ranson criteria predicts a severe course and increased mortality [7]. A limitation of this method is the requirement for 48 hours of observation before one can identify patients who have severe disease [7]. Among the various scoring systems, the APACHE II monitoring system has been considered the most reliable, with an accuracy of about 75% for the assessment of the severity of pancreatitis at admission [15–17]. This system is complex and more difficult to perform, because 12 physiologic measurements are used. It has been suggested that an APACHE II threshold score greater than 8 indicates severe pancreatitis [7].

Role of imaging

Imaging plays an important role in the management of patients who have acute pancreatitis. CT and transabdominal ultrasound are useful to confirm the diagnosis of acute pancreatitis and to rule out other causes of acute abdomen such as gastrointestinal perforation, acute cholecystitis, acute aortic dissection, and mesenteric artery occlusion. Clinically, all these entities can mimic acute pancreatitis. In established cases of acute pancreatitis, contrast-enhanced CT (CECT) is considered the criterion standard for evaluating morphologic changes of the disease, particularly in the assessment of pancreatic necrosis. CECT has become an integral part of the new classification system [5]. Other imaging modalities such as MR imaging are indicated in certain problematic clinical situations. The use of MR cholangiopancreatography (MRCP) with or without secretin administration is limited in the acute setting but now is used increasingly to evaluate the integrity of the pancreatic duct.

CT

CT is integral in the diagnosis and management of acute pancreatitis. After helping establish the diagnosis, it can exclude other causes of the patient's symptoms. In patients who have known acute pancreatitis, CECT is used to grade the severity of the disease and to detect local complications of necrosis, abscess, or pseudocysts (Fig. 1). CT can be useful in determining the underlying cause of disease, especially in identifying choledocholithiasis and biliary ductal dilatation associated with biliary pancreatitis, which ultimately guides therapeutic decision making. Last, CT is the imaging modality of choice for performing percutaneous interventions, which frequently are warranted in patients who have complications related to severe disease.

Technique

Early animal research has suggested that the administration of intravenous contrast media may exacerbate the severity of acute pancreatitis by the impaired oxygenation of the pancreatic parenchyma. These data, along with data from subsequent outcome studies in patients who had acute pancreatitis, and the risk of not using imaging have led to the routine use of CECT for this indication [18–22]. Unenhanced CT is rarely performed, although it may be indicated when there is clinical suspicion for pancreatic or intra-abdominal hemorrhage.

The use of multidetector CT (MDCT) scanners now is considered the standard of care for pancreatic imaging. By virtue of its scanning speed and

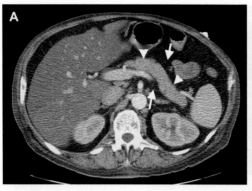 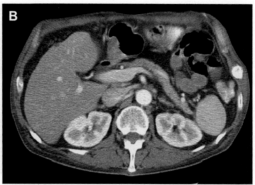

Fig. 1. Mild pancreatitis. (*A*) Axial CT helps grade disease and in this example shows very slight peripancreatic inflammatory change (*arrows*) and a featureless swollen pancreas (*arrowheads*). (*B*) Follow-up axial CT 2 weeks later shows the gland to be normal in size with resolution of inflammation.

superior resolution, MDCT permits high-quality, multiphase imaging of the pancreas in a short breathhold. This attribute is important, because often the patients being imaged are quite sick and are not able to hold their breath. The remainder of the abdomen and pelvis also can be be surveyed to study ancillary findings and related complications. Automated bolus tracking is desirable to trigger scanning in the optimal phase of contrast enhancement. In most cases of acute pancreatitis, a single-phase CECT performed in the portal venous phase is sufficient. When vascular complications are suspected, an additional arterial-phase scan can be added to the imaging protocol following a rapid bolus intravenous injection of a contrast agent. With current MDCT scanners, image data can be acquired in a volumetric fashion; hence high-quality two-dimensional (2D) and three-dimensional (3D) images can be postprocessed in any desirable plane. These postprocessed images often are crucial to relay the complex imaging findings more appropriately to the referring physician or surgeon. For a dedicated pancreas protocol study, the administration of

900 to 1000 mL of neutral oral contrast (such as water) typically is encouraged. This approach facilitates better assessment of the duodenal wall and ampullary region, especially when this region is being evaluated as the possible cause of pancreatitis. Positive contrast such as diatrizoate meglumine and diatrizoate sodium, or barium is more desirable for a routine abdomen and pelvis examination. The CT imaging parameters used in the Massachusetts General Hospital are depicted in Table 1.

More recently, MDCT is being used to evaluate regional pancreatic blood flow quantitatively. Preliminary data suggest that pancreatic perfusion measurements could be helpful in diagnosing pancreatic necrosis and also in assessing the severity of acute pancreatitis (Fig. 2) [23].

Imaging findings

CT is not necessary in a patient who has a clinical diagnosis of mild acute pancreatitis, especially if the clinical course is improving. CT findings in mild pancreatitis may be absent, or the pancreas may be enlarged or low in attenuation, indicating

Parameter	Vascular phase (40–45 seconds)	Portal venous phase (65–70 seconds)
Intravenous contrast	4–5 cm³/s	3 cm³/s
Range	Celiac through entire pancreas	Dome of diaphragm to symphysis pubis
Automated bolus Tracking	+ (150 HU threshold in the aorta at the level of celiac artery and 8–10 sec diagnostic delay)	+ (55 HU threshold in the right lobe of liver at the level of the right portal vein)
Slice thickness	1–3 mm	5 mm
Spacing	1–3 mm	5 mm
Kilovoltage peak	120–140	120–140
Milliamps	240–280	240–280
Time	0.5–0.8 seconds	0.5–0.8 seconds
Field of view	28	Based on size of patient

Table 1: CT acquisition parameters

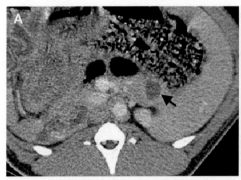
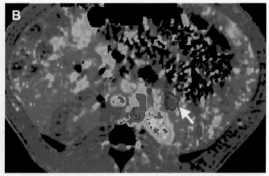

Fig. 2. CT perfusion. (*A*) Axial CT shows a small focal hypodense area of necrosis (*black arrow*) in the tail of a pig pancreas at a site of 60% ethyl alcohol injection. (*B*) The hypodense area in panel A corresponds to an area of decreased blood flow and blood volume on CT perfusion images (*white arrow*). This area demonstrated necrosis on histopathology, thus mirroring the severity of disease as seen on CT and perfusion images.

interstitial edema. CECT is the mainstay of imaging in patients who have severe acute pancreatitis. It is particularly useful in assessing pancreatic necrosis and local retroperitoneal complications.

The 1992 International Symposium on Acute Pancreatitis defined and standardized various terminologies commonly associated with acute pancreatitis [5]; these terms should be used in the radiologic report.

Acute fluid collections

Acute fluid collections occur early in the course of acute pancreatitis (within 48 hours) and consist of collections of enzyme-rich pancreatic juices that lack a wall of granulation or fibrous tissue. They usually occur in or near the pancreas and may dissect into the lesser sac, anterior pararenal spaces (most commonly left), transverse mesocolon, and the mesenteric root. These collections occur in 30% to 50% of cases, and in half of these cases they resolve without intervention. The remaining collections progress to become pseudocysts or abscesses (Fig. 3) [5,24,25].

Acute pseudocyst

A pseudocyst is a collection of pancreatic juice enclosed by a wall of fibrous or granulation tissue. Formation of a pseudocyst requires 4 or more weeks from the onset of acute pancreatitis [24]. On CT, a pseudocyst appears as a well-circumscribed, low-attenuation collection in the vicinity of the pancreas. Pseudocysts can occur in other locations such as the mediastinum [26] and usually are sterile. When there is pus in a pseudocyst, it is referred to as an "abscess" (Figs. 4 and 5).

Pancreatic abscess

A pancreatic abscess is a circumscribed intra-abdominal collection of pus, usually in proximity to the pancreas, containing little or no pancreatic necrosis, which arises as a consequence of acute pancreatitis or pancreatic trauma. Pancreatic abscesses occur later in the course of severe acute pancreatitis, often 4 weeks or more after disease onset [5]. On CECT, the wall of a pancreatic abscess may appear thick or irregular, unlike the more well-delineated, thin wall of a pseudocyst (Fig. 6).

Pancreatic necrosis

Pancreatic necrosis is focal or diffuse areas of nonviable pancreatic parenchyma and typically is associated with peripancreatic fat necrosis (Fig. 7) [5]. This definition is based on the presence of one or more focal areas of nonenhancing pancreatic parenchyma on dynamic CECT. Nonenhancing areas correspond to nonviable pancreatic tissue. Although an initial CT scan helps confirm the diagnosis of acute pancreatitis, CECT performed 48 to

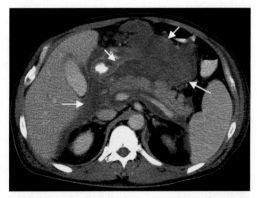

Fig. 3. Acute fluid collection. Axial CECT shows peripancreatic fluid as a result of acute pancreatitis. This finding may contain areas of fat necrosis and commonly resolves with no sequelae, although a significant portion evolve into abscess or pseudocyst.

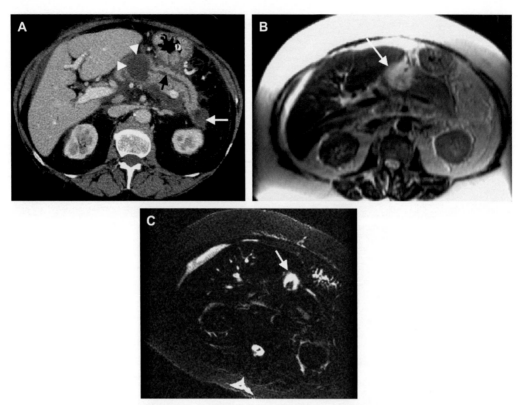

Fig. 4. Pancreatic pseudocyst. (*A*) A fairly well-defined focal fluid collection is seen in the pancreatic neck, which has a thin wall (*white arrowheads*). The pancreatic duct, which is slightly dilated, can be seen coursing directly into this fluid collection (*black arrow*). Note a second pseudocyst at the pancreatic tail (*white arrow*). (*B*) T2-weighted MR imaging and (*C*) MRCP image show the same pseudocyst containing internal debris (*white arrow*). Again, note the adjacent pancreatic duct coursing into the lesion.

72 hours after the onset of an acute attack gives more reliable information for grading purposes because necrotic areas of pancreatic parenchyma become better defined 2 to 3 days after the onset of symptoms. CT scans performed during the initial 12 hours of presentation can produce equivocal findings [7].

The unenhanced pancreas has CT attenuation values of 40 to 50 Hounsfield units (HU), although unenhanced CT generally is not performed in patients who have acute pancreatitis. A normal pancreas should demonstrate a homogeneous increase in attenuation with intravenous contrast to 100 to 150 HU. Lack of contrast enhancement or minimal contrast enhancement of less than 30 HU of a portion of the pancreas or of the entire pancreas indicates decreased tissue perfusion and correlates with the development of necrosis [7]. A crude method of diagnosing pancreatic necrosis is to compare the attenuation of the pancreas and spleen. In the absence of pancreatic necrosis, the pancreas and spleen should be similar in attenuation on a portal venous phase examination. Certain

pitfalls should be kept in mind, however, to eliminate a false-positive diagnosis. Pancreatic parenchymal enhancement often is decreased in individuals who have fatty infiltration of the gland and in patients who have pancreatic edema or interstitial pancreatitis. Likewise, commonly seen small focal intrapancreatic fluid collections can masquerade as focal necrosis. This distinction occasionally may be difficult without prior studies or follow-up imaging.

Necrotic pancreatic tissue serves as a good medium for infection, which occurs in approximately 20% to 70% of cases, usually in the second to third week following the onset of acute pancreatitis [27]. Differentiation of sterile from infected necrosis is important from a management perspective. Although crucial, distinguishing sterile from infected necrosis based on imaging findings alone is not always feasible except when the presence of gas bubbles within the collection is detected (Fig. 8). Imaging-guided percutaneous needle aspiration usually is needed to meet this objective. Infected pancreatic necrosis, when diagnosed, is an

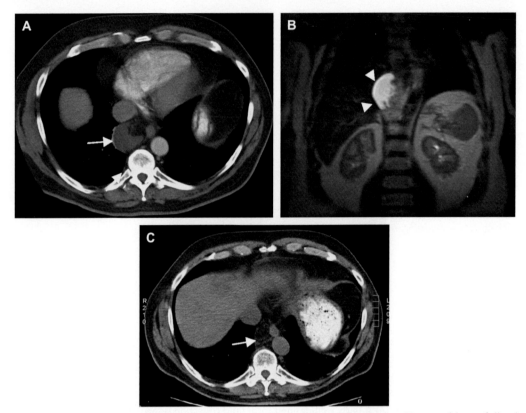

Fig. 5. Mediastinal pseudocyst. (*A*) Axial CECT shows a mediastinal fluid collection in a 59-year-old man following acute pancreatitis (*arrow*). (*B*) This fluid is seen on coronal T2-weighted MR imaging tracking superiorly from the abdomen (*arrowheads*). (*C*) The pseudocyst subsequently resolves.

indication for necrosectomy or aggressive percutaneous intervention [28–30].

Retroperitoneal fat necrosis is seen invariably in patients who have pancreatic necrosis, but the converse is not true [7]. Local complications can occur 22% of the time in patients who have peripancreatic fluid collections, in the absence of glandular necrosis [31]. Because CT cannot reliably diagnose retroperitoneal fat necrosis, it has been suggested that all heterogeneous peripancreatic collections should be considered as areas of fat necrosis until proven otherwise [7].

CT severity index

Balthazar and colleagues [32] have graded the severity of acute pancreatitis based on CT findings into five groups (A through E) (Table 2). They have found that most patients who have severe pancreatitis exhibit one or several fluid collections on initial CT scan. In their study, patients who had grade D or E pancreatitis had a mortality rate of 14% and a morbidity rate of 54%, compared with 0% mortality and 4% morbidity in patients who had grade A, B, or C pancreatitis [32].

This grading system has been refined based on the extent of pancreatic necrosis seen at imaging, and the term "CT severity index" (CTSI) is used now (Table 3) [31]. Balthazar and colleagues [31] report that patients with less than 30% necrosis seen on CT exhibit no increase in mortality, although they do show a 48% morbidity rate. Larger areas of necrosis (30%–50% and > 50%) are associated with a morbidity rate of 75% to 100% and a mortality rate of 11% to 25%. The CTSI score correlates positively with morbidity and mortality. Patients who have CTSI scores of 0 to 3 showed a 3% mortality rate and 8% morbidity rate, whereas in patients who had CTSI scores of 7 to 10, the mortality and morbidity rates were 17% and 92%, respectively [31].

Vascular complications

Vascular complications, both arterial and venous, are known to occur in patients who have severe acute pancreatitis [33]. Arterial bleeding is one of the most life-threatening complications [34], and although virtually all peripancreatic vessels can be involved, the splenic artery is the most common

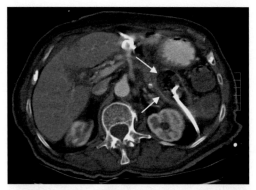

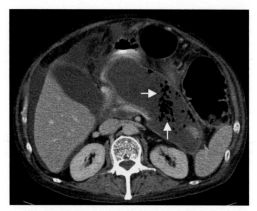

Fig. 6. Pancreatic abscess following necrotizing pancreatitis. A well-defined fluid collection with a thick enhancing rim, containing debris and air, is seen in the pancreatic tail (*arrows*). This abscess was drained successfully by percutaneous catheter placement. Surgery is an alternative treatment depending on the status of the patient and condition of the remainder of the pancreas.

Fig. 8. Pancreatic necrosis in a 38-year-old man. After initial conservative management, the patient in Fig. 7. developed fever, and a subsequent CECT examination demonstrated gas within the collection raising concern for infection/abscess (*arrows*).

because of its anatomic contiguity with the pancreas. Erosion of arteries can result in free hemorrhage from the erosion site or in the formation of a pseudoaneurysm (Fig. 9). The latter has the potential to rupture into the lesser sac, into the peritoneal cavity, or into an adjacent hollow organ. On imaging, a pseudoaneurysm can be seen as a completely or partially vascular cystic mass. In patients who have a history of acute pancreatitis, one should suspect a pseudoaneurysm when a cystic pancreatic mass demonstrates transient vascular enhancement. CT angiography and 3D reconstructions can demonstrate precisely the specific vessel involved. In addition to arterial complications, venous thrombosis in the portal-mesenteric circulation

can occur. In order of frequency, the splenic vein is involved most commonly, followed by the portal and the superior mesenteric veins (Fig. 10). When the splenic vein is involved, left-sided portal hypertension can occur with the development of gastric and mesenteric varices.

Extrapancreatic findings

In addition to peripancreatic fluid collections and vascular complications, abnormalities in other solid organs (eg, liver and spleen) occasionally may be seen at imaging. Because of the close proximity of the pancreatic tail and spleen, inflammatory processes may extend along splenic vessels into the splenic hilum. Splenic involvement in pancreatitis includes intrasplenic pseudocyst, abscess, hemorrhage, and infarction (Fig. 11). Intrasplenic hemorrhage occurs because of the erosion of small intrasplenic vessels. Blood may collect beneath the splenic capsule resulting in subcapsular hematoma. When hemorrhage is large, splenic laceration and rupture can occur and may be catastrophic. Splenic

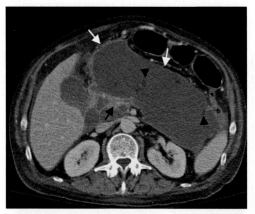

Fig. 7. Pancreatic necrosis in a 38-year-old man. Note a fluid attenuation collection in the pancreatic bed (*white arrows*) with islands of preserved fatty tissue suggestive of fat necrosis (*arrowheads*). Glandular enhancement is only seen in the head (*black arrow*).

Table 2:	Balthazar grading system
Grade	**Description**
A	Normal-appearing pancreas
B	Focal or diffuse enlargement of the pancreas
C	Pancreatic gland abnormalities accompanied by mild peripancreatic inflammatory changes
D	Fluid collection in a single location
E	Two or more fluid collections near the pancreas or gas in or adjacent to the pancreas

Table 3: **CT severity index**

CT Grade	Score	Necrosis (%)	Score
A	0	0	0
B	1	< 30	2
C	2	30–50	4
D	3	> 50	6
E	4	—	—

CT severity index (maximum score 10) = CT grade (0–4) + necrosis (0–6).

infarction can occur if inflammatory exudate compresses the splenic vasculature.

Transient hepatic enhancement can be seen in the liver, typically near the gallbladder fossa and in the left lobe [35]. It has been hypothesized that this enhancement occurs because of increased arterial blood flow, secondary to inflammation of the liver capsule and gallbladder [35]. These areas of abnormal enhancement should not be misinterpreted as primary hepatic abnormalities, such as hypervascular tumor.

The inflammatory process also can extend into the perinephric space resulting in renal and perirenal abnormalities (Fig. 12). These abnormalities include subcapsular and perirenal fluid collections and pseudocysts, and extensive inflammation around renal vessels can lead to venous compression and thrombosis [36]. There can be asymmetric enhancement of the renal parenchyma from compression of the renal artery by inflammatory exudates [36].

In rare cases, the colon can be affected by local inflammation because of the direct contact of the pancreas with the transverse colon [37]. Direct extension of the inflammatory process or pseudocyst may compress, inflame, or erode the large bowel (Fig. 13). There could be resultant bowel

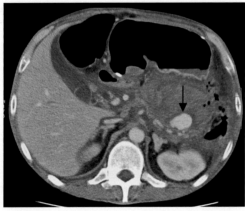

Fig. 9. Splenic artery pseudoaneurysm in a 42-year-old man after a recent episode of severe acute pancreatitis. An axial CECT image shows a high-density enhancing collection in the pancreatic bed with attenuation matching that of the aorta favoring a diagnosis of splenic artery pseudoaneurysm (*arrow*).

obstruction, ischemic necrosis, perforation, hemorrhage, or fistula formation. Large bowel involvement may present weeks or months after an attack of acute pancreatitis. Vascular thrombosis can lead to colonic ischemia.

MR imaging

MR imaging is comparable to CT in the depiction of morphologic changes from acute pancreatitis, including the extent of pancreatic necrosis and peripancreatic fluid collections [38,39]. MR imaging can be used as an alternative imaging modality in patients who cannot receive iodinated contrast media because of allergy or renal insufficiency. Patients who have acute pancreatitis often are young and require multiple follow-up CT examinations. In this regard, MR imaging has an advantage over CT,

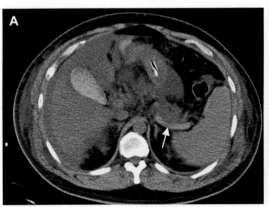
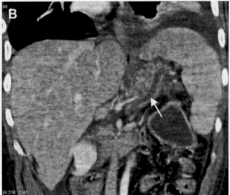

Fig. 10. Splenic vein thrombosis. (*A*) Axial noncontrast CT image shows high attenuation in the splenic vein (*arrow*). (*B*) The corresponding coronal CECT image shows lack of enhancement in the splenic vein (*arrow*).

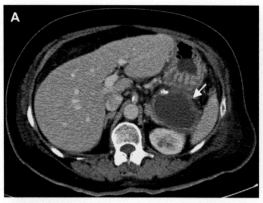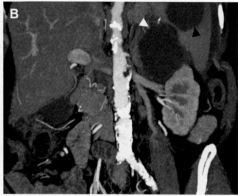

Fig. 11. Pancreatic pseudocyst in a 54-year-old man. (*A*) Axial CECT image 6 weeks after an episode of acute pancreatitis demonstrates a well-defined fluid attenuation lesion in the pancreatic tail (*white arrow*). (*B*) Coronal image from a follow-up CT examination demonstrates interval increase in the size of the pseudocyst, and a new intrasplenic pseudocyst has now appeared (*black arrowhead*). These two cysts communicate (*white arrowhead*).

because exposure to excessive ionizing radiation can be avoided.

Optimal MR imaging of the pancreas requires a 1.5 Tesla MR scanner and phased-array coils. Breath-hold gradient echo or fast spin-echo sequences in the axial and coronal places are used most commonly for imaging the pancreas. The authors' MR imaging protocol used for imaging the pancreas is outlined in Table 4.

A T2-weighted fast spin-echo sequence accurately depicts fluid collections, pseudocysts, and hemorrhage. T2-weighted images are more sensitive than

CT in the evaluation of a fluid collection's internal characteristics and therefore in the assessment of its drainability (Fig. 14) [40]. Breath-hold, T1-weighted in-phase (TR/TE: 120/4.2) and T1-weighted opposed-phase (TR/TE: 120/2.1) gradient echo sequences are useful to depict pancreatic and peripancreatic edema.

Dynamic gadolinium-diethylenetriamine pentaacetic acid –enhanced (0.1 mmol/kg body weight) MR imaging is performed using breath-hold, fat-suppressed, 3D gradient echo sequences. Images are acquired in the arterial (20–40 seconds), portal venous (70–80 seconds), and equilibrium (180 seconds) phases. Dynamic contrast-enhanced images are extremely useful for depicting viable from nonviable pancreatic parenchyma. The dynamic contrast-enhanced sequences can be used to produce excellent MR angiography images for the delineation of possible peripancreatic vascular complications.

Fig. 12. Fat necrosis/portal vein thrombosis. Coronal CECT image shows inflammatory soft tissue changes in the peripancreatic region tracking into the right perirenal space (*white arrow*) and retroperitoneum (*arrowheads*). Note a filling defect in the portal vein, consistent with thrombus (*black arrow*).

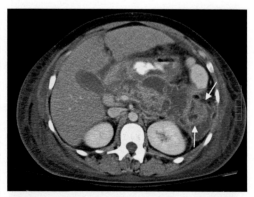

Fig. 13. Fat necrosis encasing colon. An acute fluid collection is noted tracking from the pancreatic bed into the left abdomen and surrounds the colon (*arrows*). This entity can lead to bowel fistulization with surrounding structures.

Table 4: **MR imaging parameters**

	Fast spin-echo with fat saturation	Fast spin-echo without fat saturation	T1 gradient echo (spoiled gradient recalled)	3D Dynamic pre- and postcontrast
Imaging plane	Axial	Axial	Axial	Axial
TR	4000–4500	2100	200	150
TE	68	60	Minimum	2.4
Flip angle	90	90	80	15
Field of view	36	36	36	36
Matrix	128 × 256	128 × 256	256 × 512	160 × 256
Thickness (mm)	3	3	4	4
Gap (mm)	0	0	0	Not applicable
Respiration	Triggered	Breathhold	Breathhold	Breathhold (three acquisitions)

In addition, comprehensive MR imaging of the pancreas includes MRCP, which is an excellent non-invasive technique to depict biliary and pancreatic ductal anatomy [41]. Heavily T2-weighted images are acquired that selectively display static or slow-moving fluid-filled structures. MRCP is highly sensitive and specific for diagnosing choledocholithiasis, thus limiting ERCP to those patients requiring therapeutic intervention [41–44]. In addition, MRCP accurately demonstrates pancreatic ductal abnormalities associated with pancreatitis, including ductal dilatation, disruption, or leakage [45]. Communication of a pseudocyst with the pancreatic duct can be well depicted by MRCP. In patients presenting with recurrent attacks of acute pancreatitis, MRCP is capable of identifying contributing structural anomalies such as pancreas divisum and of diagnosing pancreatic neoplasms (eg, intraductal papillary mucinous neoplasms), which also can present as recurrent disease (Fig. 15).

A conventional MRCP protocol consists of coronal thin-section images and rotating oblique-coronal thick-slab images using the 2D single-shot fast spin-echo sequence. The MR imaging parameters are detailed in Table 5. Thick-slab MRCP is obtained along rotating oblique coronal planes and displays the biliary and pancreatic ductal anatomy on one image. Thick-slab MRCP is operator dependent; thus, to obtain high-quality images, a radiologist often must monitor the study and identify complex anatomy. Multisection thin-slab MRCP in the coronal plane allows depiction of the ductal anatomy and the solid organs. These images are not suitable for multiplanar reformations, because the images are acquired in an interleaved fashion in one or more adjacent acquisitions and hence can be affected by respiratory misregistration. The recently introduced 3D MRCP provides exceptionally high-quality images of the pancreatic and biliary ductal system [46]. The 3D fast-recovery fast spin-echo MR sequence is performed in a single breath-hold and, unlike, the conventional thin-section MRCP sequence, produces images that are inherently contiguous and registered. This sequence is ideal for multiplanar reformations and rotating oblique-coronal maximum intensity projection

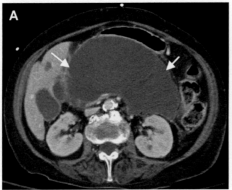 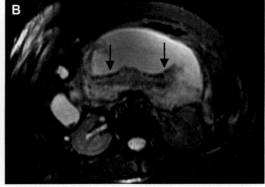

Fig. 14. Pancreatic necrosis in a 45-year-old man who had severe pancreatitis. A well-defined fluid attenuation collection in the pancreatic bed (*white arrows*) seen on (*A*) the CECT image is more complex appearing on (*B*) the corresponding T2-weighted MR image. The internal debris and necrotic tissue are better appreciated because of the superior soft tissue contrast of MR imaging (*black arrows*).

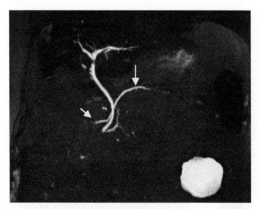

Fig. 15. Pancreas divisum. MRCP maximum intensity projection image demonstrates the dorsal pancreatic duct coursing directly to the duodenum (*white arrows*). This diagnosis can be made from the coronal 3D MRCP image when the dorsal pancreatic duct is seen "crossing over" the common bile duct, and a separate ventral duct joins the common bile duct.

reconstructions and thus offers the possibility of replacing the combined thin-section and thick-slab MRCP protocol with a single-volume acquisition. At the Massachusetts General Hospital, MRCP is performed following the intravenous administration of gadolinium. Gadolinium frequently suppresses the depiction of background structures and the renal pelves and therefore improves the depiction of the biliary tracts or main pancreatic duct in selected patients [47].

With the recent availability of secretin, functional MRCP of the pancreas is now feasible. Exogenous administration of secretin stimulates secretion of pancreatic juice, notably rich in bicarbonate, which consequently results in transient distension of the pancreatic duct [45]. This distension improves duct visualization and provides the rationale for the test. Secretin-enhanced MRCP is useful in identifying structural anomalies such as pancreas

divisum and has been useful in making an early diagnosis of ductal disruption [48–50]. Thick-slab MRCP is performed in the coronal plane before intravenous secretin administration (1 clinical unit/kg body weight, or per insert) and is repeated every 15 to 30 seconds for 10 to 15 minutes thereafter. A significant delay in acquisition of images results in obscuration of ductal detail by high signal intensity fluid entering the duodenum. Secretin MRCP also helps in assessing pancreatic ductal flow dynamics and pancreatic exocrine function, based on the degree of duodenal filling with fluid [45].

Ultrasound

The usefulness of transabdominal ultrasound in acute pancreatitis is limited. Early in the course of an episode of acute pancreatitis, ultrasound is used to evaluate biliary dilatation and also to determine presence of stones in the gallbladder and common bile duct. Limiting technical factors often relate to large body habitus and overlying bowel gas, because paralytic ileus is common in these patients. The ultrasonographic findings in acute pancreatitis can range from a normal-appearing pancreas to a diffusely enlarged hypoechoic gland (Fig. 16). One should assess the presence of intrapancreatic or peripancreatic fluid collections, particularly in the lesser sac and anterior pararenal space. Sonography cannot reliably differentiate these fluid collections from pancreatic necrosis, thus limiting its role in the assessment of disease severity.

Although a growing body of literature supports the usefulness of endoscopic ultrasound in the evaluation of various pancreatic diseases, its role is limited in patients who have acute pancreatitis. There have been reports suggesting that endoscopic ultrasound is accurate in identifying common bile duct stones [51,52]. MRCP, however, is a highly accurate, noninvasive alternative for detecting common bile duct stones measuring more than 3 mm in

Table 5: **MR cholangiopancreatography parameters**

| | 2D SSFSE | | |
	Thin section	Thick section	**3D FRFSE**
Acquisition plane	Coronal	Coronal	Coronal
TR	min	4849	1717
TE	180	874	500–600
Bandwith	62.5	31.25	19
Field of view	48	35	36
Matrix	160 × 384	256 × 256	256 × 256
Thickness (mm)	5	40	3
Gadolinium	±	±	±

Abbreviations: 2D, two-dimensional; 3D, three-dimensional; FRFSE, fast-recovery fast spin-echo; SSFSE, single-shot fast spin-echo.

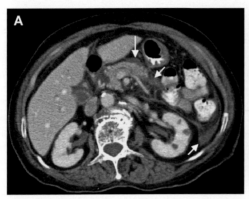
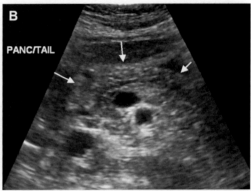

Fig. 16. Mild pancreatitis. (*A*) Mild pancreatic swelling and peripancreatic fat stranding (*arrows*) is noted on a CECT. (*B*) The gland appears relatively normal on the ultrasound performed the same day (*white arrows*).

diameter. The reported sensitivity of MRCP for the detection of common bile duct stones varies from 57% to 100%; specificity varies from 73% to 100%. With more refined techniques, the values for sensitivity and specificity values are toward the higher end of the spectrum [53]. In patients who have unexplained recurrent pancreatitis, endoscopic ultrasound may be useful in identifying occult pancreatic neoplasms not seen on thin-section MDCT or MR imaging. Likewise, fine-needle aspiration guided by endoscopic ultrasound may be needed to enable distinction of focal pancreatitis from a pancreatic neoplasm, a distinction that often is difficult on CT and MR imaging (Fig. 17).

Percutaneous cross-sectional imaging–guided interventions

Both diagnostic and therapeutic percutaneous interventions are performed on a variety of

collections in patients who have acute pancreatitis. Diagnostic aspiration for Gram stain and culture is performed on fluid collections, pseudocysts, or pancreatic necrosis when there is a clinical suspicion for infection. Percutaneous catheter drainage is indicated in patients who have established infection. Although most pseudocysts regress spontaneously, large (> 5 cm), unresolving (> 6 weeks), or symptomatic (pain, gastric outlet obstruction, or biliary obstruction) pseudocysts require drainage, which can be performed using percutaneous or endoscopic techniques. Pancreatic abscesses and infected necrosis often require multicatheter drainage either as definitive treatment or as a temporizing measure before surgery [30].

CT is the imaging modality most commonly used to guide percutaneous intervention because it demonstrates the size, location, and relationship of collections to adjacent vasculature and critical organs. As mentioned earlier, MR imaging is superior to CT

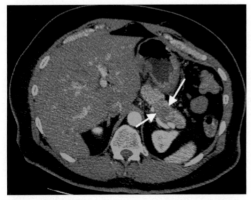

Fig. 17. Pancreatic mass simulating focal pancreatitis. Axial CECT shows a focal mass in the pancreatic tail, with mild glandular swelling (*arrows*). This patient was acutely ill and had elevated pancreatic enzymes. The mass was biopsied by endoscopic ultrasound, showing adenocarcinoma.

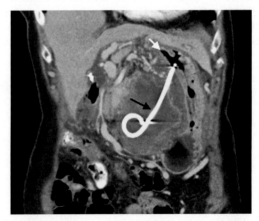

Fig. 18. Pancreatic cystogastrostomy. Coronal CT image demonstrates a cystogastrostomy tube within a pancreatic pseudocyst (*black arrow*). Note the tube coursing into the pancreatic fluid collection from the stomach (*white arrow*).

in determining the viscosity of pancreatic collections, including the presence of solid debris. Internal consistency may predict the success of percutaneous techniques in draining focal fluid and the size of the catheter necessary for successful drainage [40]. The presence of septations and lobulations also may guide the number of catheters needed to produce effective drainage. If an endoscopic drainage procedure such as cystogastrostomy is contemplated, CT is useful in determining the relationship of the relevant collection to the stomach or duodenum (Fig. 18). Ultrasound can be used as a guidance modality when there are large collections. The portable nature of ultrasound is particularly useful in the critically ill ICU patient.

Once a drainage procedure has been performed, follow-up CT is critical in assessing procedural success. Complete evacuation can be determined once drain output diminishes. Persistent collections lasting for months may suggest pancreatic ductal communication.

Summary

Acute pancreatitis can be a mild, self-limiting disease or can be severe with significant patient morbidity and mortality. The severity of the patient's condition is judged based on clinical, laboratory, and imaging criteria. CECT is the imaging modality of choice and is used to stage the severity of inflammation, detect pancreatic necrosis, and identify local complications. Percutaneous CT-guided interventions provide therapeutic options in these patients. Other cross-sectional imaging modalities including MR imaging/MRCP and ultrasound are used in specific clinical scenarios.

References

[1] Whitcomb DC. Clinical practice. Acute pancreatitis. N Engl J Med 2006;354(20):2142–50.

[2] Venneman NG, Buskens E, Besselink MG, et al. Small gallstones are associated with increased risk of acute pancreatitis: potential benefits of prophylactic cholecystectomy? Am J Gastroenterol 2005;100(11):2540–50.

[3] Sakorafas GH, Tsiotou AG. Etiology and pathogenesis of acute pancreatitis: current concepts. J Clin Gastroenterol 2000;30(4):343–56.

[4] Banks PA. Practice guidelines in acute pancreatitis. Am J Gastroenterol 1997;92(3):377–86.

[5] Bradley EL 3rd. A clinically based classification system for acute pancreatitis. Summary of the International Symposium on Acute Pancreatitis, Atlanta (GA), September 11 through 13, 1992. Arch Surg 1993;128(5):586–90.

[6] Banks PA. A new classification system for acute pancreatitis. Am J Gastroenterol 1994;89(2):151–2.

[7] Balthazar EJ. Acute pancreatitis: assessment of severity with clinical and CT evaluation. Radiology 2002;223(3):603–13.

[8] Dervenis C, Johnson CD, Bassi C, et al. Diagnosis, objective assessment of severity, and management of acute pancreatitis. Int J Pancreatol 1999;25(3):195–210.

[9] McKay CJ, Imrie CW. The continuing challenge of early mortality in acute pancreatitis. Br J Surg 2004;91(10):1243–4.

[10] Kloppel G, VonGerkan R, Dreyer T. Pathomorphology of acute pancreatitis: analysis of 367 autopsy cases and through surgical specimens. In: Gyr KE, Singler MV, Sarles H, editors. Pancreatitis: concepts and classifications. Amsterdam (The Netherlands): Elsevier Science Publishers; 1984. p. 29–35.

[11] Leger L, Chiche B, Louvel A. Pancreatic necrosis and acute pancreatitis. World J Surg 1981;5(3):315–7.

[12] Ranson JH, Rifkind KM, Roses DF, et al. Objective early identification of severe acute pancreatitis. Am J Gastroenterol 1974;61(6):443–51.

[13] Blamey SL, Imrie CW, O'Neill J, et al. Prognostic factors in acute pancreatitis. Gut 1984;25(12):1340–6.

[14] Agarwal N, Pitchumoni CS. Simplified prognostic criteria in acute pancreatitis. Pancreas 1986;1(1):69–73.

[15] Knaus WA, Draper EA, Wagner DP, et al. APACHE II: a severity of disease classification system. Crit Care Med 1985;13(10):818–29.

[16] Larvin M, McMahon MJ. APACHE-II score for assessment and monitoring of acute pancreatitis. Lancet 1989;2(8656):201–5.

[17] Wilson C, Heath DI, Imrie CW. Prediction of outcome in acute pancreatitis: a comparative study of APACHE II, clinical assessment and multiple factor scoring systems. Br J Surg 1990;77(11):1260–4.

[18] Foitzik T, Bassi DG, Schmidt J, et al. Intravenous contrast medium accentuates the severity of acute necrotizing pancreatitis in the rat. Gastroenterology 1994;106(1):207–14.

[19] Foitzik T, Bassi DG, Fernandez-del Castillo C, et al. Intravenous contrast medium impairs oxygenation of the pancreas in acute necrotizing pancreatitis in the rat. Arch Surg 1994;129(7):706–11.

[20] Schmidt J, Hotz HG, Foitzik T, et al. Intravenous contrast medium aggravates the impairment of pancreatic microcirculation in necrotizing pancreatitis in the rat. Ann Surg 1995;221(3):257–64.

[21] Uhl W, Roggo A, Kirschstein T, et al. Influence of contrast-enhanced computed tomography on course and outcome in patients with acute pancreatitis. Pancreas 2002;24(2):191–7.

[22] Hwang TL, Chang KY, Ho YP. Contrast-enhanced dynamic computed tomography does not aggravate the clinical severity of patients with severe acute pancreatitis: reevaluation of the effect of

intravenous contrast medium on the severity of acute pancreatitis. Arch Surg 2000;135(3): 287–90.

[23] Bize PE, Platon A, Becker CD, et al. Perfusion measurement in acute pancreatitis using dynamic perfusion MDCT. AJR Am J Roentgenol 2006;186(1):114–8.

[24] Bradley EL III, Gonzalez AC, Clements JL Jr. Acute pancreatic pseudocysts: incidence and implications. Ann Surg 1976;184(6):734–7.

[25] Siegelman SS, Copeland BE, Saba GP, et al. CT of fluid collections associated with pancreatitis. AJR Am J Roentgenol 1980;134(6):1121–32.

[26] Yamamura M, Iki K. Mediastinal extension of a pancreatic pseudocyst. Pancreatology 2004; 4(2):90.

[27] Paulson EK, Vitellas KM, Keogan MT, et al. Acute pancreatitis complicated by gland necrosis: spectrum of findings on contrast-enhanced CT. AJR Am J Roentgenol 1999;172(3):609–13.

[28] Buchler MW, Gloor B, Muller CA, et al. Acute necrotizing pancreatitis: treatment strategy according to the status of infection. Ann Surg 2000;232(5):619–26.

[29] Buchler P, Reber HA. Surgical approach in patients with acute pancreatitis. Is infected or sterile necrosis an indication–in whom should this be done, when, and why? Gastroenterol Clin North Am 1999;28(3):661–71.

[30] Shankar S, vanSonnenberg E, Silverman SG, et al. Imaging and percutaneous management of acute complicated pancreatitis. Cardiovasc Intervent Radiol 2004;27(6):567–80.

[31] Balthazar EJ, Robinson DL, Megibow AJ, et al. Acute pancreatitis: value of CT in establishing prognosis. Radiology 1990;174(2):331–6.

[32] Balthazar EJ, Ranson JH, Naidich DP, et al. Acute pancreatitis: prognostic value of CT. Radiology 1985;156(3):767–72.

[33] Vujic I. Vascular complications of pancreatitis. Radiol Clin North Am 1989;27(1):81–91.

[34] Burke JW, Erickson SJ, Kellum CD, et al. Pseudoaneurysms complicating pancreatitis: detection by CT. Radiology 1986;161(2):447–50.

[35] Arita T, Matsunaga N, Takano K, et al. Hepatic perfusion abnormalities in acute pancreatitis: CT appearance and clinical importance. Abdom Imaging 1999;24(2):157–62.

[36] Mortele KJ, Mergo PJ, Taylor HM, et al. Renal and perirenal space involvement in acute pancreatitis: spiral CT findings. Abdom Imaging 2000; 25(3):272–8.

[37] Gardner A, Gardner G, Feller E. Severe colonic complications of pancreatic disease. J Clin Gastroenterol 2003;37(3):258–62.

[38] Ward J, Chalmers AG, Guthrie AJ, et al. T2-weighted and dynamic enhanced MRI in acute pancreatitis: comparison with contrast enhanced CT. Clin Radiol 1997;52(2):109–14.

[39] Saifuddin A, Ward J, Ridgway J, et al. Comparison of MR and CT scanning in severe acute

pancreatitis: initial experiences. Clin Radiol 1993;48(2):111–6.

[40] Morgan DE, Baron TH, Smith JK, et al. Pancreatic fluid collections prior to intervention: evaluation with MR imaging compared with CT and US. Radiology 1997;203(3):773–8.

[41] Sica GT, Braver J, Cooney MJ, et al. Comparison of endoscopic retrograde cholangiopancreatography with MR cholangiopancreatography in patients with pancreatitis. Radiology 1999;210(3): 605–10.

[42] Fulcher AS, Turner MA. MR pancreatography: a useful tool for evaluating pancreatic disorders. Radiographics 1999;19(1):5–24.

[43] Fulcher AS, Turner MA, Zfass AM. Magnetic resonance cholangiopancreatography: a new technique for evaluating the biliary tract and pancreatic duct. Gastroenterologist 1998;6(1):82–7.

[44] Fulcher AS, Turner MA, Capps GW, et al. Half-Fourier RARE MR cholangiopancreatography: experience in 300 subjects. Radiology 1998;207(1): 21–32.

[45] Matos C, Cappeliez O, Winant C, et al. MR imaging of the pancreas: a pictorial tour. Radiographics 2002;22(1):e2.

[46] Sodickson A, Mortele KJ, Barish MA, et al. Three-dimensional fast-recovery fast spin-echo MRCP: comparison with two-dimensional single-shot fast spin-echo techniques. Radiology 2006; 238(2):549–59.

[47] Kanematsu M, Matsuo M, Shiratori Y, et al. Thick-section half-Fourier rapid acquisition with relaxation enhancement MR cholangiopancreatography: effects of i.v. administration of gadolinium chelate. AJR Am J Roentgenol 2002; 178(3):755–61.

[48] Hellerhoff KJ, Helmberger H 3rd, Rosch T, et al. Dynamic MR pancreatography after secretin administration: image quality and diagnostic accuracy. AJR Am J Roentgenol 2002;179(1):121–9.

[49] Fukukura Y, Fujiyoshi F, Sasaki M, et al. Pancreatic duct: morphologic evaluation with MR cholangiopancreatography after secretin stimulation. Radiology 2002;222(3):674–80.

[50] Arvanitakis M, Delhaye M, De Maertelaere V, et al. Computed tomography and magnetic resonance imaging in the assessment of acute pancreatitis. Gastroenterology 2004;126(3):715–23.

[51] Chak A, Hawes RH, Cooper GS, et al. Prospective assessment of the utility of EUS in the evaluation of gallstone pancreatitis. Gastrointest Endosc 1999;49(5):599–604.

[52] de Ledinghen V, Lecesne R, Raymond JM, et al. Diagnosis of choledocholithiasis: EUS or magnetic resonance cholangiography? A prospective controlled study. Gastrointest Endosc 1999; 49(1):26–31.

[53] Kim JH, Kim MJ, Park SI, et al. MR cholangiography in symptomatic gallstones: diagnostic accuracy according to clinical risk group. Radiology 2002;224(2):410–6.

RADIOLOGIC
CLINICS
OF NORTH AMERICA

Radiol Clin N Am 45 (2007) 461–483

Review of CT Angiography of Aorta

Tongfu Yu, MD[a], Xiaomei Zhu, MD[a], Lijun Tang, MD[a],
Dehang Wang, MD[a],*, Nael Saad, MB, BCh[b]

During the past decade CT angiography (CTA) has become a standard noninvasive imaging modality for the depiction of vascular anatomy and pathology. The quality and speed of CTA examinations have increased dramatically as CT technology has evolved from one-channel spiral CT systems to multichannel (4-, 8-, 10- and 16-slice) spiral CT systems. Sixty-four multidetector row CT (MDCT) became available in 2004 [1–4]. The imaging modality most commonly used for diagnosis of aortic disease is CT, followed by transesophageal echocardiography, MR imaging, and aortography. If multiple imaging is performed, the initial imaging technique most frequently used is CT [5].

CT techniques

Examination protocols

CTA of the aorta using four-slice scanners produces images with a lower spatial resolution and a relatively longer scan time than those produced using scanners with 16 or more slices. The spatial resolution needed to render diagnostic images of the smaller branches of the aorta and of intimal tears becomes feasible with the latter scanners. The scan should cover the area from a level 3 cm above the aortic arch to the level of the femoral heads. Typical protocols for 4-, 16- and 64-slice scanners for aortic CTA are given in Table 1.

[a] Radiological Department of the First Affiliated Hospital of Nanjing Medical University, Nanjing, Jiangsu 210029, China
[b] Department of Imaging Sciences, University of Rochester Medical Center, Rochester, NY, USA
* Corresponding author.
E-mail address: Wangdehang@hotmail.com (D. Wang).

doi:10.1016/j.rcl.2007.04.010

Table 1: Scan protocols for CT angiography of the entire aorta with a range of 100 cm for different scanners

Scanner	Rotation time (s)	Collimation	Table feed (mm/s)	Slice thickness (mm)	Slice interval (mm)	Duration (s)	Number of images
4-slice	0.5	4 × 2.5 mm	30	3	1.5	33	667
	0.8	4 × 2.5 mm	19	3	1.5	53	667
16-slice	0.5	16 × 1.5 mm	48	2	1.2	21	833
64-slice	0.33	32 × 0.6 mm × 2	48	1	0.8	21	1250

Currently the standard tube voltage for CTA is 120 kV. The tube current should be approximately 120 mAs, and automated dose modulation should be used. A tube voltage of 100 kV increases the contrast-to-noise ratio because of effective X-ray absorption by iodine at lower tube voltages, which improves the quality of images and reduces the radiation exposure to patients by 35% in comparison with 120 kV at a constant tube current [6]. CTA of the abdominal aorta performed at a low voltage results in higher attenuation in the aorta with reduced radiation dose and without degrading the diagnostic image quality. The volume of iodinated contrast medium can be reduced by lowering the voltage during CTA [7,8].

The beating of the heart results in both circular and perpendicular motion of the aorta that is most pronounced near the heart. Pseudodissection of the thoracic aorta, a well-known pitfall, occurs predominantly at the right anterior and left posterior aortic circumference (Fig. 1) [9]. Multiplanar reconstruction of images from contrast-enhanced or unenhanced helical CT provides evidence of motion artifacts [10]. Hofmann and colleagues [11] recommended the use of retrospective ECG gating for imaging of the heart, the aortic root, and the ascending aorta, especially when motion artifacts may influence the diagnosis critically (eg, when aortic dissection is suspected); however, an ECG-gated scan increases the radiation dose to the patient. Morgan-Hughes and colleagues [12] suggested that in patients who have slower heart rates (≤ 70 beats per minute), a reconstruction window should be centered at 75% of the R-R interval and that in patients who have faster heart rates (> 70 beats per minute) the construction window should be centered at 50% of the R-R interval. ECG-assisted MDCT shows a significant reduction of motion artifacts for the entire thoracic aorta compared with non–ECG-assisted MDCT [9].

Protocols for administration of contrast medium

High-quality CTA of the aorta requires sufficient contrast enhancement. An intra-arterial target threshold higher than 200 Hounsfield units (HU) produces adequate aortic enhancement for a diagnostic study [13]. As blood and the contrast media travel downstream, gradual mixing of the central and peripheral parts of the lumen occurs; to compensate for this dilution effect, a high-contrast delivery rate should be used to reach the target threshold. In addition, the reduction in the volume of contrast material for a given

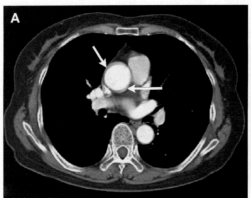 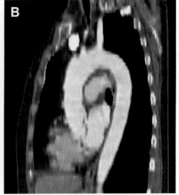

Fig. 1. (A) The motion of the heart transfers motion to the right anterior and left posterior walls of the ascending aorta (*white arrows*), which mimics aortic dissection. (B) Sagittal multiplanar reformation reconstruction shows evidence of motion artifact.

iodine dose may reduce adverse hemodynamic effects, especially in large patients [14]. Therefore, contrast media with a high iodine concentration (350–400 mg/mL) should be used at a flow rate of 3 to 4 mL/s to reach the target threshold [3]. Uniform vascular contrast enhancement with a reduced volume of contrast medium, which is desirable in CTA and essential for steady-state quantification of blood volume, can be achieved by using an exponentially decelerated method for injecting contrast medium [15].

Another challenge of aortic CTA is scan synchronization, which is determined by several factors including the transit of contrast medium bolus in the aorta, the start of the scan, and the table feed. Factors that influence the pattern of the arterial enhancement include the volume of contrast medium, the injection rate, and the iodine concentration [16,17]. Adjusting the volume of contrast medium according to the patient's weight can result in a predictable degree of aortic enhancement, but in clinical practice a fixed amount is applied [18]. A saline chaser usually is used in CTA performed by 16-row CT, especially in CTAs examining the vessels of the thorax. A saline chaser can facilitate the use of a smaller volume of contrast medium, decrease the streak artifacts in the superior vena cava, and produce a uniform enhancement pattern without affecting the maximal enhancement in the main arteries [19–21]. The time to peak aortic enhancement depends mainly on the injection rate; increasing the injection rate leads to a proportional increase in arterial enhancement regardless of the iodine concentration and volume of the contrast medium [22]. Effective opacification of the thoracic aorta is achieved better by injecting a contrast medium with a high iodine concentration at injection rates of 3 mL/s or more [23].

The start of the scan can be determined by one of three methods: using a fixed delay time, using a delay time determined by a peak enhancement time obtained from a test bolus, or triggered by bolus tracking [13]. Awai and colleagues [24] showed that in a protocol using a fixed injection duration, the time of arterial phase CT scanning may remain unchanged; thus, the scanning protocol can be specified easily because the aortic peak enhancement time and the period during which contrast enhancement is 200 HU or greater are almost constant. The authors did not specify the time value for a fixed injection duration, however [24]. Because scan times become shorter with the use of faster MDCT scanners, bolus timing is essential to make the full use of the contrast media. Automated bolus tracking is used more often than the test-bolus technique because it is easier to use, is more efficient, and reduces the total contrast medium dose [25]. Also, with the bolus-tracking protocol, scanning is performed during the plateau of attenuation, which may offer a more homogenous enhancement in the aorta and less pooling of contrast material in the right side of the heart [26]. Another important consideration with regards to synchronization of the contrast bolus and the scan is the table feed. The table feed of 64-slice scanners, sometimes up to 7 cm/s, may result in the scan overriding the bolus if a proximal stenosis is present. A lower table feed may result in the bolus overtaking the scan if there is peripheral vasodilatation. These two circumstances will affect the quality of the aortic CTA. Thomas and Bernhard [25] recommend using a fixed table feed of 40 to 48 mm/s combined with bolus tracking to perform aortic CTA.

Postprocessing techniques

CTA of the aorta using modern CT scanners produces several hundred images per study. This volume of data makes a comprehensive review of all axial images virtually impossible, and postprocessing techniques providing three-dimensional volumetric images are a prerequisite for efficient interpretation of the CTA and for reporting the findings to referring physicians. An important point for all postprocessing techniques is that they should not be rendered from the entire data set, because doing so would reduce the spatial resolution substantially. The aorta should be divided into segments to exploit the high Z-axis resolution inherent in the data set. Volume rendering is not without its disadvantages, however: skeletal structures may overlap vessels, and vessel wall calcifications may obscure underlying stenotic lesions. Maximum intensity projection (MIP) is a projection without depth information. MIP images of vessels are similar to digital subtraction angiography images, with the advantage that any desired projection can be visualized from a single data acquisition set. Overlapping bones that completely obscure the view of the artery may be resolved by thin-slab MIP images or bone-removal techniques. Thin-slab MIP images are performed in a short time and depict a particular vascular segment but lack a comprehensive overview of the entire vascular bed. A threshold of 200 to 300 HU is selected for bone removal, and a few reference points are set in bones at different positions. Despite the relatively long postprocessing time, the authors of this article consider MIP with bone removal the best way of displaying CTAs because of the excellent image quality. Curved multiplanar reformation is a technique that can be used if the vascular lumen travels along the long axis. Curved multiplanar reformation is an excellent adjunct to MIP reconstructions whenever extensive calcifications obscure the view of the lumen on MIP images.

CT angiography is noninvasive, is substantially less expensive than conventional digital subtraction angiography, and allows three-dimensional visualization of vessels from any angle from a single set of data acquisition [26,27]. Another advantage of CTA over digital subtraction angiography is the ability to show the shape, size, and density of the vascular wall and the adjacent organs. Compared with CTA, the major disadvantages of conventional angiography are cost, failure to detect intramural hematoma (IMH), and excessive time required for the examination [10]. CTA also has some disadvantages, which include lack of dynamic information and a somewhat poor visualization of small collaterals. Because of the use of contrast media, the most common complications during general CT examinations are allergic reactions and contrast extravasation, and quite a few cases of iatrogenic intravenous air embolism have been reported in the literature [28].

Anatomy

The aorta consists of an ascending segment, a transverse segment or arch, and a descending segment. The ascending aorta is approximately 5 cm long and has two distinct segments. The lower segment is the aortic root, which begins at the level of the aortic valve and extends to the sinotubular junction. This portion of the ascending aorta is the widest and measures about 3.5 cm in diameter. The ascending aorta extends to the origin of the innominate artery. The aortic arch begins at the innominate artery and ends at the ligamentum or ductus arteriosum. The innominate, left carotid, and left subclavian arteries arise from the aortic arch. The point at which the aortic arch joins the descending aorta is called the "aortic isthmus." The aortic arch is usually on the left side. The descending aorta begins at the ligamentum or ductus, and its proximal portion may appear slightly dilated, ending at the twelfth intercostal space [29].

The thoracic portion of the aorta is a continuation of the aortic arch as it descends through the thoracic cavity to the diaphragm. The descending aorta in the thoracic cavity gives off branches to the organs and muscles of the thoracic region. These branches include pericardial arteries, bronchial arteries for systemic circulation to the lungs; esophageal arteries, which supply the esophagus as it passes through the mediastinum; segmental posterior intercostal arteries supplying the intercostal muscles and other structures of the thoracic wall; and superior phrenic arteries supplying blood to the diaphragm.

The abdominal portion of the aorta is the segment of the aorta between the diaphragm and the level of the fourth lumbar vertebra, where it divides into the right and left common iliac arteries. Three major unpaired arteries supply blood to the abdominal organs. The first, a short and thick celiac trunk, divides immediately into three arteries: the left gastric, splenic, and common hepatic arteries. The next unpaired vessel is the superior mesenteric artery. It arises anteriorly from the abdominal portion of the aorta, just below the celiac trunk, supplying blood to the small intestine (except for a portion of the duodenum), the cecum, the appendix, the ascending colon, and the proximal two thirds of the transverse colon. The third unpaired vessel is the inferior mesenteric artery. It arises just before the iliac bifurcation. The inferior mesenteric artery supplies the distal one third of the transverse colon, the descending colon, the sigmoid colon, and the rectum. Variations of the abdominal aorta branches are common, and sometimes a multiplicity of variations may be present. Knowledge of these variations allows clinicians to identify and protect these branches during surgical procedures [30].

The abdominal aorta also gives rise to some important paired arteries. Small inferior phrenic arteries that supply the diaphragm are the first vessels arising from the abdominal portion of the aorta. The next major paired vessels are the paired renal arteries that carry blood to the kidneys. Smaller suprarenal arteries, located just above the renal arteries, supply the adrenal glands. The gonadal arteries are small, paired vessels that arise from the abdominal portion of the aorta, just below the renal arteries. Several lumbar arteries branch posteriorly from the abdominal portion of the aorta throughout its length and supply the muscles and the spinal cord in the lumbar region. In addition, an unpaired middle sacral artery arises from the posterior terminal portion of the abdominal portion of the aorta to supply the sacrum and coccyx. The abdominal portion of the aorta terminates in the posterior pelvis as it bifurcates into the right and left common iliac arteries. These vessels pass downward approximately 5 cm on their respective sides and terminate by dividing into the internal and external iliac arteries (**Fig. 2**) [31].

Congenital anomalies

A multitude of congenital anomalies may affect various portions of the aorta. Examples of these anomalies are described in the following sections.

Interrupted aortic arch

Interrupted aortic arch is defined as a separation between the ascending and descending aortas [32–36], and the classification is based on the site of interruption. Interrupted aortic arch has been classified into three types (A, B, and C) based on

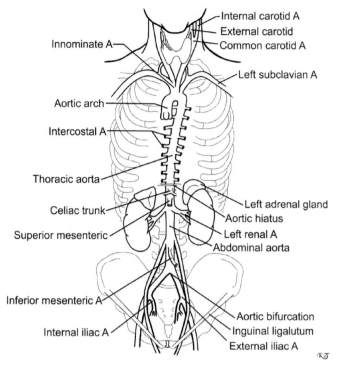

Internal carotid A
External carotid
Common carotid A
Innominate A
Left subclavian A
Aortic arch
Intercostal A
Thoracic aorta
Left adrenal gland
Celiac trunk
Aortic hiatus
Superior mesenteric
Left renal A
Abdominal aorta
Inferior mesenteric A
Internal iliac A
Aortic bifurcation
Inguinal ligalutum
External iliac A

Fig. 2. The anatomy of the aorta.

the site of aortic interruption. In type A, the interruption occurs distal to the origin of the left subclavian artery. In type B, the interruption occurs distal to the origin of the left common carotid artery. In type C, the interruption occurs proximal to the origin of the left common carotid artery.

In any of the three types, the right subclavian artery may arise normally or abnormally; the two most common abnormal sites are distal to the left subclavian artery (aberrant right subclavian artery) and from the right ductus arteriosus (isolated right subclavian artery). Type B interruptions account for about two thirds of cases, type A occurs in about one third of cases, and type C occurs in less than 1% of cases. CTA examination can show the direct signs of the three types and even the subtypes [29].

In addition to the type of interrupted aortic arch, evaluation of the distance between the proximal and distal segments, the size of a patent ductus arteriosus, the narrowest dimension of the left ventricular outflow tract, and other cardiac structural abnormalities are important for surgical planning. Three-dimensional reconstruction of the aorta and the branches is very useful in this regard. A right-sided descending aorta with aortic interruption is almost always associated with DiGeorge syndrome.

Coarctation of the aorta

There are two types of coarctation of the aorta: tubular and localized coarctation. The latter is more

common. In classic coarctation, the narrowing is located just distal to the left subclavian artery and has male predilection (Fig. 3) [32–35,37]. Coarctation at or immediately proximal to the left subclavian artery is rare and compromises the left subclavian artery. An aberrant right subclavian artery may arise at or below the coarctation. An external indentation

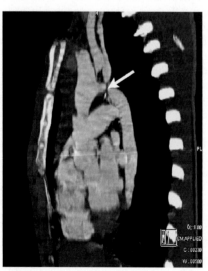

Fig. 3. Sagittal reformatted CT image demonstrating a membranous septation (*arrow*) distal to the left subclavian artery in a patient who has a classic aortic coarctation.

that involves all but the ventral portion of the coarctation corresponds internally to the ridge. The aorta just distal to the coarctation typically is dilated. Uniform narrowing of the aortic arch (tubular hypoplasia) can be seen frequently in neonates and usually is associated with other cardiac anomalies. Localized coarctation and tubular hypoplasia may coexist or may occur independently. Localized coarctation can be asymptomatic and detected incidentally, but it occasionally may present with headaches caused by hypertension or claudication caused by decreased blood flow. Depending on the severity, surgical correction is needed when patients are 3 to 5 years of age. Polson and colleagues [38] reported that coarctation of the aorta is associated with hypertension and abnormalities of blood pressure control that persist after repair and suggest that infants who have coarctation already show signs of pathologic adjustment of autonomic cardiovascular homeostasis. Proper imaging is of vital importance for the depiction and quantification of ascending aortic ectasia, aortic arch hypoplasia, recoarctation, or the formation of a local aneurysm or pseudoaneurysm at the previous site of coarctation [39,40]. MDCT and MR imaging are similarly useful for noninvasive evaluation of the thoracic aorta in patients who have coarctation. CTA can define the extent and location of the coarctation as well as associated cardiac anomalies. It is important to measure the diameter of the aorta, especially after treatment to assess stability of the repair and detect complications early. The slices for the measurements should be manually adjusted separately for each aortic level to get an oblique plane that is strictly perpendicular to the course of the aorta. Hager and colleagues [41] suggested that in explaining the diameter differences, one should consider the nature of the changes in the diameter of an aging aorta, which grows roughly 1 mm per year.

A diverticulum of Kommerell is characterized by an ectatic infundibulum at the origin of an anomalous right subclavian artery that originates distal to the left subclavian artery in a left-sided arch configuration. In this anomaly, the infundibular origin may become aneurysmal and often exhibits circumferential atherosclerotic changes. The vessel, which most often courses posterior to the esophagus, may create an extrinsic compression on the esophagus and result in the clinical syndrome of dysphagia lusorum [42].

Right aortic arch

Patients who have a right-sided aortic arch are usually asymptomatic. An aberrant left subclavian artery in association with a right-sided aortic arch is the most common type of right-arch anomaly. It is rare and is associated with congenital heart disease. Five percent of patients who have an aberrant left subclavian artery develop compression symptoms caused by a tight vascular ring. Mirror imaging branching, which is the second most common right-arch anomaly, frequently is symptomatic and is associated with congenital heart disease (Fig. 4). The third most common, but rare, presentation is a right aortic arch with isolated left subclavian artery associated with congenital subclavian steal syndrome presenting with diminished pulse in left upper extremity. CTA can visualize the right aortic arch and various branching patterns directly and evaluate the associated heart disease correctly.

Aortic aneurysm

Aneurysm of the aorta is defined as a permanent localized dilatation of the aorta, at least 50% greater than normal and involving all three wall layers [43]. The lesser degree of dilatation generally is referred to as "ectasia." Most aneurysms of the thoracic aorta are atherosclerotic in origin. Other causes are infection (mycotic aneurysms) and cystic medial necrosis (annuloaortic ectasia) [44]. Frequent comorbidities include hypertension, coronary artery disease, obstructive pulmonary disease, and congestive heart failure. Atherosclerotic aneurysms typically are fusiform in shape and are more common in the descending aorta, with a high incidence of concomitant abdominal aortic aneurysm. In Marfan syndrome, aneurysms most commonly occur in the proximal portion of the ascending aorta, involving the aortic root and resulting in a pear-shaped aorta [45]. Important imaging features of aortic aneurysms are the maximum diameter, the length, and involvement of major branch vessels. The aneurysmal thoracic aorta grows at an average rate of 1 mm per year with a high risk for natural complications (rupture or dissection) at 6 cm for the ascending aorta and 7 cm for the descending aorta [46]. The yearly risk of any occurrence of rupture, dissection, or death in a patient who has a thoracic aneurysm larger than 6 cm in diameter is greater than 14% [46]. As is the case with abdominal aortic aneurysms (AAAs), the risk of rupture for thoracic aneurysms increases with size, and the 5-year rupture rate is fivefold higher for aneurysms larger than 6 cm in diameter [47]. In asymptomatic patients, risk/benefit analysis in a large population study supports that thoracic aneurysms larger than 6.5 cm be repaired electively, with the threshold for Marfan's disease or familial TAAs being more than 6 cm [46]. Crawford and DeNatale [48] classified thoracoabdominal aneurysms based on the anatomic location. Type I involves the descending thoracic aorta below the subclavian vessels and the upper abdominal

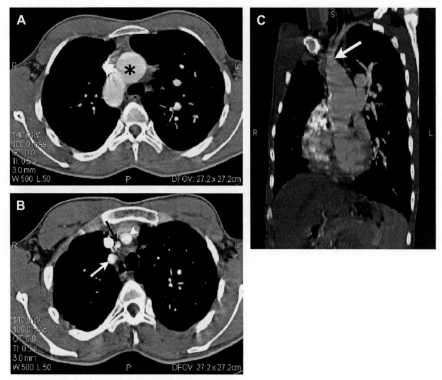

Fig. 4. (*A*) Axial CT image demonstrating a right aortic arch (*asterisk*). (*B*) The right common carotid (*black arrow*) and the right subclavian (*white arrow*) arteries have separate origins at the aortic arch. There is a common trunk (*arrowhead*) of the left common carotid and left subclavian arteries. (*C*) Coronal reformatted image demonstrates a saccular aneurysm of the ascending aorta. The origin of the common trunk of the left common carotid artery and left subclavian artery is also seen (*arrow*).

aorta. Type II involves most of the descending aorta and most of the abdominal aorta below the diaphragm. Type III involves the lower portion of the thoracic aorta. Type IV aneurysms begin at the diaphragm and extend caudally. Type II and type III AAAs are the most difficult to repair. Type II aneurysms have the highest risk for spinal cord injury and renal failure. Overall, up to 13% of all patients in whom an aortic aneurysm is diagnosed have multiple aneurysms; 25% to 28% of those who have thoracic aortic aneurysms have concomitant abdominal aortic aneurysms.

The incidence and prevalence of AAA, a common pathology in the elderly, is increasing [49]. Although most AAAs remain asymptomatic, their increase in size may lead to spontaneous rupture, which is associated with a mortality rate ranging from 66% to 95%. Forty percent to 50% of patients who have ruptured AAA die before they reach the hospital, and the overall mortality rate is greater than 90% [50]. Several studies indicated the necessity of mass screening for AAA [51,52]. AAA screening of men aged 65 to 75 years reduces AAA-related mortality [53]. Indeed, the Screening AAAs Very Effectively (SAAAVE) Act was passed by Congress and received Presidential approval. It went into effect at

the beginning of 2007 and offers an ultrasound screening as part of the "Welcome to Medicare" physical examination for patients older than 65 years who join Medicare. Most AAAs are asymptomatic, not detectable on physical examination, and silent until discovered during radiologic testing for other reasons. Tobacco use, hypertension, a family history of AAA, and male sex are clinical risk factors for the development of an aneurysm [54]. In contrast, pseudoaneurysms of the abdominal aorta usually are iatrogenic (eg, prior graft repair of an AAA or a complication of inferior vena cava filter placement or orthotopic heart transplant procedure) (Fig. 5) [55–57].

Aortic rupture

Rupture of an AAA involves complete loss of aortic wall integrity and is a surgical emergency requiring immediate repair (Fig. 6). The mortality rate approaches 90% if rupture occurs outside the hospital [54]. AAA rupture is a complicated and multifactorial event, dependent upon the maximum diameter, expansion rate, diastolic pressure, wall stress and strength, asymmetry, saccular index, intraluminal thrombus, and change in stiffness. Clearly, one cannot rely on one or two simple factors alone to

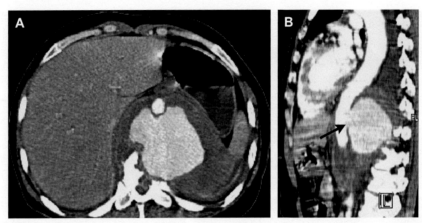

Fig. 5. (A) Axial CT image in a patient who has a chronic aortic pseudoaneurysm. The thick pseudocapsule formed by blood and fibrotic tissue is invading the thoracic vertebrae resulting in bone resorption. (B) Sagittal reformatted CT image demonstrates a narrow neck connecting the aorta and the sac of the pseudoaneurysm (arrow).

determine the risk of rupture accurately [58]. The site of rupture usually involves the posterior wall of the aorta [59]. The CT features of retroperitoneal rupture are discontinuity of the rim of calcification in the aneurysm wall, well-defined soft tissue density adjacent to the aorta, concealed psoas muscle, and displaced viscera. Extravasation of contrast medium from aortic lumen is a definite sign of aortic rupture [60,61]. Contained rupture is characterized more frequently by a relatively well-defined soft tissue density adjacent to the aorta. Rupture of an aortic aneurysm is preventable in most cases by close surveillance and the recognition of physical and imaging findings that place patients at a higher risk for rupture. Early detection reduces mortality because repair is elective rather than emergent [62].

Infection

Infection is estimated to complicate about 0.7% to 2.6% of aortic aneurysms [63]. The infectious agent can reach the artery either by contiguous spread of an adjacent infectious process (Fig. 7) or by traumatic and/or iatrogenic inoculation. Risk factors for development of a mycotic aneurysm include arterial trauma, various immunocompromised states (diabetes mellitus, malignancy, alcoholism, collagen vascular disease, AIDS, steroid use), concurrent sepsis, endocarditis, and congenital cardiovascular defects [64]. Cross-sectional imaging is a valuable tool that helps identify adjacent findings such as a periaortic soft tissue mass, stranding, and/or fluid (Fig. 8). Compared with the natural history of arteriosclerotic aneurysm, relatively rapid progression of disease was a feature that was present when sequential examinations were obtained [65]. In addition to demonstrating the size and extent of the aneurysm, a CT scan also demonstrates leak and perianeurysmal hemorrhage. Because almost 90% of arteriosclerotic aneurysms are located in the

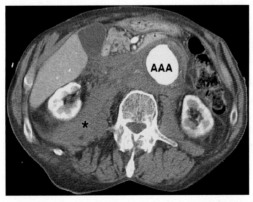

Fig. 6. Axial CT image demonstrating an abdominal aortic aneurysm that has ruptured retroperitoneally with resultant hematoma (asterisk).

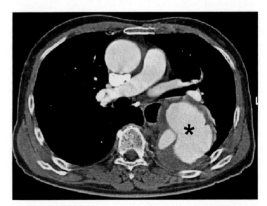

Fig. 7. Axial CT image in a patient who has tuberculosis in the posterior segment of the lower lobe of the left lung. A pseudoaneurysm (asterisk) of the descending thoracic aorta has developed because of necrosis of the aortic wall.

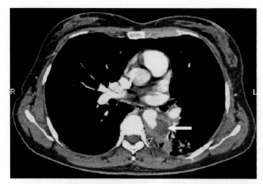

Fig. 8. Axial CT image demonstrating a mycotic aneurysm of the descending thoracic aorta with periaortic soft-tissue mass (*arrowhead*) and fluid (*arrow*).

infrarenal aorta, the majority of infected aneurysms are found in this location.

Management of abdominal aortic aneurysm

Surgical intervention is worthwhile when the aneurysm is at least 5.5 cm in diameter, or greater than 4.5 cm with an increase of 0.5 cm in the 6 months before intervention [66]. Asymptomatic patients who have an AAA should be medically optimized before repair. Symptomatic aneurysms require urgent surgical attention. There is a paradigm shift in the treatment of AAAs with endovascular aortic repair. Endovascular aortic repair has been shown to have lower morbidity and mortality rates than open surgical repair, in addition to a reduced hospital stay [66].

CT techniques

Three-dimensional CT or volume rendering (VR) CT reconstruction is an invaluable tool for evaluating aortic aneurysm size, location, extent, visceral aortic branches, and aortoiliac tortuosity [67] in addition to performing measurements for preoperative planning of stent-graft repair [68]. Characteristics and measurements of the abdominal aorta and its branches that make it suitable for endovascular stent grafting include an aneurysm neck (the portion of the infrarenal abdominal aorta between the lowest renal artery and the proximal aspect of the aneurysm) that is cylindrical in shape, at least 1.5 cm in length, free of thrombus and excessive plaque, and relatively straight in orientation to the long axis of the aneurysm. Iliac artery features are similar to those of the neck, including a small degree of tortuosity and disease-free lumens. The maximal diameter of the neck and iliac arteries suitable for endovascular aortic repair varies according to the commercial graft device used [69]. Some authors consider VR images more reliable than axial CT images for the detection of renal and iliac artery involvement in an AAA [70].

Aortic dissection

Aortic dissection is a potentially catastrophic cardiovascular disease associated with high morbidity and mortality that mandates emergent treatment. Advances in the understanding of this disease have established that survival generally is better in patients who have lesions limited to the descending aorta than in patients who have lesions involving the ascending aorta. Acute aortic dissection is the most common cause of aortic emergency. Factors predisposing patients to aortic dissection include hypertension (the most important), Marfan syndrome (Fig. 9), Turner syndrome, other connective tissue diseases, congenital aortic valvular defects, aortic coarctation, aortic aneurysm, infection and other causes of aortitis, and pregnancy. Cocaine use also has been associated with aortic dissection.

Aortic dissection is classified according to the extent of involvement of the aorta. The Stanford system classifies the dissection into two types. Type A, which accounts for about 75% of the total dissections, affects only the ascending aorta or the aortic arch, regardless of the site of the intimal tear; Type B affects the descending aorta [71]. Because the Stanford system is based on whether the dissection needs to be corrected surgically, it has superseded the original DeBakey system that classified aortic dissection into three types (with types I and II equivalent to type A in the Stanford system) (Fig. 10).

Aortic dissection may be acute or chronic, depending on its clinical manifestation. Dissection is considered acute if the onset of symptoms occurred less than 2 weeks at the time of presentation and is considered chronic if the onset of symptoms occurred more than 2 weeks before presentation. Seventy-five percent of deaths from aortic dissection occur within 2 weeks of the initial manifestation of symptoms. Mean plasma levels of thrombin-antithrombin complex and D-dimer decrease in correlation with the morphologic regressive changes. Serial measurement of D-dimer and thrombin-antithrombin complex is useful to predict morphologic changes in chronic aortic dissection and has been proposed as a method to follow-up patients who have aortic dissection [72]. Aortic dissection with extension into a common carotid artery (Fig. 11) can cause ischemic stroke, and acute aortic dissection sometimes can result in acute aortic obstruction, which frequently causes life-threatening organ ischemia [65,73].

Acute type A aortic dissection can have fatal complications including extension to the pericardium, the pleural space, the coronary arteries, and/or the aortic valvular ring, so it should be repaired immediately [73]. A risk-prediction model with control

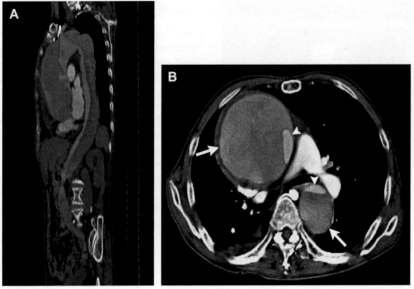

Fig. 9. (*A*) Axial CT image in a patient who has a type A aortic dissection. The true lumen (*arrowhead*) is smaller and of higher density than the false lumen (*arrow*). (*B*) Coronal reformatted image demonstrates extension of the dissection flap into the innominate and right common carotid arteries (*arrow*).

for age and gender showed hypotension/shock (odds ratio [OR] 23.8; *P* < .0001), absence of chest/back pain on presentation (OR 3.5; *P* = .01), and branch vessel involvement (OR 2.9; *P* = .02), collectively named "the deadly triad," to be independent predictors of in-hospital death for patients who have type B dissection.

Type B aortic dissections usually are managed conservatively with aggressive blood pressure control. Complicated type B aortic dissections (eg,

containing rupture, occlusion of major branch, extension, or enlargement) may require surgical management, which at times may be emergent (eg, rupture, enlargement); other complications (eg, intractable pain, visceral malperfusion) may allow more time for medical/interventional management. Early and midterm results show endovascular repair to be effective in treatment of acute type B aortic dissections [74,75]. Surgical repair should be performed if the aortic diameter enlarges or if a new

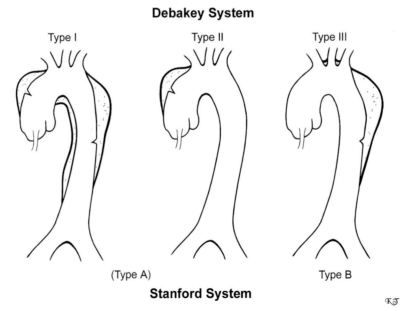

Fig. 10. The DeBakey and Stanford systems for classifying aortic dissection.

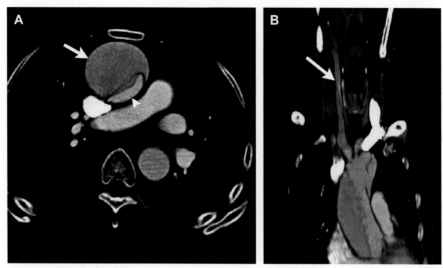

Fig. 11. (*A*) Sagittal reformatted CT image demonstrating a type A aortic dissection involving the entire length of the aorta in a patient who has Marfan syndrome. (*B*) Axial CT image at the level of the main pulmonary artery showing involvement of the ascending and descending thoracic aorta. The larger cavity is the false lumen with a lower density (*arrows*); the true lumen is smaller with a higher density (*arrowheads*).

complication appears during the chronic phase [76]. Patients who have type B or surgically treated type A dissections may develop vascular complications such as mesenteric or peripheral arterial ischemia, which cannot be managed medically. Aortic fenestration is a method for decompressing the hypertensive false lumen by creating a hole in the distal part of the dissection flap to address this complication [77]. In type B aortic dissections, the affected aortas have shown a high incidence of enlargement during the follow-up period. Eijun and colleagues [78] reported that age greater than 60 years and the presence of blood flow in the false lumen during the follow-up period are the only two significant risk factors predisposing to an increase in the diameter of the aorta, and the thoracic aorta grows at a faster rate than the abdominal aorta. These results suggest that the segment with the largest diameter does not always show the fastest rate of growth. Familiarity with these results is useful for following-up patients who have type B aortic dissection [75–76].

CT findings

CT scans performed before and after the injection of contrast medium are mandatory in patients suspected of having aortic dissection. Unenhanced CT is useful in evaluating the aorta in patients suspected of having an aortic dissection. Occasionally, on unenhanced CT scans one may see a calcified intima with internal displacement (Fig. 12). This finding may be confused with an aneurysm with calcified mural thrombus. The density of the lumen is useful to differentiate the two conditions: an

aortic dissection has a hypodense lumen and an aortic aneurysm with a calcified mural thrombus has a hyperdense lumen.

An intimal flap separating the true lumen from the false lumen is the hallmark of aortic dissection on contrast-enhanced CT (Figs. 12 and 13). Distinguishing the true and false lumens on CTA is of paramount importance when endovascular therapy is considered, because the endograft must be deployed in the true lumen. This consideration is less significant with open surgical repair. CT characteristics that aid in the identification of the false lumen include the presence of slender linear areas of low attenuation within the false lumen corresponding to residual ribbons of the media incompletely sheared away during the dissection process. This manifestation known as the "cobweb sign" is specific to the false lumen. Two other useful indicators of the false lumen are a larger cross-sectional area and the beak sign. The beak sign is the cross-sectional imaging manifestation of the wedge of hematoma that cleaves a space for the propagation of the false lumen [79]. On most contrast-enhanced CT scans, the lumen that is continuous with the undissected portion of the aorta usually can be identified as the true lumen. Circumferential dissection of the intimal layer can produce an intimo-intimal intussusception, an unusual type of aortic dissection, which subsequently invaginates like a windsock. This type of intimal tear usually begins near the coronary orifices. An aortic aneurysm with intraluminal thrombus may be difficult to distinguish from a dissection with a thrombosed false lumen. The fact that a dissection generally has a spiral shape

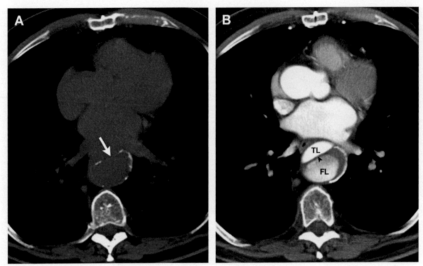

Fig. 12. (A) Unenhanced axial CT image demonstrates displacement of the calcified intima (*arrow*), which corresponds to the intimal flap (*arrowhead*) on (B) the contrast-enhanced CT. The true lumen (*TL*) is brightly enhancing; the false lumen (*FL*) is partially enhancing to a lesser degree because of slower flow and thrombosis.

with a smooth inner border, whereas a thrombus tends to maintain a constant circumferential relationship with the aortic wall with an irregular inner border, can help in differentiating between the two. Furthermore, intimal calcification occurring in an aortic aneurysm typically is located at the periphery of the aorta.

CTA in patients suspected of having an aortic dissection or IMH helps identify the site of an entry tear (the most proximal split in the intimal flap or an ulcerlike projection within the IMH on enhanced CT). Involvement of an aortic arch branch vessel, pericardial effusion, and aortic arch anomalies

also should be examined carefully. Any remnant entry tear may increase the possibility of enlargement of the false lumen as a late complication.

Intramural hematoma

IMH may be an early stage or a variant of aortic dissection [80]. In contrast to typical aortic dissection, in which there is an intimal tear, IMH is caused by a spontaneous hemorrhage from the vasa vasorum of the medial layer, which weakens the media without an intimal tear. IMH accounts for approximately 13% of acute aortic dissection. Because

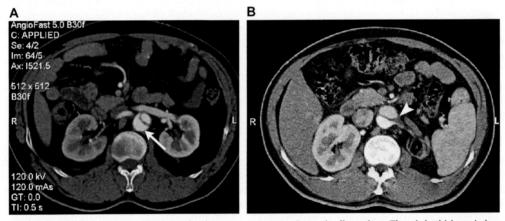

Fig. 13. (A) Axial CT image in a patient who has an acute type B aortic dissection. The right kidney is less enhanced than the left kidney because of slower blood flow through the right renal artery that originates from the false lumen of the aorta (*arrow*). (B) Axial CT image in a different patient demonstrating a chronic type B aortic dissection. Long-standing decreased perfusion to the left kidney resulting from obstruction of the left renal artery origin (*arrowhead*) by the dissection flap has caused atrophy of the left kidney. The right kidney shows compensatory hypertrophy.

IMH and typical dissection have similar clinical manifestations and risk factors, IMH is commonly classified according to the Stanford system for classification of aortic dissection. Some authors recommend that IMH of Stanford type A should be treated surgically [81]; others have suggested that, because of the high mortality and morbidity associated with aortic surgery, conservative medical treatment with frequent imaging follow-up may be a rational management option [82]. Song and colleagues [82] hypothesized that the absence of an intimal tear and the lack of continuous blood flow in IMH probably indicates a better clinical outcome than in typical aortic dissection. Gerber and colleagues [65] suggested that one indication for endovascular repair may include an IMH in the descending aorta with or without a penetrating atherosclerotic ulcer (PAU).

The difficulty with this pathology is that the exact origin of the intramural bleeding cannot always be verified easily [83]. Ganaha and colleagues [83] suggested that both symptoms and radiologic findings (eg, recurrent pain, pleural effusion, and the size and depth of the ulcerlike projection) may be predictive of disease progression. Early diagnosis and prompt treatment are critical in improving the outcome of patients who have IMH.

The growth patterns of type B aortic dissection and type B IMH are somewhat different. In patients who have type B IMH, the affected aortas do not have a high incidence of enlargement during the follow-up period but tend to increase in size after 1 year. An initial diameter of 40 mm or greater and the presence of blood flow in the false lumen are important risk factors for enlargement during the follow-up period [84]. Several investigators have attempted to assess the usefulness of CT findings for predicting the progression of aortic IMH to aortic dissection. The maximum aortic diameter (> 50 mm), estimated on the basis of the initial CT scan, is the most important predictive factor of progression in type A IMH. Findings in type A IMH, such as thick hematoma with compression of the true lumen, pericardial effusion, or, less important, pleural effusion, were useful for predicting progression to aortic dissection [80]. A large hematoma may indicate active bleeding from the ruptured vasa vasorum, which may result in increased weakening of the intima of the affected aorta. If the IMH progresses to typical dissection, especially in type A IMH, emergent treatment is mandatory. Patients who have type A IMH develop ulcerlike projections significantly more often than do patients who have type B IMH. These ulcerlike projections, which represent new areas of intimal disruption, can progress to aneurysm formation or overt aortic dissection [85,86].

CT findings

It is important to perform unenhanced CT as the first imaging evaluation when aortic dissection is suspected, because contrast material within the vessel may obscure IMH. On unenhanced CT scans, characteristic findings include a cuff or crescent of high attenuation and internal displacement of intimal calcification. The crescent-shaped area of high attenuation in the aortic wall corresponds to a hematoma in the medial layer, which may or may not compress the aortic lumen. The density of the IMH often is higher than that of the normal lumen. Intimal calcifications also may be displaced by IMH.

IMH is characterized by the absence of both an intimal flap and blood flow within its substance. Unlike the false lumen in typical aortic dissection, which has various degrees of enhancement from one patient to another, the crescent-shaped area of IMH does not enhance after administration of contrast material (Fig. 14). The relationship of IMH and the thrombosed false lumen with the aortic wall is an important factor in their differentiation. IMH maintains a constant circumferential relationship with the aortic wall, but the thrombosed false lumen tends to spiral longitudinally around the aorta.

Atherosclerotic disease

Atherosclerosis arterial occlusive disease (PAU) is a significant disease in the elderly and has been shown to progress rapidly after menopause in women [87]. Atheromatosis of the thoracic aorta has been recognized as a major source of stroke or systemic embolism [88]. Complex atherosclerotic aortic debris is a marker for generalized atherosclerosis and well-established atherosclerotic and cardioembolic mechanisms of cerebral ischemia [89]. Therefore it is important to demonstrate the changes atherosclerosis makes to the main arteries.

A PAU is an ulceration of atheromatous plaque that has eroded the inner, elastic layer of the aortic wall, reached the medial layer, and produced a hematoma in the media. Involvement of the media sometimes can be complicated by aneurysmal dilatation or, less frequently, by rupture (Figs. 15 and 16) [90]. Some authors have theorized that most saccular aneurysms are caused by a PAU [85]. Unlike typical aortic dissection, PAUs most often occur in elderly patients who have severe underlying atherosclerosis. Sometimes, a PAU with IMH may occur in a nonemergent or nondissection setting. These ulcers typically involve the aortic arch and descending thoracic aorta and rarely occur in the ascending aorta, where rapid blood flow from the

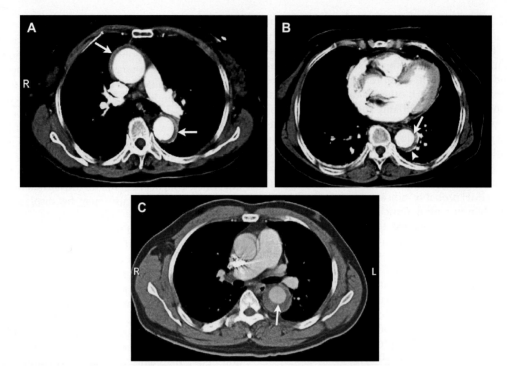

Fig. 14. (*A*) Axial CT image in a patient who has a type A IMH involving the ascending and descending thoracic aorta. Curvilinear hypodensities correspond to the IMH (*arrows*). (*B*) Axial CT image in a patient who has a type B IMH (*arrow*) with calcified aortic adventitia (*arrowhead*). (*C*) Axial CT image in a patient who has a type B IMH with extensive hematoma (*arrow*) circumferentially within the wall of aorta.

left ventricle provides protection against atherosclerosis. They therefore can be distinguished easily from type A aortic dissection or type A IMH. Rarely, type B aortic dissection can occur as a late complication of a PAU.

The initial therapy for PAU is medical management similar to management for type B aortic dissection. Surgery is performed in patients who have hemodynamic instability, persistent pain, aortic rupture, distal embolization, or rapid enlargement of the aortic diameter. It is important to emphasize that surgical repair of a PAU generally is more complicated and extensive than surgical repair of typical type B aortic dissection, because much of the aortic wall may have been damaged by ulceration and may have to be replaced. Consequently, aortic grafting for PAU may be associated with higher morbidity (eg, increased risk of paraplegia) because of a greater compromise of the blood supply to the spinal cord during surgery.

Patients who are asymptomatic and are found incidentally to have a PAU should undergo the same CT follow-up as those who have thoracic aortic aneurysms, because one third of ulcerlike lesions may progress, resulting in mild interval aortic enlargement [85]. When rupture and mediastinal hemorrhage occur, it is difficult to differentiate between a ruptured aneurysm and a complicated atherosclerotic ulcer by imaging findings. In both cases, immediate surgical treatment is required. Tatsumi and colleagues [91] suggested that fluorodeoxyglucose positron emission tomography/CT may detect the metabolic activity of atherosclerotic changes, which may be useful for monitoring the progress of the atherosclerotic lesions. PAUs typically are located in the descending and abdominal aorta, which are severely atherosclerotic. In contrast, in classic aortic dissection, most intimal disruptions also are related to mechanical stress and usually occur at the ascending aorta or aortic arch. The progression of intimal disruption may be more common in IMH than in PAU [79].

CT findings

In PAU, extensive atherosclerosis and IMH of variable extent are visible on unenhanced CT scans. Frequently the IMH is focal because of medial fibrosis caused by atherosclerosis. Displaced intimal calcifications are often present.

At CTA, the ulcerlike projection appears as a localized blood-filled pouch protruding into the thrombosed lumen of the aorta, showing the same degree of contrast enhancement as the aortic lumen. The appearance of the lesion is similar to that of a peptic ulcer (Fig. 16). Lesions can be single or multiple. PAU often is associated with thickening

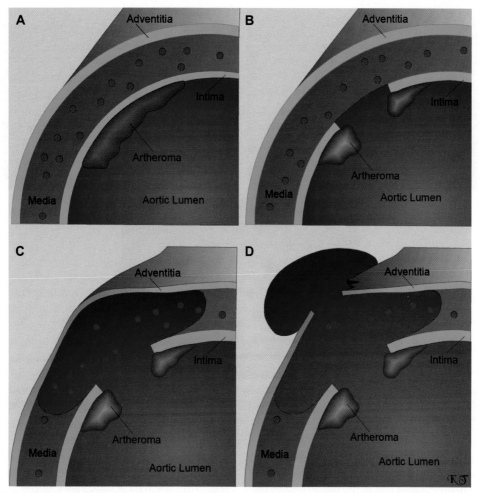

Fig. 15. The four stages in the formation of a penetrating atherosclerotic ulcer. (*A*) Aortic atheroma. (*B*) Benign intimal plaque ulceration contained in the intima. (*C*) Medial hematoma with potential adventitial false aneurysm. (*D*) Transmural rupture.

of the aortic wall, which appears enhanced. Atheromatous ulcers that are confined to the intimal layer sometimes have a radiologic appearance similar to that of PAU. Therefore, particular care should be taken in making a diagnosis of PAU if the lesions are discovered incidentally in an asymptomatic patient and if associated focal IMH is absent [92].

Traumatic aortic injury

MDCT angiography is very sensitive in detecting traumatic vascular injuries. To make full use of MDCT, a well-adjusted scanning protocol consisting a thin collimation and bolus tracking after injection of intravenous contrast medium is needed. Chest CTA is an excellent initial imaging tool because of its high sensitivity and ease of performance in the trauma patient suspected of having an aortic injury. Sometimes, however, artifacts and other limitations require the use of conventional

aortography for further evaluation [93]. Aortic transaction is the cause of 16% of all deaths from motor vehicle collisions. Eighty-five percent of patients sustaining an aortic transaction die before reaching the hospital. Of the remaining survivors, 50% die within 24 hours [94].

Acute aortic injury may result in incomplete rupture, complete rupture, traumatic aortic dissection, and acute traumatic IMH [95]. CT findings of aortic injury include blood within the mediastinum, deformities of the aortic contour, intimal flaps, thrombus or debris protruding into the aortic lumen, the presence of a pseudoaneurysm, or an abrupt tapering of the diameter of the descending aorta compared with the ascending aorta (pseudo-coarctation) [96].

Incomplete rupture

A combination of traction, torsion, and hydrostatic forces created by differential deceleration of

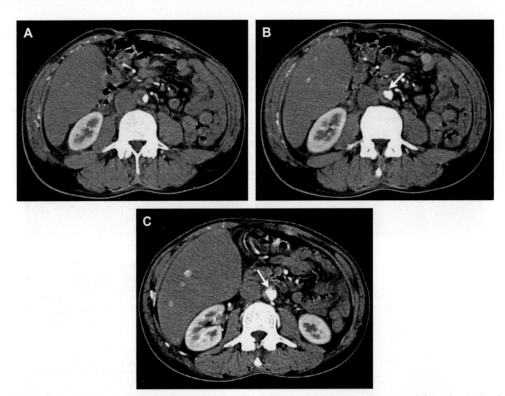

Fig. 16. Aortic changes caused by atherosclerosis in different stages. (*A*) Aortic atheroma. (*B*) Benign intimal plaque ulceration (*white arrow*) contained in the intima. (*C*) Medial hematoma (*white arrow*) with potential adventitial false aneurysm.

thoracic structures can result in aortic rupture. Incomplete rupture of the aorta is caused by a limited partial circumferential tear in the intima and/or the media of the aortic wall [97,98]. CT findings typically consist of a saccular outpouching demarcated from the aortic lumen by a collar, usually with a periaortic hematoma (Fig. 17). Because of the fresh hematoma, the density usually is a little higher than that of the soft tissue adjacent to the aorta in the unenhanced CT scan. A thin layer of the adventitia and neighboring tissue form the outer wall of the pseudoaneurysm, which requires emergent treatment by stent grafting or open surgical repair to avoid progression to a complete rupture that carries a higher mortality rate.

Complete rupture

In severe aortic injury, the forces mentioned previously can cause complete transection when the tear extends from the intima and media into the adventitial layer [97–99]. This injury results in massive mediastinal and pleural hemorrhage, usually leading to hypovolemic shock and, ultimately, death. In approximately 90% of patients who sustain blunt traumatic aortic injuries and survive to be transferred to a hospital, the complete rupture

occurs at the anteromedial aspect of the aortic isthmus distal to the origin of the left subclavian artery (Fig. 18). The typical appearance of the ruptured isthmus on contrast-enhanced CT is a sleeve of subadventitial contrast medium. CT also accurately shows hemomediastinum and hemothorax, which may be indirect signs of a blunt traumatic aortic injury. Although thoracic aortic transections remain a highly lethal injury, hemodynamically stable patients have a low operative mortality, and spinal cord injury is decreased by the use of adjuvant perfusion techniques that maintain distal aortic perfusion during cross-clamping of the aorta [100].

Traumatic aortic dissection

Aortic dissection is less common in the setting of blunt thoracic trauma than with the complete or incomplete rupture of the aorta [101,102]. Acute hypertension and steepness of the pulse wave along with the rapid deceleration force sustained by the aorta may cause intimal tears and assist in the distal propagation of the dissection [102]. The CT signs of traumatic aortic dissection are similar to those of the nontraumatic type, with other associated traumatic injuries, including pulmonary contusions [103].

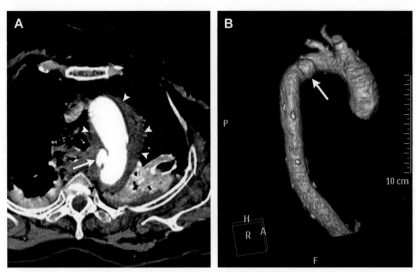

Fig. 17. (*A*) Axial CT image demonstrating a contained traumatic aortic transection. A pseudoaneurysm (*arrow*) has formed at the site of the aortic wall disruption, and the arch is surrounded by a hematoma (*arrowheads*). (*B*) A three-dimensional volume-rendered image from a right lateral projection shows the pseudoaneurysm (*arrow*) at the aortic isthmus.

Traumatic acute intramural hematoma

An IMH is referred to as a dissection that lacks an intimo-medial tear, which is the hallmark of a typical dissection [104,105]. In patients who have traumatic acute IMH, the thickening of the aortic wall generally is circular. Acute IMH weakens the aorta and may progress either to rupture of the aortic wall externally, leading to a pseudoaneurysm, or to inward disruption of the intimal layer, leading to a communicating aortic dissection. MDCT angiography has been reported to approach a sensitivity of 100% and a negative predictive value of 100% in detecting IMH [106]. IMHs usually are hyperattenuating on unenhanced CT and hypoattenuating compared with the vessel lumen on contrast-enhanced CT. Identification of the intima can be used to differentiate an acute IMH from a mural thrombus. A mural

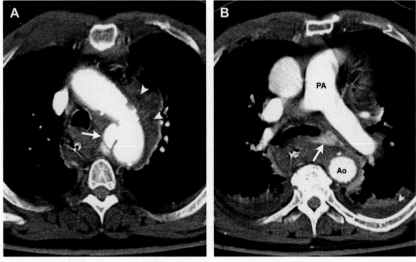

Fig. 18. (*A*) Axial CT image demonstrating a traumatic aortic transection. A pseudoaneurysm (*arrow*) has formed at the site of the aortic wall disruption, and the arch is surrounded by a hematoma (*arrowheads*). (*B*) Axial CT image at the level of the pulmonary artery (*PA*) shows extensive mediastinal hematoma with extravasated contrast material (*arrow*) indicating a noncontained aortic transection. Ao, descending thoracic aorta.

thrombus lies on top of the intima, which frequently is calcified, whereas an IMH is subintimal [105]. Periaortic hematoma near the level of the aortic isthmus is an indirect sign of aortic injury and has been identified as a common and suggestive finding of aortic rupture. Periaortic hematoma near the level of the diaphragmatic crura is an insensitive but relatively specific sign for thoracic aortic injury after blunt trauma [107].

Postoperative changes

Endovascular stent grafting is an established therapeutic option for abdominal aortic aneurysms. Recently, it has emerged as a less invasive therapeutic alternative for aneurysms and dissections of the descending thoracic aorta [108]. Endograft therapy for thoracic aortic disease can be performed safely in elderly patients with no significant increase in perioperative morbidity or mortality compared with younger patients. If the proximal landing zone, defined as the distance from the origin of the left subclavian artery to the entry tear of the dissection or the proximal aspect of the descending aortic aneurysm, is less than 5 mm, covering the left subclavian artery with graft fabric lengthens the proximal fixation site and should minimize proximal endoleaks. Because of the collateral blood flow from the right vertebral artery, circle of Willis, carotid arteries, and the vessels around the thoracic wall and the shoulder, the coverage of the left subclavian artery does not result in ischemic disease [109,110]. Kern and colleagues [111] advocate endograft therapy, when anatomically possible, as the treatment of choice for thoracic aortic disease in elderly patients. Reduction in sac diameter after endovascular aneurysm repair is considered a definite indication of treatment success. If the diameter remains static, it is unclear whether the treatment has succeeded (because it has arrested growth) or failed (because there has been no shrinkage). Although early results compare favorably with those of conventional open surgery, several procedure-related complications have been described, such as stent-graft dislodgment, migration, stent fracture, collapse of the stent, changes in the size and shape of the aorta, and arterial wall injury [112–115].

Migration

Because the attachment sites are not sutured, there may be movement at the aortic or iliac attachments or at points of connection within modular grafts.

Pseudoaneurysm

Arterial wall injury can result in acute retrograde aortic dissection or pseudoaneurysm formation, mandating urgent surgical repair. Although pseudoaneurysm formation at conventional anastomotic sites is a recognized complication, it rarely is seen with endografts [114].

Endoleak

Persistent blood flow in the aortic aneurysm sac outside the stent graft is called an "endoleak" (Fig. 19). The term was coined to distinguish this perigraft blood flow from aortic rupture with retroperitoneal or intraperitoneal leak. There are four types of endoleak. Type I endoleak is related to the stent graft device itself and is caused by an insufficient seal between the proximal portion of the endograft and the aortic wall or between the distal portion of the endograft and the iliac artery wall. Type II endoleak is retrograde flow from collateral branches (lumbar, inferior mesenteric, and accessory renal arteries). Type III endoleak is cause by fabric tears, graft wall defect, or modular disconnection or disintegration. Type IV endoleak is flow through the graft assumed to be associated with graft wall porosity, that is, endotension [65]. The most common branches causing type II endoleak are the fourth lumbar arteries and the inferior mesenteric artery. Endoleak is recognized by the accumulation of contrast medium in the aneurysm sac outside the stent graft. Contrast-enhanced MDCT performed during the arterial phase is the method of choice for detecting endoleaks, although some slow-filling side branch endoleaks may not be seen until a later phase after contrast medium injection. If the sac remains pressurized because of blood flow, it may enlarge and rupture.

Stenosis

Aortic stenosis, or narrowing of the aortic lumen, has many causes. It may be caused by coarctation or pseudocoarctation of the aorta, midaortic dysplastic syndrome, atherosclerosis, Takayasu arteritis, aortic dissection, various intra-aortic and periaortic diseases, or surgical aortic repair [116]. The impedance of blood flow through the stenotic segment may lead to the development of collateral arterial pathways that vary according to the location of stenosis [117]. The site of aortic stenosis varies according to the disease or condition that caused the stenosis. Stenosis of the proximal descending thoracic aorta is typical of congenital coarctation, stenosis of the thoracoabdominal aortic junction occurs in dysplastic midaortic syndrome, and stenosis of the abdominal aorta often is secondary to atherosclerosis [115]. In Takayasu arteritis—aortic dissection caused by intra-aortic and periaortic diseases or aortic stenosis—stenosis can occur in any part of the vessel. Thickening of the vessel wall in

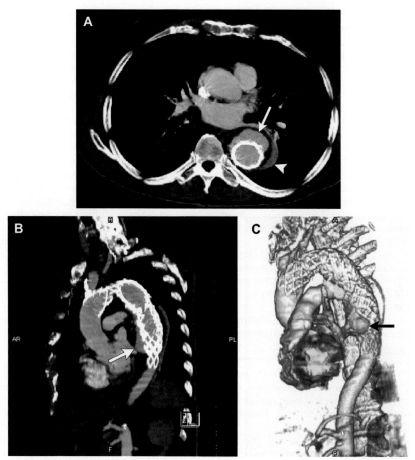

Fig. 19. Endoleak after endovascular aortic repair. (*A*) Axial CT image demonstrates an irregular isodensity around the circular stent within the descending thoracic aorta corresponding to the endoleak (*white arrow*). The native wall of aorta is thickened (*white arrowhead*), and the aorta is a little dilated. (*B*) Sagittal reformatted and (*C*) three-dimensional volume-rendered images also demonstrate the endoleak (*arrows*).

Takayasu arteritis is an early sign of the disease and leads to stenosis, thrombosis, and sometimes to aneurysm formation [118].

Summary

CTA has become a standard noninvasive imaging method for depicting vascular anatomy and pathology during the past decade. It is the most frequently used technique when multiple imaging is needed. The quality and speed of CTA is superior to that of other imaging modalities, and it is cheaper and less invasive. CTA of the aorta has proven to be superior to conventional arteriography in diagnostic accuracy in several applications. It allows three-dimensional visualization from any angle and in any direction. Proper imaging is of vital importance in diagnosing several cardiac anomalies, such as interrupted aortic arch, coarctation of the aorta, abdominal aortic aneurysm, aortic rupture, aortic

dissection, IMH, atherosclerotic arterial occlusive disease, and traumatic aortic injury. For example, in aortic dissection, an intimal flap that separates the true lumen from the false lumen is a typical finding on contrast CT scan. Accurate differentiation between the true and false lumen is important for placement of an endovascular stent. In traumatic aortic injury, multidetector CTA is useful for detecting complications of vascular emergencies of the aorta.

References

[1] Schoenhagen P, Halliburton SS, Stillman AE, et al. Non-invasive imaging of coronary arteries: current and future role of multidetector row CT. Radiology 2004;232:7–17.
[2] Lepor NE, Madyoon H, Friede G. The emerging use of 16- and 64-slice computed tomography coronary angiography in clinical cardiovascular practice. Rev Cardiovasc Med 2005;6:47–53.

[3] Flohr TG, Schoepf UJ, Kuettner A, et al. Advances in cardiac imaging with 16-section CT systems. Acad Radiol 2003;10:386–401.

[4] Kuettner A, Beck T, Drosch T, et al. Imaging quality and diagnostic accuracy of non-invasive coronary imaging with 16-detector slice spiral computed tomography with 188ms temporal resection. Heart 2005;91:938–41.

[5] Suzuki T, Mehta RH, Ince H, et al. Clinical profiles and outcomes of acute type B aortic dissection in the current Era: lessons from the International Registry of Aortic Dissection (IRAD). Circulation 2003;108:312–7.

[6] Wintersperger B, Jakobs T, Herzog P, et al. Aorto-iliac multidetector-row CT angiography with low kV settings: improved vessel enhancement and simultaneous reduction of the radiation dose. Eur Radiol 2005;15:334–41.

[7] Kalva SP, Sahani DV, Hahn PF, et al. Using the K-edge to improve contrast conspicuity and to lower radiation dose with a 16-MDCT: a phantom and human study. J Comput Assist Tomogr 2006;30:391–7.

[8] Strocchi S, Vite C, Callegari L, et al. Optimisation of multislice computed tomography protocols in angio-CT examinations. Radiol Med (Torino) 2006;111:238–44.

[9] Roos JE, Willmann JK, Weishaupt D, et al. Thoracic aorta: motion artifact reduction with retrospective and prospective electrocardiography-assisted multi-detector row CT. Radiology 2002;222:271–7.

[10] Yoshida S, Akiba H, Tamakawa M, et al. Thoracic involvement of type A aortic dissection and intramural hematoma: diagnostic accuracy—comparison of emergency helical CT and surgical findings. Radiology 2003;228:430–5.

[11] Hofmann LK, Kelly HZ, Philip C, et al. Electrocardiographically gated 16-section CT of the thorax: cardiac motion suppression. Radiology 2004;233:927–33.

[12] Morgan-Hughes GJ, Owens PE, Marshall AJ, et al. Thoracic aorta at multi-detector row CT: motion artifact with various reconstruction windows. Radiology 2003;228:583–8.

[13] Macari M, Israel GM, Berman P, et al. Infrarenal abdominal aortic aneurysms at multi-detector row CT angiography: intravascular enhancement without a timing acquisition. Radiology 2001;220:519–23.

[14] Shigeki I, Mitsuru I, Masataka A, et al. Multiphase contrast-enhanced CT of the liver with a multislice CT scanner: effects of iodine concentration and delivery rate. Radiat Med 2005;23(1):61–9.

[15] Bae KT, Tran HQ, Heiken JP. Uniform vascular contrast enhancement and reduced contrast medium volume achieved by using exponentially decelerated contrast material injection method. Radiology 2004;231:732–6.

[16] Brink JK. Contrast optimization and scan timing for single and multidetector-row computed tomography. J Comput Assist Tomogr 2003;27:s3–8.

[17] Feyter PJ, Krestin GP, editors. Computed tomography of the coronary arteries. Abingdon (UK): Taylor & Franics; 2005.

[18] Cademartiri F, Luccichenti G, Marano R, et al. Spiral CT-angiography with one, four, and sixteen slice scanners. Technical note. Radiol Med (Torino) 2003;106:269–83.

[19] Hopper KD, Mosher TJ, Kasales CJ, et al. Thoracic spiral CT: delivery of contrast material pushed with injectable saline solution in a power injector. Radiology 1997;205:269–71.

[20] Cademaritiri F, mollet N, van der Lugt A, et al. Non-invasive 16-row multislice coronary angiography: usefulness of saline chaser. Eur Radiol 2004;14:178–83.

[21] Tatsugami F, Matsuki M, Kani H, et al. Effect of saline pushing after contrast material injection in abdominal multidetector computed tomography with the use of different iodine concentrations. Acta Radiol 2006;47(2):192–7.

[22] Han JK, Kim AY, Lee KY, et al. Factors influencing vascular and hepatic enhancement at CT: experimental study on injection protocol using a canine model. J Comput Assist Tomogr 2000;24:400–6.

[23] Fenchel S, Fleiter TR, Aschoff AJ, et al. Effect of iodine concentration of contrast media on contrast enhancement in multislice CT of the pancreas. Br J Radiol 2004;77:821–30.

[24] Awai K, Hiraishi K, Hori Sl. Effect of contrast material injection duration and rate on aortic peak time and peak enhancement at dynamic CT involving injection protocol with dose tailored to patient weight. Radiology 2004;230:142–50.

[25] Thomas A, Bernhard M. New trends in multidetector computed tomography angiography of peripheral arteries. Advances in MDCT—an international literature review service. 2005;2(2):1–6.

[26] Cademartiri F, Nieman K, Lugt AV, et al. Intravenous contrast material administration at 16-detector row helical CT coronary angiography: test bolus versus bolus-tracking technique. Radiology 2004;233:817–23.

[27] Catalano C, Fraioli F, Laghi A, et al. Infrarenal aortic and lower-extremity arterial disease: diagnostic performance of multi-detector row CT angiography. Radiology 2004;231:555–63.

[28] Imai S, Tamada T, Gyoten M, et al. Iatrogenic venous air embolism caused by CT injector—from a risk management point of view. Radiat Med 2004;22:269–71.

[29] Goo HW, Park Is, Ko JK, et al. CT of congenital heart disease: normal anatomy and typical pathologic conditions. Radiographics 2003;23:S147–65.

[30] Ucerler H, Asli Aktan Ikiz Z. Multiplicity of the variations in ventral branches of abdominal aorta. Ital J Anat Embryol 2006;111(1):15–22.

[31] Van De Graaff. Human anatomy. 6th edition. New York: The McGraw–Hill Companies; 2001. p. 574–83.

[32] Kawano T, Ishii M, Takagi J, et al. Three-dimensional helical computed tomographic angiography in neonates and infants with complex heart disease. Am Heart J 2000;139:654–60.

[33] Moon Y, Kim YM, Kim TH, et al. Congenital anomalies of aortic arch: CT angiography. J Korean Radiol Soc 2001;44:51–8.

[34] Freedom RM, Mawson JB, Yoo SJ, et al. Congenital heart disease: textbook of angiocardiography. Armonk (NY): Futura; 1997.

[35] Didier D, Ratib O, Beghetti M, et al. Morphologic and functional evaluation of congenital heart disease by magnetic resonance imaging. J Magn Reson Imaging 1999;10:639–55.

[36] Roche KJ, Krinsky G, Lee VS, et al. Interrupted aortic arch: diagnosis with gadolinium-enhanced 3D MRA. J Comput Assist Tomogr 1999; 23:197–202.

[37] Haramati LB, Glickstein FS, Issenberg HF, et al. MR imaging and CT of vascular anomalies and connections in patients with congenital heart disease: significance in surgical planning. Radiographics 2002;22:337–49.

[38] Polson JW, McCallion N, Waki H, et al. Evidence for cardiovascular autonomic dysfunction in neonates with coarctation of the aorta. Circulation 2006;113:2844–50.

[39] Marx GR. "Repaired" aortic coarctation in adults: not a "simple" congenital heart defect. J Am Coll Cardiol 2000;35:1003–6.

[40] Kaminishi Y, Kono Y, Kato M, et al. Late pseudoaneurysm formation after patch angioplasty of coarctation of the aorta; report of a case. Kyobu Geka 2006;59:407–9.

[41] Hager A, Kaemmerer H, Rapp-Bernhardt U, et al. Diameters of the thoracic aorta throughout life as measured with helical computed tomography. J Thorac Cardiovasc Surg 2002;123:1060–6.

[42] Malloy PC, Richard HM 3rd. Thoracic angiography and intervention in trauma. Radiol Clin North Am 2006;44(2):239–49, viii.

[43] Gotway MB, Dawn SK. Thoracic aorta imaging with multislice CT. Radiol Clin North Am 2003;41(3):521–43.

[44] Mitchell RS, Dake MD, Sembra CP, et al. Endovascular stent-graft repair of thoracic aortic aneurysms. J Thorac Cardiovasc Surg 1996;111(5): 1054–62.

[45] Tatli S, Mortele KJ, Breen EL, et al. Local staging of rectal cancer using combined pelvic phased-array and endorectal coil MRI. J Magn Reson Imaging 2006;23(4):534–40.

[46] Elefteriades JA. Natural history of thoracic aortic aneurysms: indications for surgery, and surgical versus nonsurgical risks. Ann Thorac Surg 2002; 74:S1877–80 [discussion: S1892–8].

[47] Perko MJ, Norgaard M, Herzog TM, et al. Unoperated aortic aneurysm: a survey of 170 patients. Ann Thorac Surg 1995;59:1204–9.

[48] Crawford ES, DeNatale RW. Thoracoabdominal aortic aneurysm: observations regarding the natural course of the disease. J Vasc Surg 1986;3(4):578–82.

[49] Hello CL, Koskas F, Cluze LP, et al. French women from multiplex abdominal aortic aneurysm Families should be screened. Ann Surg 2005;242:739–44.

[50] Beebe HG, Kritpracha B. Screening and preoperative imaging of candidates for conventional repair of abdominal aortic aneurysm. Semin Vasc Surg 1999;12:300–5.

[51] Ashton HA, Buxton MJ, Day NE, et al. Multicentre Aneurysm Screening Study Group. Multicentre Aneurysm Screening Study (MASS) into the effect of abdominal aortic aneurysm screening on mortality in men: a randomized controlled trial. Lancet 2002;360:1531–9.

[52] Beard JD. Screening for abdominal aortic aneurysm. Br J Surg 2003;90:515–6.

[53] Fleming C, Whitlock EP, Beil TL, et al. Screening for abdominal aortic aneurysm: a best-evidence systematic review for the U.S. preventive services task force. Ann Intern Med 2005;142:203–11.

[54] Upchurch GR, Schaub TA. Abdominal aortic aneurysm. Am Fam Physician 2006;73:1198–204.

[55] Kapoor V, Kanal El, Fukui MB, et al. Vertebral mass resulting from a chronic-contained rupture of an abdominal aortic aneurysm repair graft. AJNR Am J Neuroradiol 2001;22:1775–7.

[56] Medina CR, Indes J, Smith C. Endovascular treatment of an abdominal aortic pseudoaneurysm as a late complication of inferior vena cava filter placement. J Vasc Surg 2006;43(6):1278–82.

[57] Palanichamy N, Gregoric ID, La Francesca S, et al. Mycotic pseudo-aneurysm of the ascending thoracic aorta after cardiac transplantation. J Heart Lung Transplant 2006;25(6):730–3.

[58] Kleinstreuer C, Li LH. Analysis and computer program for rupture-risk prediction of abdominal aortic aneurysms. Biomed Eng Online 2006;5:19.

[59] Ando M, Igari T, Yokoyama H, et al. CT features of chronic contained rupture of an abdominal aortic aneurysm. Ann Thorac Cardiovasc Surg 2003;9:274–8.

[60] Dorrucci V, Dusi R, Rombola G, et al. Contained rupture of an abdominal aortic aneurysm presenting as obstructive jaundice: report of a case. Surg Today 2001;31:331–2.

[61] Tuma MA, Hans SS. Rupture of abdominal aortic aneurysm with tear of inferior vena cava in a patient with prior endograft. J Vasc Surg 2002;35:798–800.

[62] Patel SN, Kettner NW. Abdominal aortic aneurysm presenting as back pain to a chiropractic clinic: a case report. J Manipulative Physiol Ther 2006;29(5):409, e1–7.

[63] Oderich GS, Panneton JM, Bower TC, et al. Infected aortic aneurysms: aggressive presentation, complicated early outcome, but durable results. J Vasc Surg 2001;34:900–8.

[64] Sungjin Oh, Young WY, Gil JJ, et al. Spontaneous disruption of mycotic aneurysm involving innominate artery. J Korean Med Sci 2003;18: 589–91.

[65] Gerber M, Immer FF, Do DD, et al. Endovascular stent-grafting for diseases of the descending thoracic aorta. Swiss Med Wkly 2003;133: 44–51.

[66] Drury D, Michaels JA, Jones L, et al. Systematic review of recent evidence for the safety and efficacy of elective endovascular repair in the management of infrarenal abdominal aortic aneurysm [review]. Br J Surg 2005;92(8): 937–46.

[67] Wolf YG, Tillich M, Lee WA, et al. Impact of aortoiliac tortuosity on endovascular repair of abdominal aortic aneurysms: evaluation of 3D computer-based assessment. J Vasc Surg 2001; 34:594–9.

[68] Kato K, Ishiguchi T, Maruyama K, et al. Accuracy of plastic replica of aortic aneurysm using 3D-CT data for transluminal stent-grafting: experimental and clinical evaluation. J Comput Assist Tomogr 2001;25:300–4.

[69] Whitaker SC. Imaging of abdominal aortic aneurysm before and after endoluminal stent-graft repair [review]. Eur J Radiol 2001;39(1):3–15.

[70] Fukuhara R, Ishiguchi T, Ikeda M, et al. Evaluation of abdominal aortic aneurysm for endovascular stent-grafting with volume-rendered CT images of vessel lumen and thrombus. Radiat Med 2004;22:332–41.

[71] Khan IA, Nair CK. Clinical diagnostic and management perspectives of aortic dissection. Chest 2002;122:311–28.

[72] Iyano K, Kawada T, Aiba M, et al. Correlation of hemostatic molecular markers and morphology of the residual false lumen in chronic aortic dissection. Ann Thorac Cardiovasc Surg 2004;10: 106–12.

[73] Shimazaki Y, Minowa T, Watanabe T, et al. Acute aortic dissection with new massive cerebral infarction—a successful repair with ligature of the right common carotid artery. Ann Thorac Cardiovasc Surg 2004;10:64–6.

[74] Daitoku K, Fukui K, Tamo W, et al. Emergency small-sized stent placement following aortic true lumen obliteration of Stanford type B acute aortic dissection. Kyobu Geka 2006;59:445–8.

[75] Xu SD, Huang FJ, Yang JF, et al. Endovascular repair of acute type B aortic dissection: early and mid-term results. J Vasc Surg 2006;43(6): 1090–5.

[76] Sueyoshi E, Sakamoto I, Hayashi K, et al. Growth rate of aortic diameter in patients with type B aortic dissection during the chronic phase. Circulation 2004;110(Suppl II):256–61.

[77] Hartnell GG, Gates J. Aortic fenestration: a why, when, and how-to guide. Radiographics 2005; 25(1):175–89.

[78] Eijun S, Ichiro S, Kuniaki H, et al. Growth rate of aortic diameter in patients with Type B aortic dissection during the chronic phase. Circulation 2004;110(Suppl 2):256–61.

[79] LePage M, Quint LE, Sonnad SS, et al. Aortic dissection: CT features that distinguish true lumen from false lumen. AJR Am J Roentgenol 2001;177:207–11.

[80] Choi SH, Choi SJ, Kim JH, et al. Useful CT findings for predicting the progression of aortic intramural hematoma to overt aortic dissection. J Comput Assist Tomogr 2001;25:295–9.

[81] Rerkpattanapipat P, Jacobs LE, Makornwattana P, et al. Meta-analysis of 143 reported cases of aortic intramural hematoma. Am J Cardiol 2000;86: 664–8.

[82] Song JK, Kim HS, Kang DH, et al. Different clinical features of aortic intramural hematoma versus dissection involving the ascending aorta. J Am Coll Cardiol 2001;37:1604–10.

[83] Ganaha n, Fumikiyo n, Miller n, et al. Prognosis of aortic intramural hematoma with and without penetrating atherosclerotic ulcer: a clinical and radiological analysis. Circulation 2002; 106:342–8.

[84] Sueyoshi E, Sakamoto I, Uetani, et al. MCT analysis of the growth rate of aortic diameter affected by acute type B intramural hematoma. AJR Am J Roentgenol 2006;186(6 Suppl 2): S414–20.

[85] Quint LE, Williams DM, Francis IR, et al. Ulcer-like lesions of the aorta: imaging features and natural history. Radiology 2001;218:719–23.

[86] Sueyoshi E, Matsuoka Y, Imada T, et al. New development of an ulcerlike projection in aortic intramural hematoma: CT evaluation. Radiology 2002;224:536–41.

[87] Welty FK. Cardiovascular disease and dyslipidemia in women. Arch Intern Med 2001;161: 514–22.

[88] Casella G, Greco C, Perugini E, et al. [Atheromatosis of the thoracic aorta and risk of stroke]. G Ital Cardiol (Rome) 2006;7(5):309–16 [in Italian].

[89] Petty GW, Khandheria BK, Meissner I, et al. Population-based study of the relationship between atherosclerotic aortic debris and cerebrovascular ischemic events. Mayo Clin Proc 2006; 81(5):609–14.

[90] Castañer Eva, Andreu M, Gallardo X, et al. CT in nontraumatic acute thoracic aortic disease: typical and atypical features and complications. Radiographics 2003;23:S93–110.

[91] Tatsumi M, Cohade C, Nakamoto Y, et al. Fluorodeoxyglucose uptake in the aortic wall at PET/CT: possible finding for active atherosclerosis. Radiology 2003;229:831–7.

[92] Hayashi H, Matsuoka Y, Sakamoto I, et al. Penetrating atherosclerotic ulcer of the aorta: imaging features and disease concept. Radiographics 2000;20:995–1005.

[93] Bruckner BA, DiBardino DJ, Cumbie TC, et al. Critical evaluation of chest computed tomography scans for blunt descending thoracic

aortic injury. Ann Thorac Surg 2006;81(4): 1339–46.

[94] Trerotola SO. Can helical CT replace aortography in thoracic trauma. Radiology 1995;197: 13–5.

[95] Alkadhi H, Wildermuth S, Desbiolles L, et al. Vascular emergencies of the thorax after blunt and iatrogenic trauma: multi-detector row CT and three-dimensional imaging. Radiographics 2004;24:1239–55.

[96] Kuhlman JE, Pozniak MA, Collins J, et al. Radiographic and CT findings of blunt chest trauma: aortic injuries and looking beyond them. Radiographics 1998;18:1085–106.

[97] Wintermark M, Wicky S, Schnyder P. Imaging of acute traumatic injuries of the thoracic aorta. Eur Radiol 2002;12:431–42.

[98] Macura KJ, Corl FM, Fishman EK, et al. Pathogenesis in acute aortic syndromes: aortic aneurysm leak and rupture and traumatic aortic transection. AJR Am J Roentgenol 2003;181: 303–7.

[99] Richens D, Field M, Neale M, et al. The mechanism of injury in blunt traumatic rupture of the aorta. Eur J Cardiothorac Surg 2002;21:288–93.

[100] Crestanello JA, Zehr KJ, Mullany CJ, et al. The effect of adjuvant perfusion techniques on the incidence of paraplegia after repair of traumatic thoracic aortic transections. Mayo Clin Proc 2006;81(5):625–30.

[101] Mimasaka S, Yajima Y, Hashiyada M, et al. A case of aortic dissection caused by blunt chest trauma. Forensic Sci Int 2003;132:5–8.

[102] Bashar AH, Kazui T, Washiyama N, et al. Stanford type A aortic dissection after blunt chest trauma: case report with a reflection on the mechanism of injury. J Trauma 2002;52:380–1.

[103] Yokoyama S, Maeda Y, Maisawa K, et al. Ascending aortic dissection associated with pulmonary contusion caused by blunt trauma. Kyobu Geka 2006;59(5):383–6.

[104] Vilacosta I, Roman JA. Acute aortic syndrome. Heart 2001;85:365–8.

[105] Macura KJ, Corl FM, Fishman EK, et al. Pathogenesis in acute aortic syndromes: aortic dissection, intramural hematoma, and penetrating atherosclerotic aortic ulcer. AJR Am J Roentgenol 2003;181:309–16.

[106] Dyer DS, Moore EE, Ilke DN, et al. Thoracic aortic injury: how predictive is mechanism and is chest-computed tomography a reliable screening tool? A prospective study of 1,561 patients. J Trauma 2000;48:673–82 [discussion: 682–3].

[107] Wong H, Gotway MB, Sasson AD, et al. Periaortic hematoma at diaphragmatic crura at helical CT: sign of blunt aortic injury in patients with mediastinal hematoma. Radiology 2004; 231:185–9.

[108] Fattori R, Napoli G, Lovato L, et al. Descending thoracic aortic diseases: stent-graft repair. Radiology 2003;229:176–83.

[109] Lawlor Dk, Michael O, Thomas LF, et al. Endovascular management of traumatic thoracic aortic injuries. Can J Surg 2005;48(4):293–7.

[110] Fu WG, Dong ZH, Wang YQ, et al. Strategies for the insufficiency of the proximal landing zoom during endovascular thoracic aortic repair. Chin Med J (Engl) 2005;118(13):1066–71.

[111] Kern JA, Matsumoto AH, Tribble CG, et al. Thoracic aortic endografting is the treatment of choice for elderly patients with thoracic aortic disease. Ann Surg 2006;243(6):815–20 [discussion: 820–3].

[112] Bethuyne N, Bove T, Van den Brande P, et al. Acute retrograde aortic dissection during endovascular repair of a thoracic aortic aneurysm. Ann Thorac Surg 2003;75:1967–9.

[113] Kato N, Hirano T, Kawaguchi T, et al. Aneurysmal degeneration of the aorta after stent-graft repair of acute aortic dissection. J Vasc Surg 2001;34:513–8.

[114] Chen FH, Shim WH, Chang BC, et al. False aneurysms at both ends of a descending thoracic aortic stent-graft: complication after endovascular repair of a penetrating atherosclerotic ulcer. J Endovasc Ther 2003;10:249–53.

[115] Mestres G, Maeso J, Fernandez V, et al. Symptomatic collapse of a thoracic aorta endoprosthesis. J Vasc Surg 2006;43(6):1270–3.

[116] Carmen Sebastia, Sergi Quiroga, Rosa Boye', et al. Aortic stenosis: spectrum of diseases depicted at multisection CT. Radiographics 2003; 23:S79–91.

[117] Yurdakul M, Tola M, Ozdemir E, et al. Internal thoracic artery-inferior epigastric artery as a collateral pathway in aortoiliac occlusive disease. J Vasc Surg 2006;43(4):707–13.

[118] Quemeneur T, Hachulla E, Lambert M, et al. Takayasu arteritis. Presse Med 2006;35(5 Pt 2): 847–56.

ELSEVIER
SAUNDERS

RADIOLOGIC
CLINICS
OF NORTH AMERICA

Radiol Clin N Am 45 (2007) 485–497

MR Imaging of the Aorta

Ichiro Sakamoto, MD*, Eijun Sueyoshi, MD, Masataka Uetani, MD

- Comparison with CT
- Basic technical considerations
  Black-blood vascular imaging
  Bright-blood vascular imaging
  Contrast-enhanced MR angiography
- Aortic disease

- *Aortic aneurysm*
- *Aortic dissection*
- *Intramural hematoma*
- *Penetrating atherosclerotic ulcer*
- *Takayasu arteritis*
- References

Acquired disease of the aorta is widespread. In the past invasive angiography was required to depict structural abnormalities. Recent advances in noninvasive imaging methods, such as CT and MR imaging, have replaced most of invasive angiographic procedures, thus decreasing the cost and morbidity of diagnosis [1–8]. With its ability to delineate the intrinsic contrast between blood flow and vessel wall and to acquire images in multiple planes, MR imaging provides a high degree of reliability in the diagnosis of aortic diseases. Because of its noninvasive nature, MR imaging can be performed repeatedly, allowing the progression of the aortic disease to be evaluated over time. This article reviews and illustrates present MR imaging methods for evaluation of the aorta. Common diseases of the aorta also are discussed with a focus on their unique morphologic and functional features and characteristic MR imaging findings. Knowledge of pathologic conditions of common aortic diseases and proper MR imaging techniques enables accurate and time-efficient aortic evaluation.

Nevertheless, MR imaging has several distinct advantages over CT. First, MR imaging does not require the use of ionizing radiation. Because of the lack of radiation, MR imaging can be performed for repeatedly the follow-up of the patient without concern for radiation exposure. Second, unlike CT angiography, MR angiography dose not require the use of nephrotoxic iodinated contrast material. Nephrotoxicity is a particularly relevant issue, because patients who have acquired aortic disease frequently suffer from renal insufficiency. In particular, MR angiography has advantages for patients undergoing endovascular treatment. Preprocedural planning using MR angiography excludes concerns related to iodine load and impaired renal function, thus enabling same-day or close performance of endovascular treatment [7]. Finally, cine MR imaging can be performed for dynamic evaluation of blood flow without using contrast material. Particularly, cine phase-contrast (cine PC) imaging can be used to determine flow velocity and direction. These cine MR techniques can be used to evaluate valvular and cardiac function.

Comparison with CT

Compared with MR angiography, CT angiography has the advantages of general availability and ease of performance, especially in urgent cases.

Basic technical considerations

Several different MR imaging techniques are used to depict the arteries. These techniques include

Department of Radiology and Radiation Biology, Nagasaki University Graduate School of Biomedical Sciences, 1-7-1 Sakamoto, Nagasaki 852-8501, Japan
* Corresponding author.
E-mail address: ichiro-s@net.nagasaki-u.ac.jp (I. Sakamoto).

doi:10.1016/j.rcl.2007.04.007

black-blood imaging (conventional spin echo, fast spin echo), bright-blood imaging (time-of-flight imaging, PC imaging), and contrast-enhanced MR angiography. Recent advances in fast imaging, such as steady state free precession (SSFP) and subsecond contrast-enhanced MR angiography, enable quick examinations for initial screening evaluations of the aorta within several minutes. These improvements in MR technology and the aforementioned advantages of MR imaging over CT evaluation have increased the role of MR angiography, even in the evaluation of some acute conditions.

Black-blood vascular imaging

The aorta can be well illustrated using black blood methods, namely, ECG-gated spin echo or fast spin echo, that exploit the inherent contrast between rapidly flowing blood and the aortic wall [7,9–12]. Unlike bright blood imaging, luminal signal void occurs because of the movement of spins and dephasing of turbulent flow. Spin echo imaging still constitutes the basis of any aortic study because this technique provides the best anatomic details of the aortic wall and pathologic conditions. Usually, a conventional study of the aorta in the axial plane is acquired first to display the orientation of the great arteries and to visualize mural lesions optimally perpendicular to their long axes. A main consideration in spin echo imaging is that each section corresponds to a different cardiac phase. Diastolic slow flow and entry or exit slice phenomena may produce high signal in the aortic lumen, which is difficult to differentiate from mural thrombus. Usually, T2-weighted imaging is of little usefulness in the study of the aorta because the low signal-to-noise ratio and the long acquisition time affect the image quality, mainly through motion artifact. With spin echo imaging the aortic caliber and also the vessel wall and perivascular tructures can be evaluated. Wall thickness can be demonstrated readily on T1-weighted imaging, and edema is seen as hyperintense intramural signal on T2-weighted imaging. Mural hyperenhancement of the vessel wall on T1-weighted images after injection of contrast material is considered to indicate active inflammation. ECG-gated double inversion recovery fast spin echo is a more recent black-blood method that allows breathhold acquisition [13]. By applying a nonselective inversion pulse followed by a section-selective inversion pulse, double inversion recovery fast spin echo provides better suppression of the signal from flowing blood (Fig. 1). This technique, however, is substantially less efficient in terms of scan time than fast spin echo technique because it is a sequential-slice imaging sequence.

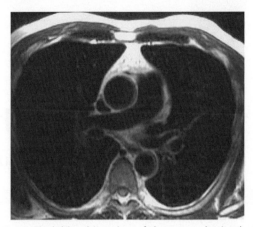

Fig. 1. Black-blood imaging of the aorta obtained at the level of the right pulmonary artery. Note the excellent suppression of the luminal blood signal and demonstration of the vessel wall. The image was obtained in 12 seconds with cardiac gating and breathholding.

Bright-blood vascular imaging

Several bright-blood techniques can be performed without the need for contrast agents [7,14–17]. One of the oldest techniques is the time-of-flight (TOF) effect, which is based on the phenomenon of flow-related enhancement of spins entering into a partially saturated imaging section. These unsaturated spins give more signal than surrounding stationary spins. With the two-dimensional (2D) technique, multiple thin, sequential sections are acquired by using a flow-compensated gradient echo (GRE) sequence. The acquired sections are viewed individually or are reformatted with the maximum intensity projection (MIP) technique to obtain a three-dimensional (3D) image. TOF imaging has several limitations [18,19]: (1) complex flow pattern producing loss of signal caused by intravoxel dephasing may mimic disease; (2) vessels not perpendicular to the acquired section plane may cause low signal intensity; (3) retrograde flow in collateral vessels may be saturated also, obscuring the true level of steno-occlusive lesions. Although arterial signal can be improved with cardiac gating, imaging times become long, and arterial signal on TOF MR angiography often remains inhomogeneous and unreliable for proper depiction of the aorta and its branches. Because of the long imaging times and aforementioned limitations, TOF imaging is being replaced rapidly with contrast-enhanced MR angiography.

The TOF effect can be useful when acquired in a 2D cine mode, for example, cine gradient echo (cine GRE) [7]. Cine GRE images are acquired with ECG gating, thus resulting in high temporal resolution throughout the cardiac cycle, and can be displayed in cine format. The recently introduced SSFP (commercially known as "true fast imaging with steady precession (FISP)," "fast imaging employing steady state acquisition (FIESTA)," or "balanced fast field echo (FFE)" technique, with shorter TE and TR sequences, has become more widely available [16,17]. On SSFP, intraluminal signal generally is very high and homogenous even in cases of turbulent flow because this sequence depends mainly on a function of the T2/T1 ratio. Hence, in urgent situations, SSFP can be used to demonstrate quickly aortic abnormalities such as an intimal flap and a false lumen in aortic dissection.

One critical advantage of flow-based bright-blood techniques is the ability to perform a functional assessment of blood flow [7,20,21]. On cine GRE, turbulent flow produces rapid spin dephasing and results in flow jets extending distal to or downstream from the lesion, thus providing additional information in many pathologic conditions such as coarctation of the aorta, aortic valve insufficiency, and aortic dissection. Particularly in aortic dissection, the detection of entry and reentry sites is a special capability of this method that can be helpful in planning surgical and endovascular treatment. With the use of newer fast GRE pulse sequences with an ultrashort TR and TE, a flow jet may not be present despite the presence of a significant flow disturbance. The very short TE times may be insufficient for a sizable flow jet to form on this faster sequence. In cases of high suspicion, standard GRE sequences can be performed during free breathing (Fig. 2) [7]. The longer TE will allow

intravoxel dephasing to develop, and a flow jet should be seen if flow is turbulent.

Cine PC is another bright-blood technique that can be used for dynamic evaluation of blood flow [7,22,23]. Cine PC depends on the phase shifts that flowing protons experience as they travel along the gradient field. The data obtained with cine PC are processed into two sets of images: magnitude and phase-contrast. PC images display the direction of flow as bright or dark pixels, with their relative signal intensity representing their velocity. Hence, PC images can be used to assess flow direction, which may be important information for proper identification of a vascular structure or for quantifying blood flow.

Contrast-enhanced MR angiography

Contrast-enhanced MR angiography, which first was described for imaging of aortoiliac disease in 1993, is the most widely accepted method for comprehensive evaluation of the aortic disease [18,24–26]. This technique can provide images that have high spatial resolution with a single breathhold and therefore is suitable for the depiction of aortic abnormalities such as aneurysm, dissection, penetrating atherosclerotic ulcer, and Takayasu arteritis.

Contrast-enhanced MR angiography uses the T1-shortening effect of a gadolinium-based contrast agent. By using a gadolinium chelate contrast agent, the T1 of blood is shortened so that the blood appears bright irrespective of flow patterns or velocities. Because signal enhancement and overall image quality of contrast-enhanced MR angiography depend on the intra-arterial concentration of the

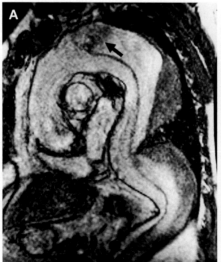 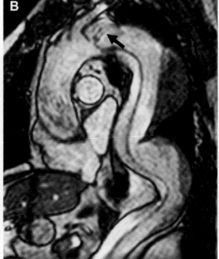

Fig. 2. Cine MR imaging in a patient who has aortic dissection. (*A*) Sagittal cine MR imaging obtained with standard GRE pulse sequence and during free breathing more clearly reveals a flow jet (*arrows*) through the entry than (*B*) that obtained with SSFP sequence and during breathholding.

contrast agent, the correct timing of imaging after contrast material injection is crucial. Because image contrast depends mainly on central k-space data, collection of the central lines of k space during the plateau phase of arterial enhancement is essential for optimal contrast-enhanced MR angiography [27]. The authors use 10 to 20 mL of contrast material delivered at a rate of 2 to 3 mL/s followed by 20 mL of saline solution delivered at the same rate. The dosage and delivery rate of the contrast material should be adjusted in individual patients, with special attention to the acquisition time. Several methods are used to determine the optimal delay between the start of intravenous contrast material injection and the start of image acquisition. Timing methods commonly used include injection of a test bolus using a small amount of contrast material, automatic triggering, and MR fluoroscopy [28–30].

Imaging interpretation usually is done with the aid of a computer workstation on which individual source images are analyzed and postprocessing techniques, such as multiplanar volume reformation, MIP reformation, and volume rendering of the images, are performed. MIP images, in particular, can be obtained quickly, resemble catheter angiograms, and permit a 3D appreciation of anatomy (Fig. 3).

Aortic disease

Aortic aneurysm

An aortic aneurysm is defined as a localized or diffuse dilatation involving all layers of the aortic wall

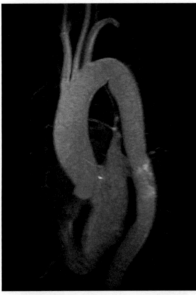

Fig. 3. 3D contrast-enhanced MR angiography of the thoracic aorta. Oblique sagittal MIP image clearly depicts the entire thoracic aorta and branch vessels from the aortic arch.

and exceeding the expected aortic diameter by a factor of 1.5 or more [11]. Most thoracic and abdominal aneurysms are atherosclerotic in nature. Other causes of aortic aneurysms include infection, inflammation, syphilis, and cystic medial necrosis. Atherosclerotic aneurysms usually are fusiform, although saccular aneurysms are encountered occasionally.

The major goal in imaging an aortic aneurysm is the exact evaluation of the maximal diameter, the length, and involvement of major branch vessels [31]. All these features can be identified and characterized with MR imaging. Additionally, because the measurements are reproducible, MR imaging frequently can be used as a follow-up tool for monitoring the progression of disease. To obtain consistent results, vessel dimensions should be measured at the same anatomic locations on two subsequent examinations. Use of the sagittal or oblique sagittal plane allows accurate assessment of the location and extent of the aneurysm and avoids partial volume effects. 3D contrast-enhanced MR angiography is most suitable for depicting the location, extent, and exact diameter. This technique can provide precise topographic information concerning the extent of an aneurysm and its relationship to the aortic branches [24,26,32,33]. Although the resolution of contrast-enhanced MR angiography remains lower than that of multidetector CT, this technique is useful, especially in patients who have contraindications to iodinated contrast material. It is essential to recognize that measurement should be obtained from source images where the vessel wall is visible, because MIP images represent a cast of the lumen alone (Fig. 4). Standard spin echo images also are helpful in evaluating changes in the aortic wall and periaortic structures. Area of high signal intensity on spin echo images within the thrombus and aortic wall may indicate instability of the aneurysm (Figs. 5 and 6) [8]. Aneurysms caused by a bacterial infection result in fragility of the vessel wall, thus causing saccular outpouching that most commonly involves the suprarenal portion of the aorta. In this condition, MR imaging can demonstrate the aneurysm itself and also wall thickening and periaortic abscess (Fig. 7) [34,35]. Inflammatory abdominal aortic aneurysm is a variant of atherosclerotic aneurysm, characterized by inflammatory and/or fibrotic changes in the periaortic lesions. In this condition, MR imaging shows homogenous periaortic tissue with sparing of the posterior aspect of the aorta. This periaortic tissue shows variable enhancement after injection of contrast material, based on the degree of inflammation and fibrosis (Fig. 8) [36,37]. Reduction in the thickness of periaortic tissue after surgical repair or endovascular stent grafting is seen occasionally.

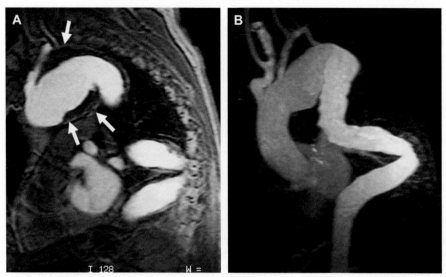

Fig. 4. 3D contrast-enhanced MR angiography in a patient with aortic arch aneurysm. (*A*) Source image of 3D contrast-enhanced MR angiography more clearly depicts involvement of the left subclavian artery by an aortic arch aneurysm than (*B*) the MIP image. Arrows in panel A indicates the aortic arch aneurysm with mural thrombus. As described in this article, in aneurysms with a large volume of mural thrombus, accurate evaluation of the branch vessel involvement by the aneurysm is difficult or impossible by MIP images alone.

If an aneurysm involves the ascending aorta or sinuses of Valsalva, concomitant aortic valve disease can be evaluated using cine MR technique. As described in the literature, the ability of contrast MR angiography to visualize the Adamkiewicz artery provides information that is important in planning the surgical repair of an aneurysm, thus avoiding postoperative neurologic deficit secondary to spinal cord ischemia [38,39].

Aortic dissection

Aortic dissection is a life-threatening condition requiring prompt diagnosis and treatment. This condition occurs when blood dissects into the media of the aortic wall through an intimal tear. Classification of aortic dissections has been based traditionally on anatomic location (Stanford or DeBakey classification) and time from onset. The 14-day period after onset has been designated as the acute

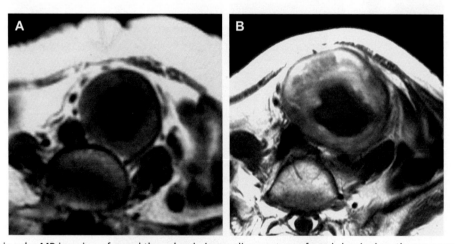

Fig. 5. Spin echo MR imaging of mural thrombus in impending rupture of an abdominal aortic aneurysm. (*A*) T1-weighted spin echo MR image obtained 24 months before impending rupture shows infrarenal abdominal aortic aneurysm with mural thrombus of homogenous low intensity. (*B*) T1-weighted spin echo MR image obtained at the time of impending rupture reveals an interval enlargement of the abdominal aortic aneurysm. A partial area of high signal intensity is also noted within the mural thrombus. In this case, a small amount of periaortic hemorrhage and hemorrhage into the mural thrombus were found at surgery.

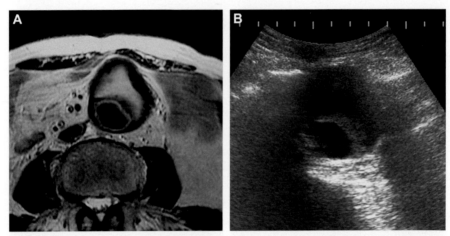

Fig. 6. Spin echo MR imaging of liquefactive thrombus in abdominal aortic aneurysm. (A) Most of mural thrombus is markedly high in signal intensity on T2-weighted spin echo images. (B) The area of high signal intensity in the mural thrombus is anechoic on ultrasound, indicating liquefaction of the thrombus.

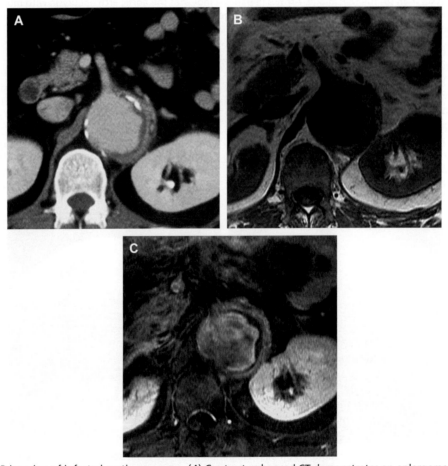

Fig. 7. MR imaging of infected aortic aneurysm. (A) Contrast-enhanced CT demonstrates an enlargement of the suprarenal abdominal aorta with a small amount of periaortic tissue adjacent to anterior to left lateral aspect of the aorta. Hyperenhancement of the periaortic tissue is also noted. T1-weighted spin echo MR images (B) before and (C) after injection of contrast material show the suprarenal abdominal aortic aneurysm with inhomogeneous hyperenhancement of the periaortic tissue.

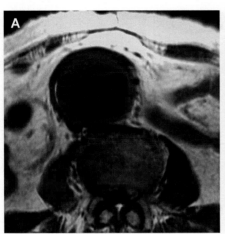 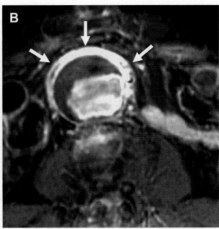

Fig. 8. MR imaging of inflammatory abdominal aortic aneurysm. (*A*) T1-weighted spin echo MR image shows infrarenal abdominal aortic aneurysm and periaortic tissue with sparing of posterolateral aspect of the aorta. (*B*) T1-weighted spin echo MR image after contrast material injection shows homogenous hyperenhancement of the periaortic tissue (*arrows*), indicating periaortic fibrosis and inflammation.

phase, because morbidity and mortality rates are highest (15%–25%), and surviving patients typically stabilize during this period. The Stanford classification simply distinguishes aortic dissection, irrespective of the site of the entry tear, into type A if the ascending aorta is involved or type B if the ascending aorta is spared. This classification is based fundamentally on prognostic factors: type A dissection necessitates urgent surgical repair, but most type B dissections can be managed conservatively. Hence, accurate recognition of anatomic details of the dissection with imaging is essential for successful management [40].

In dissection, the diagnostic goals of imaging are a clear anatomic delineation of the intimal flap and its extension and the detection of the entry and re-entry sites and branch vessel involvement. With current technology, MR imaging is the most accurate tool for detection of these features of the dissection. High spatial and contrast resolution and multiplanar acquisition provide excellent sensitivity and specificity of the disease and functional information with a totally noninvasive approach. In a patient suspected of having aortic dissection, the MR imaging examination usually begins with spin echo black-blood sequences that depict the intimal flap as a linear structure (Fig. 9). The true lumen can be differentiated from the false lumen because the true lumen shows a signal void, whereas the false lumen shows higher signal intensity indicative of turbulent flow [41]. High signal intensity of pericardial effusion indicates a bloody component and is considered a sign of impending rupture of the ascending aorta into the pericardial space.

In stable patients, adjunctive GRE sequences or PC images can be performed to identify aortic insufficiency and intimal tear sites and to differentiate slow flow from thrombus in the false lumen (see Fig. 9). Further diagnostic refinement has been reported by gadolinium-enhanced 3D MR angiography in the diagnosis of aortic dissection and definition of its anatomic details [42]. Because 3D MR angiography is acquired rapidly without the need of ECG triggering, this technique can be performed even in severely ill patients. The lack of nephrotoxicity and other adverse effects enables the use of gadolinium in patients who have renal failure or low cardiac output. The analysis of gadolinium-enhanced 3D MR angiography should not be restricted to viewing MIP images, because MIP images occasionally fail to show the intimal flap (Fig. 10). Hence, it also should include a complete evaluation of reformatted images in all three planes to confirm or improve spin echo information and exclude artifacts. Combining the spin echo images with gadolinium-enhanced 3D MR angiography images completes the diagnosis and anatomic definition [43].

Intramural hematoma

Intramural hematoma is an atypical form of dissection without flow in the false lumen or a discrete intraluminal flap [44,45]. Intramural hematoma usually results from spontaneous rupture of the aortic wall vasa vasorum or from a penetrating atherosclerotic ulcer. Because the clinical signs and symptoms and the prognosis of this condition do not differ from classic aortic dissection, its standard

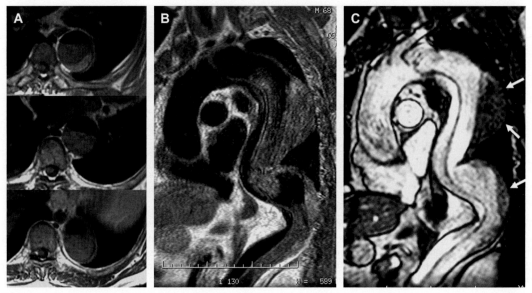

Fig. 9. MR imaging of aortic dissection. (*A*) Axial and (*B*) oblique sagittal spin echo images of type B dissection show a linear structure in the descending thoracic aorta, indicating the dissection flap. The true lumen is narrowed by compression of a dilated false lumen. Note the higher signal intensity in the false lumen, indicating turbulent flow and/or thrombus in the false lumen. Turbulent flow in the false lumen cannot be differentiated from thrombus using spin echo techniques alone. (*C*) On oblique sagittal cine MR imaging with SSFP technique, flowing blood in the false and true lumens is visualized as high intensity and partial thrombus in the false lumen as low intensity (*arrows*).

treatment is considered to be similar to that of classic aortic dissection [44]. Complete resolution of the aortic hematoma is seen occasionally, but complications such as fluid extravasation with pericardial, pleural, and periaortic hematoma or aortic rupture may occur at the time of the onset or during the follow-up period.

Intramural hematoma can be identified as crescentic thickening of the aortic wall with abnormal signal intensity. Because of the short T1 relaxation time of fresh blood, differentiation from the adjacent mediastinal fat may be difficult. In such circumstances, precontrast fat saturation images can be helpful in differentiating intramural hematoma

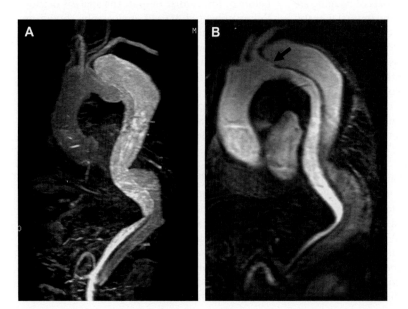

Fig. 10. 3D contrast-enhanced MR angiography of aortic dissection. (*A*) The anatomic details of the dissected aorta are difficult to recognize on the MIP image of 3D contrast-enhanced MR angiography alone. (*B*) Oblique sagittal reformatted image clearly depicts the intimal flap and also the entry site (*arrow*).

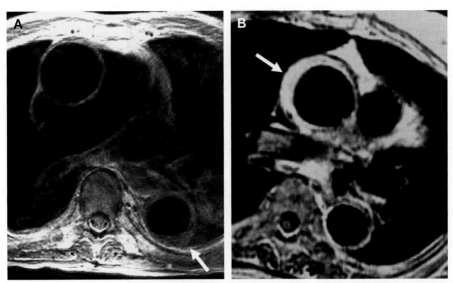

Fig. 11. Spin echo MR imaging of intramural hematoma. (*A*) On a T1-weighted spin echo MR image obtained 2 days after the onset, intramural hematoma of the descending thoracic aorta shows intermediate signal intensity (*arrow*) caused by the presence of oxyhemoglobin (acute stage). (*B*) In another patient, in a T1-weighted spin echo MR image obtained 40 days after the onset, an intramural hematoma of the ascending thoracic aorta shows high signal intensity (*arrow*) caused by the presence of methemoglobin (subacute stage).

from surrounding mediastinal fat. Moreover, MR imaging may allow the assessment of the age of hematoma on the basis of the different degradation products of hemoglobin. T1-weighted spin echo MR imaging may show intermediate signal intensity caused by the presence of oxyhemoglobin in the acute stage and high signal intensity caused by the presence of methemoglobin in the subacute stage (Fig. 11) [8,46]. The progression of intramural hematoma to overt dissection and rupture has been reported in 32% of the cases, particularly when the ascending aorta is involved.

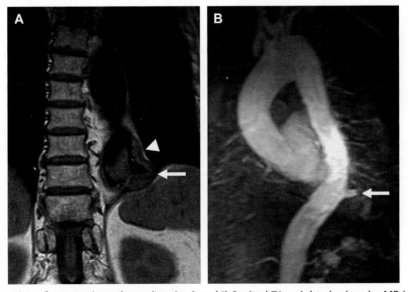

Fig. 12. MR imaging of penetrating atherosclerotic ulcer. (*A*) Sagittal T1-weighted spin echo MR image and (*B*) MIP image of 3D contrast-enhanced MR angiography clearly depict a penetrating atherosclerotic ulcer in the midportion of the descending thoracic aorta (*arrow*). Note mural thickening with intermediate signal intensity (*arrowhead* in A) indicating the formation of intramural hematoma.

A　　　　　**B**

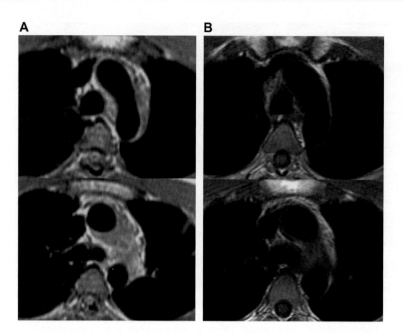

Fig. 13. Improvement of aortic wall thickening in early-phase Takayasu arteritis. T1-weighted spin echo MR images obtained (*A*) before and (*B*) after steroid therapy demonstrate marked reduction of the aortic wall thickening after the therapy.

Penetrating atherosclerotic ulcer

Penetrating atherosclerotic ulcer is characterized by ulceration of an atherosclerotic plaque that disrupts the intima [47,48]. The ulcerated atheroma may extend into the media, resulting in an intramural hematoma, or it may penetrate through the media and form a saccular pseudoaneurysm with the risk of transmural aortic rupture. Penetrating atherosclerotic ulcer usually affects elderly individuals who have hypertension and extensive aortic atherosclerosis. It typically is located in the descending aorta, but locations in the aortic arch or in the abdominal aorta have been reported occasionally. Penetrating atherosclerotic ulcer should be considered a distinct entity with different management and prognosis, although clinical features of this condition may be similar to those of aortic dissection. Persistent pain, hemodynamic instability, and signs of expansion are indications for surgical treatment, but asymptomatic patients can be managed medically and followed up with imaging. The diagnostic MR imaging finding in penetrating atherosclerotic ulcer is a craterlike outpouching extending beyond the contour of the aortic lumen [48–50]. Mural thickening with high or intermediate signal intensity on spin echo sequences indicates the formation of intramural hematoma. On MR angiography, the penetrating atherosclerotic ulcer is recognized readily as a contrast-filled outpouching with a jagged edge (Fig. 12). The disadvantage of MR imaging, compared with CT, is its inability to visualize dislodgment of intimal calcification, frequently seen in penetrating atherosclerotic ulcer.

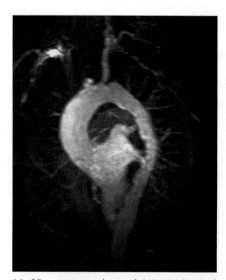

Fig. 14. 3D contrast-enhanced MR angiography of late-phase Takayasu arteritis. MIP image of 3D contrast-enhanced MR angiography shows occlusion of the right brachiocephalic and right common carotid arteries and mild stenosis of the orifice of the left subclavian artery. Note the irregular and diffuse narrowing of the proximal segment of the thoracic descending aorta.

Takayasu arteritis

Takayasu arteritis is an idiopathic large vessel vasculitis affecting the aorta and its major branches as well as pulmonary arteries. The cause of Takayasu arteritis is still unknown, although an autoimmune

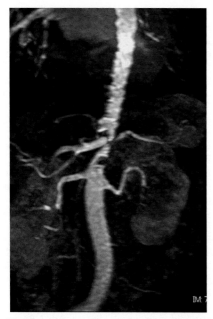

Fig. 15. 3D contrast-enhanced MR angiography of late-phase Takayasu arteritis. MIP image of 3D contrast-enhanced MR angiography shows marked and irregular narrowing of the abdominal aorta. This stenosing type of late-phase Takayasu arteritis is known as "atypical coarctation of the aorta."

mechanism has been suspected. The arteritis is most common in Japan and other Asian countries, although it now is known worldwide. Women are affected about 10 times more often than men. Young women are particularly susceptible to the disease. Steno-occlusive lesions are characteristics of this disorder, but dilated forms are also common. Fever, malaise, easy fatigability, weakness of the upper extremity, dizziness, headache, and syncope are the symptoms frequently mentioned.

There are many synonyms including "aortitis syndrome," "aortic arch syndrome," "pulseless disease," and "young female arteritis."

Angiography used to be the reference standard for delineating the vascular abnormalities, but CT and MR imaging now are considered to be alternative noninvasive techniques [51–53]. In fact, they provide more information about vascular changes in Takayasu arteritis. In particular, the thickness of the vessel wall is better demonstrated by these new modalities. MR imaging provides direct imaging in the axial, sagittal, and coronal planes, with good contrast resolution between the arterial lumen and its wall without use of contrast material.

The significant finding of acute-phase Takayasu arteritis is wall thickening of the aorta and its branches and the pulmonary arteries, which can be visualized better with multisectional scanning by MR imaging. Wall thickening of the vertically positioned aorta can be seen best on axial images; the horizontal portion of the right pulmonary artery can be evaluated best in the coronal and sagittal planes. Dramatic reduction of wall thickening in the aorta and pulmonary artery following steroid therapy may be documented by MR imaging (Fig. 13) [54].

In the late occlusive phase, 3D contrast-enhanced MR angiography can reveal short- or long-segment stenoses in the descending thoracic and abdominal aorta and major branch vessels (Fig. 14). The stenosing variety of late-phase Takayasu arteritis is known as "atypical coarctation of the aorta" (Fig. 15). Pulmonary arterial involvement (which as an incidence of approximately 70%) can also be depicted by 3D contrast-enhanced MR angiography or contrast-enhanced MR perfusion imaging (2D fast spoiled GRE sequence with single-slice technique) (Fig. 16) [55].

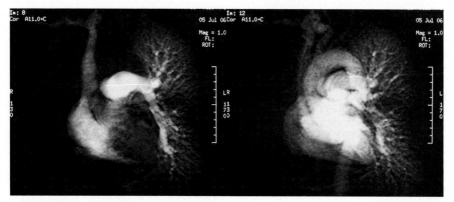

Fig. 16. Contrast-enhanced MR perfusion imaging of the lung in a patient who has late-phase Takayasu arteritis. Serial subtracted MR images of contrast-enhanced MR perfusion imaging of the lung show occlusion of the right main trunk of the pulmonary artery and a perfusion defect in the middle lung field of the left lung.

References

[1] Flamm SD, VanDyke CW, White RD. MR imaging of the thoracic aorta. Magn Reson Imaging Clin N Am 1996;4:217–35.

[2] Leung DA, Debatin JF. Three-dimensional contrast-enhanced MRA of the thoracic vasculature. Eur Radiol 1997;7:981–9.

[3] Krinsky G, Reuss PM. MR angiography of the thoracic aorta. Magn Reson Imaging Clin N Am 1998;6:293–320.

[4] Reddy GP, Higgins CB. MR imaging of the thoracic aorta. Magn Reson Imaging Clin N Am 2000;8:1–15.

[5] Ho VB, Corse WR, Hood MN, et al. MRA of the thoracic vessels. Semin Ultrasound CT MR 2003;24:192–216.

[6] Tatli S, Lipton MJ, Davison BD, et al. MR imaging of aortic and peripheral vascular disease. Radiographics 2003;23:S59–78.

[7] Czum JM, Corse WR, Ho VB. MR angiography of the thoracic aorta. Magn Reson Imaging Clin N Am 2005;13:41–64.

[8] Russo V, Renzulli M, Buttazzi K, et al. Acquired diseases of the thoracic aorta: role of MRI and MRA. Eur Radiol 2006;16:852–65.

[9] Glazier HS, Gutierrez FR, Levitt G, et al. The thoracic aorta studied by MR imaging. Radiology 1985;157:149–55.

[10] Gomes AS. MR imaging of congenital anomalies of the thoracic aorta and pulmonary arteries. Radiol Clin North Am 1989;27:1171–81.

[11] Fattori R, Nienaber CA. MRI of acute and chronic aortic pathology: pre-operative and postoperative evaluation. J Magn Reson Imaging 1999;10:741–50.

[12] Russo V, Renzulli M, Palombara CL, et al. Congenital diseases of the thoracic aorta: role of MRI and MRA. Eur Radiol 2006;16:676–84.

[13] Simonetti OP, Finn JP, White RD, et al. "Black blood" T2-weighted inversion recovery MR imaging of the heart. Radiology 1996;199:49–57.

[14] Pelc LR, Pelc NJ, Rayhill SC, et al. Arterial and venous blood flow: noninvasive quantification with MR imaging. Radiology 1992;185:809–12.

[15] Rebergen SA, van der Wall EE, Doornbos J, et al. Magnetic resonance measurement of velocity and flow: technique, validation, and cardiovascular application. Am Heart J 1993;126:1439–56.

[16] Earls JP, Ho VB, Foo TK, et al. Cardiac MRI: recent progress and continued challenges. J Magn Reson Imaging 2002;16:111–27.

[17] Pereles FS, McCarthy RM, Baskaran V, et al. Thoracic aortic dissection and aneurysm: evaluation with nonenhanced true FISP MR angiography in less than 4 minutes. Radiology 2002;223:270–4.

[18] Prince MR, Yucel EK, Kaufman JA, et al. Dynamic gadolinium-enhanced three-dimensional abdominal MR arteriography. J Magn Reson Imaging 1993;3:877–81.

[19] McCauley TR, Monib A, Dickey KW, et al. Peripheral vascular occlusive disease: accuracy and reliability of time-of-flight MR angiography. Radiology 1994;192:351–7.

[20] Didier D, Ratib O, Friedli B, et al. Cine gradient-echo MR imaging in the evaluation of cardiovascular disease. Radiographics 1993;13:561–73.

[21] Ho VB, Kinney JB, Sahn DJ. Contributions of newer MR imaging strategies for congenital heart disease. Radiographics 1996;16:43–60.

[22] Niezen RA, Doombos J, van der Wall EE, et al. Measurement of aortic and pulmonary flow with MRI at rest and during physical exercise. J Comput Assist Tomogr 1998;22:194–201.

[23] Powell AJ, Maier SE, Chung T, et al. Phase-velocity cine magnetic resonance imaging measurement of pulsatile blood flow in children and young adults: in vitro and in vivo validation. Pediatr Cardiol 2000;21:104–10.

[24] Prince MR, Narasimham DL, Jacoby WT, et al. Three dimensional gadolinium-enhanced MR angiography of the thoracic aorta. Am J Roentgenol 1996;166:1387–97.

[25] Krinsky G, Rofsky N, Flyer M, et al. Gadolinium-enhanced three dimensional MR angiography of acquired arch vessels disease. Am J Roentgenol 1996;167:981–7.

[26] Krinsky G, Rofsky N, De Corato DR, et al. Thoracic aorta: comparison of gadolinium-enhanced three dimensional MR angiography with conventional MR imaging. Radiology 1997;202:183–93.

[27] Svensson J, Petersson JS, Stahlberg F, et al. Image artifacts due to a time-varying contrast medium concentration in 3D contrast-enhanced MRA. J Magn Reson Imaging 1999;10:919–28.

[28] Hany TF, Mckinnon GC, Leung DA, et al. Optimization of contrast timing for breath-holding three-dimensional MR angiography. J Magn Reson Imaging 1997;7:551–6.

[29] Foo TK, Saranathan M, Prince MR, et al. Automated detection of bolus arrival and initiation of data acquisition in fast, three-dimensional, gadolinium-enhanced MR angiography. Radiology 1997;203:275–80.

[30] Riederer SJ, Bernstein MA, Breen JF, et al. Three-dimensional contrast-enhanced MR angiography with real-time fluoroscopic triggering: design specifications and technical reliability in 330 patient studies. Radiology 2000;215:584–93.

[31] Bonser RS, Pagano D, Lewis ME, et al. Clinical and patho-anatomical factors affecting expansion of thoracic aortic aneurysms. Heart 2000;84:277–83.

[32] Debatin JF, Hany TF. MR-based assessment of vascular morphology and function. Eur Radiol 1998;8:528–39.

[33] Neimatallah MA, Ho VB, Dong Q, et al. Gadolinium-based 3D magnetic resonance angiography of the thoracic vessels. J Magn Reson Imaging 1999;10:758–70.

[34] Sueyoshi E, Sakamoto I, Kawahara Y, et al. Infected abdominal aortic aneurysm: early CT findings. Abdom Imaging 1998;23:645–8.

[35] Macedo TA, Stanson AW, Oderich GS, et al. Infected aortic aneurysms: imaging findings. Radiology 2004;231:250–7.

[36] Berletti R, D'Andrea P, Cavagna E, et al. Inflammatory and fibrotic changes in the periaortic regions: integrated US, CT and MR imaging in three cases. Radiol Med 2002;103:427–32.

[37] Anbarasu A, Harris PL, McWilliams RG. The role of gadolinium-enhanced MR imaging in the preoperative evaluation of inflammatory abdominal aortic aneurysm. Eur Radiol 2002;12:S192–5.

[38] Nijenhuis RJ, Jacobs MJ, van Engelshoven JM, et al. MR angiography of the Adamkiewicz artery and anterior radiculomedullary vein: postmortem validation. AJNR Am J Neuroradiol 2006; 27:1573–5.

[39] Yoshioka K, Niinuma H, Ehara S, et al. MR angiography and CT angiography of the artery of Adamkiewicz: state of the art. Radiographics 2006;26:S63–73.

[40] Cigarroa JE, Isselbacher EM, DeSanctis RW, et al. Diagnostic standard and new direction. N Engl J Med 1993;328:35–43.

[41] Chang JM, Friese K, Caputo GR, et al. MR measurement of blood flow in the true and false channel in chronic aortic dissection. J Comput Assist Tomogr 1991;15:418–23.

[42] Fisher U, Vossherich R, Kopka L, et al. Dissection of the thoracic aorta: pre- and postoperative findings of turbo-FLASH MR images in the plane of the aortic arch. Am J Roentgenol 1994;163: 1069–72.

[43] Bogaert J, Meyns B, Rademakers FE, et al. Follow-up of aortic dissection: contribution of MR angiography for evaluation of the abdominal aorta and its branches. Eur Radiol 1997;7:695–702.

[44] Nienaber CA, von Kodolitsch Y, Petersen B, et al. Intramural hemorrhage of the thoracic aorta: diagnosis and therapeutic implications. Circulation 1995;92:1465–72.

[45] Ganaha F, Miller DC, Sugimoto K, et al. Prognosis of aortic intramural hematoma with and without penetrating atherosclerotic ulcer:

a clinical and radiological analysis. Circulation 2002;106:342–8.

[46] Murray JG, Manisali M, Flamm SD, et al. Intramural hematoma of the thoracic aorta: MR imaging findings and their prognostic implications. Radiology 1997;204:349–55.

[47] Stanson AW, Kazmier FJ, Hollier LH, et al. Penetrating atherosclerotic ulcers of the thoracic aorta: natural history and clinicopathologic correlations. Ann Vasc Surg 1986;1:15–23.

[48] Hayashi H, Matsuoka Y, Sakamoto I, et al. Penetrating atherosclerotic ulcer of the aorta: imaging features and disease concept. Radiographics 2000;20:995–1005.

[49] Macura KJ, Szarf G, Fishman EK, et al. Role of computed tomography and magnetic resonance imaging in assessment of acute aortic syndromes. Semin Ultrasound CT MR 2003;24:232–54.

[50] Yucel EK, Steinberg FL, Egglin TK, et al. Penetrating aortic ulcers: diagnosis with MR imaging. Radiology 1990;177:779–81.

[51] Matsunaga N, Hayashi K, Sakamoto I, et al. Takayasu arteritis: protean radiologic manifestations and diagnosis. Radiographics 1997;17: 579–94.

[52] Matsunaga N, Hayashi K, Okada M, et al. Magnetic resonance imaging features of aortic diseases. Top Magn Reson Imaging 2003;14:253–66.

[53] Nastri MV, Baptista LP, Baroni RH, et al. Gadolinium-enhanced three-dimensional MR angiography of Takayasu arteritis. Radiographics 2004;24: 773–86.

[54] Tanigawa K, Eguchi K, Kitamura Y, et al. Magnetic resonance imaging detection of aortic and pulmonary artery wall thickening in acute stage of Takayasu arteritis: improvement of clinical and radiologic findings after steroid therapy. Arthritis Rheum 1992;35:476–80.

[55] Sueyoshi E, Sakamoto I, Ogawa Y, et al. Diagnosis of perfusion abnormality of the pulmonary artery in Takayasu's arteritis using contrast-enhanced MR perfusion imaging. Eur Radiol 2006;16:1551–6.

ELSEVIER
SAUNDERS

RADIOLOGIC
CLINICS
OF NORTH AMERICA

Radiol Clin N Am 45 (2007) 499–512

Multidetector Row CT of Small Bowel Obstruction

Adnan Qalbani, MD*, David Paushter, MD,
Abraham H. Dachman, MD

- Small bowel anatomy
- CT technique
- Sensitivity of CT in small bowel obstruction and related findings
- Problem solving: the key questions
- Extrinsic processes

- Intrinsic and intraluminal processes
- Conditions mimicking small bowel obstruction
- Special techniques and future modalities
- Summary
- References

State-of-the-art multidetector row CT (MDCT) technology has revolutionized abdominal imaging. With widespread use of 16-detector row scanners and the availability of 40- and 64-detector scanners, rapid acquisition of scan data has become routine and has added significantly to CT diagnosis and evaluation of many conditions. CT now plays a primary role in evaluation of the small bowel in general and of small bowel obstruction (SBO) in particular, because of the availability of high-quality multiplanar reformations. Clinical and abdominal plain-film differentiation of simple obstruction, closed-loop obstruction, and strangulation of bowel is unreliable but is critical for patient management. Specifically, a trial of conservative management for uncomplicated obstruction has become increasingly accepted as standard treatment, as opposed to early surgical intervention. The ability of CT to determine if bowel obstruction is present, to localize the obstructive site, to determine the degree of obstruction, to diagnose the presence of closed-loop obstruction, and to identify ischemia or perforation of the involved bowel is well established.

Multiplanar reformation and three-dimensional (3D) MDCT techniques, which optimize the visualization of bowel and adjacent anatomic structures, are particularly helpful in delineating anatomy and identifying an obstructive transition point with greater reliability and confidence. Furthermore, the speed of the MDCT examination optimizes the evaluation of the patient who has closed-loop obstruction or bowel ischemia because artifacts caused by bowel motility and respiratory and patient motion are minimized. In addition, multiphase imaging can be performed to evaluate blood flow in the arterial and venous phases.

In this article, the usefulness of MDCT in the evaluation of SBO and related conditions in adults is illustrated, and the benefits of advanced CT applications are emphasized.

Small bowel anatomy

The small intestine extends from the pylorus to the ileocecal valve and is involved primarily in nutrient absorption. Anatomic details vary by location, however, and may explain many of the

The University of Chicago, MC 2026, 5841 S. Maryland Ave., Chicago, IL 60637, USA
* Corresponding author.
E-mail address: adnan.qalbani@uchospitals.edu (A. Qalbani).

0033-8389/07/$ – see front matter © 2007 Elsevier Inc. All rights reserved.
radiologic.theclinics.com

doi:10.1016/j.rcl.2007.04.006

aspects of small bowel pathology, thereby contributing to focused imaging interpretation. The duodenum is the first and typically the shortest segment. It is almost entirely retroperitoneal, lacks mesentery, and is accessible to endoscopy and minimally invasive diagnostic and therapeutic interventions. Obstruction can occur in the duodenum but is less common in adults than in children and infants.

The jejunum and ileum are loosely considered the upper two fifths and lower three fifths of the remaining small bowel, respectively. Although there is no exact point of transition between the structures, specialization of function and anatomic differences exist. A common 15-cm fan-shaped mesentery anchors the jejunum and ileum to the posterior abdominal wall, allowing individual loops relatively free mobility [1]. This mobility permits the small bowel to distend and twist and helps explain the mechanism of SBO in some cases such as volvulus and internal hernias.

Jejunum is characterized by increased vascularity, larger and thicker folds, and larger intestinal villi than the ileum. Whereas the ileum has an abundance of lymphoid follicles, they are nearly absent in the proximal jejunum. The caliber of the jejunum is about 4.0 cm, slightly larger that of the ileum (3.75 cm) [1]. Fig. 1 illustrates these differences between jejunum and ileum on CT and shows normal contrast enhancement of the small bowel wall seen when a negative contrast agent is used.

Four layers form the small intestinal wall: the most superficial serosal layer, a muscularis layer composed of thin longitudinal and thick circumferential smooth muscle, the strong submucosa, and the complex mucous membrane. The mucous membrane consists of circular folds, intestinal villi, glands, and lymphoid tissue [1]. The valvulae conniventes are important from an imaging perspective because they retain their structure during distention. This feature allows confidence in determining

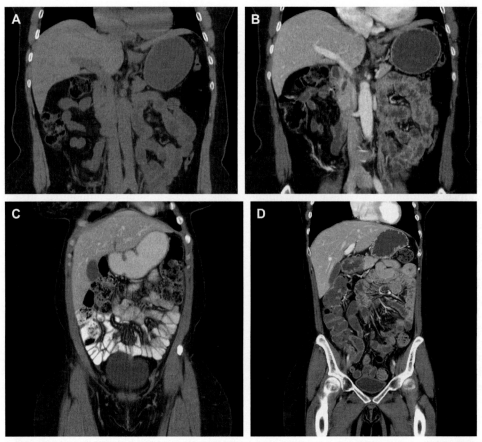

Fig. 1. Normal small bowel features on CT. Panels A and B show normal jejunum (*A*) before and (*B*) after intravenous contrast administration with a negative oral contrast agent filling the bowel lumen. (*C*) Normal opacified loops of ileum with distinctly less prominent folds than jejunum. (*D*) With intravenous contrast and negative oral contrast agent, normal jejunum can be distinguished from normal ileum.

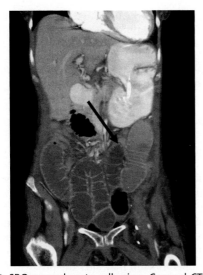

Fig. 2. SBO secondary to adhesion. Coronal CT demonstrates the transition zone (*arrow*) in a patient with an adhesion status post abdominal aortic aneurysm repair. The circular folds in the proximal ileum are well seen despite marked distension.

whether a significantly dilated loop of bowel represents small or large intestine (Fig. 2).

The superior mesenteric artery supplies the jejunum and ileum. Distal branches travel between serosal and muscularis layers with significant anastomoses and a submucosal plexus supplying the villi. The venous return parallels the arterial supply, returning blood to the portal vein through the superior mesenteric vein. A complex lymphatic system is also an important aspect of small intestinal function [1].

CT technique

The authors use 16-, 40-, and 64-detector MDCT scanners. Reformatted axial and coronal images are provided routinely. If needed, 3D images and slabs of various thicknesses can be reconstructed.

Practices vary by institution with regard to administration of oral contrast in the setting of possible SBO. Some investigators have deemed oral contrast unnecessary in this evaluation, because the bowel is likely to be dilated and fluid filled [2]. The authors prefer to use positive oral contrast in this setting as

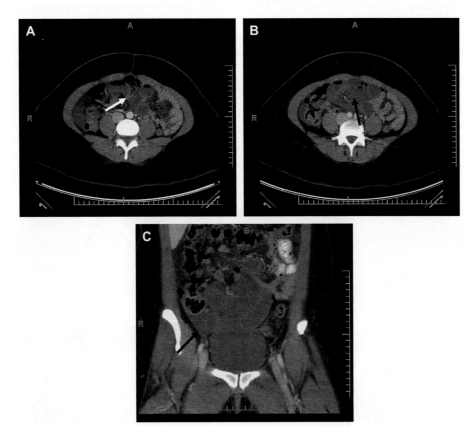

Fig. 3. Closed loop SBO. (*A, B*) Axial CT images demonstrate a dilated bowel loop with proximal (*arrow, 3A*) and distal (*arrow, 3B*) narrowing. (*C*) Coronal CT image shows the dilated loops with surrounding mesenteric congestion and fluid indicating possible strangulation. Closed loop obstruction was confirmed at surgery and the nonviable ischemic loop of small bowel was resected.

tolerated by the patient because oral contrast is help-ful in determining if an obstruction is complete. For the same reason, they also prefer that nasoenteric suction be discontinued for some time before the scan. Enteric fluid dilutes oral contrast as it prog-resses distally. This dilution effect indicates how much fluid was present in the lumen before the ad-ministration of oral contrast. Analysis of the dilution effect on CT can be particularly helpful in patients whose plain-film radiograph did not show any gas-filled dilated loops (so-called "gasless abdomen"). It also can help in localizing the point of obstruction because the small bowel loops containing more di-lute contrast are distal relative to those with more dense oral contrast. This phenomenon is present in many of the figures in this article.

An opposing viewpoint has been promoted by Maglinte and colleagues [3]. They deem oral con-trast unnecessary if SBO is evident on plain-film ra-diographs because contrast is unlikely to reach the obstruction and may make evaluation of bowel wall thickening difficult if it does reach the obstruc-tion. They do not use oral contrast in the emergent setting because of the ensuing delay in performing the CT examination. If ischemia is suspected, they use water as the enteric contrast agent because pos-itive contrast interferes with vascular 3D reconstruc-tions. In general, water is better tolerated than positive contrast in all patients, particularly those who have SBO or ileus [3].

In the absence of contraindications, intravenous contrast medium is used routinely, because it assists in the evaluation of bowel wall and mucosa, possi-ble associated inflammatory or neoplastic pro-cesses, and mesenteric vasculature. In patients suspected of having ischemic bowel, scans should be performed in the arterial and venous phases to search for occluded arteries and veins, to depict vas-cular anatomy, and to assess bowel wall perfusion.

Sensitivity of CT in small bowel obstruction and related findings

Abdominal plain-film radiographs have a sensitivity of approximately 66% in surgically proven cases of SBO [4]. In addition, the specificity of plain-film ra-diographs is diminished by disorders such as dif-fuse ileus and proximal mechanical colonic obstructions, which may simulate SBO. Neverthe-less, the abdominal plain-film radiograph con-tinues to be an appropriate starting point in the assessment of possible SBO. It can be obtained rap-idly, has a relatively low cost, and is sensitive in identifying pneumoperitoneum. The presence of pneumoperitoneum may alter the protocol for the administration of oral contrast medium; only wa-ter-soluble contrast medium should be used, with little or no delay in obtaining the scan.

MDCT findings in patients who have SBO can dictate the need for either surgical intervention or close follow-up. Mallo and colleagues [5] reviewed seven studies of the CT diagnosis of complete bowel obstruction defined by surgical findings and re-vealed the following parameters: sensitivity 92%, specificity 93%, positive predictive value (PPV) 91%, and negative predictive value (NPV) 93%. The same group reviewed 11 studies reporting on CT diagnosis of ischemia in the setting of SBO and found sensitivity of 83%, specificity of 92%, PPV of 79%, and NPV of 93%. Based on patient clinical review, they concluded that a CT finding of partial SBO is likely to represent a clinical condi-tion that will resolve with conservative management.

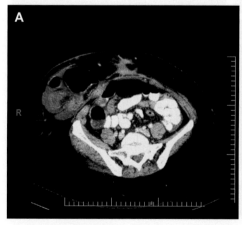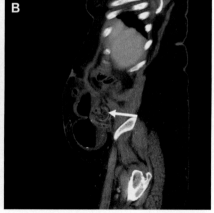

Fig. 4. Incarcerated peristomal hernia with closed loop obstruction. (*A*) Axial CT image showing small bowel wall thickening and free fluid in the hernia sac of a patient with small bowel obstruction. (*B*) Sagittal view showing a "swirl sign" (*arrows*) involving the vasculature supplying the herniated loops. At surgery, the incarcerated loops of bowel were congested but viable, and no resection was needed.

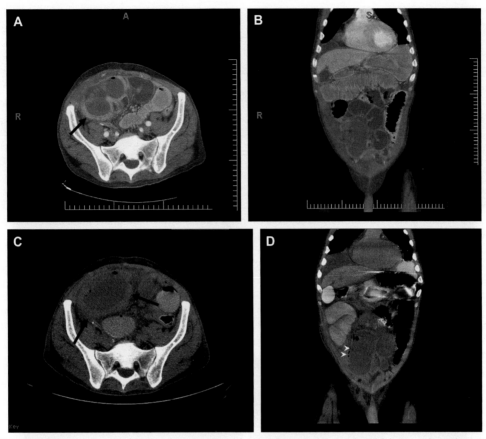

Fig. 5. SBO with early ischemic changes progressing to frank ischemia. (*A*) Axial and (*B*) coronal are the initial CT scan showing changes of SBO that do not identify a definite cause. Adjacent ascites and bowel wall thickening (*arrow*) were worrisome for possible ischemia. (*C*) Axial and (*D*) coronal are without intravenous contrast 8 days later and show considerable bowel wall thickening (*arrows*) and pneumatosis intestinalis (*white arrowheads*). Laparotomy was performed with segmental small bowel resection. Pathology confirmed mucosal ischemia and areas of full thickness necrosis as well as organizing serosal adhesions.

Scaglione and colleagues [6] retrospectively reviewed 120 cases over a 3-year period of patients who had closed-loop obstruction and who underwent surgical management within 2 to 6 hours of CT diagnosis. They demonstrated a PPV of 100% for CT in identifying ischemic complications in the setting of closed-loop obstruction and a NPV of 73%.

Recent MDCT data using multiplanar reformations have not demonstrated significantly improved sensitivity and specificity for diagnosing SBO or its complications relative to evaluation of transverse images alone [7]. The use of coronal reformations has, however, been shown to increase confidence of the radiologist in the following areas: excluding SBO, diagnosing SBO, and demonstrating abnormal bowel wall enhancement [7]. In addition, clinicians generally are appreciative of the more familiar anatomy demonstrated with multiplanar reformation and 3D sequences.

Problem solving: the key questions

Management issues are at the core of imaging in SBO. Historically, acute SBO was operated on relatively early. Because experience has demonstrated a low mortality for simple obstruction and the ability of some obstructions to resolve with conservative management, early surgery now is performed more selectively. The most important goal of MDCT is to identify cases in which surgery should not be delayed because of potential complications that increase mortality.

When present, classic clinical and plain-film radiographic findings are diagnostic for SBO. Vague examination findings and atypical presentations are common, however. In one study, obstruction was not supported on abdominal radiographs read by experienced gastrointestinal radiologists in 34% of surgically proven cases of SBO [4]. In addition, Maglinte and colleagues [3] point out from

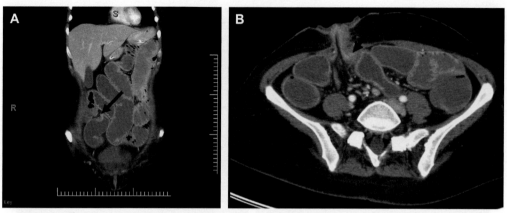

Fig. 6. SBO at ostomy site. (*A*) Coronal and (*B*) axial CT images demonstrate high-grade small bowel obstruction with transition zone at the ostomy site (*arrows*).

their review of the surgical literature that simple mechanical obstruction is not differentiated reliably from strangulation by using clinical, laboratory, or radiographic findings. MDCT generally is diagnostic in such cases and also provides critical information for management, whether or not the fundamental diagnosis of obstruction is in doubt.

Once the diagnosis of SBO has been established, one should grade the severity of the obstruction and search for a cause. Complete obstruction

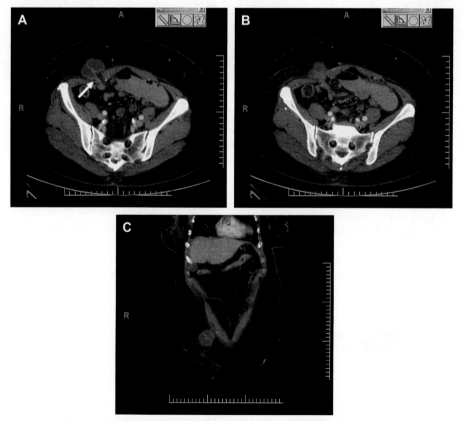

Fig. 7. Incarcerated incisional hernia. Partial SBO secondary to incarceration of small bowel loops in the right lower quadrant's anterior wall. (*A,B*) Axial CT images demonstrate the transition zone (*arrow*). (*C*) The coronal image shows proximal dilated loops. The hernia occurred at a trocar site for previous surgical procedure. Incarceration was confirmed at surgery, but the bowel loop was viable. Note the small amount of ascites in the left lower quadrant (*arrowheads*).

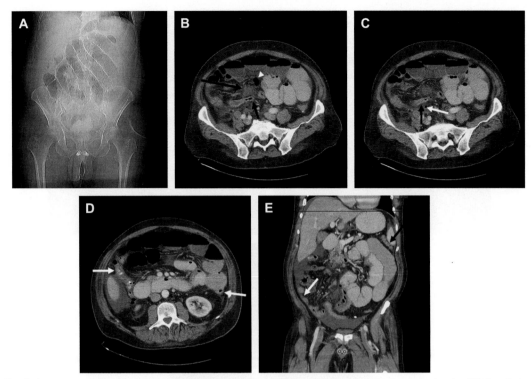

Fig. 8. Acute appendicitis with associated SBO. 65 year old man presented with abdominal pain. (*A*) Scout view showing multiple, centrally located, dilated loops of small bowel. (*B,C*) Axial CT images show the inflamed appendix (*short arrow*) with focal fluid (*long arrow*) and extraluminal gas (*arrowhead*) near tip consistent with perforation. This follow-up examination shows free fluid increased from three days earlier. Surgery confirmed partial SBO at site of abscess. (*D*) Axial and (*E*) coronal CT images show dilated loops of small bowel with decompressed colon (*arrows*). Also note contrast in proximal small bowel is denser than the more distal bowel caused by a dilutional effect as contrast progresses distally and suggesting relative stasis of fluid closer to the site of obstruction.

generally is an indication for surgery, whereas simple and uncomplicated partial SBO (as discussed later) can be managed conservatively with a period of observation, intravenous hydration, and nasogastric/enteric suction because the obstruction may resolve without surgery.

The next step is determining whether the obstruction is simple or a closed-loop obstruction. Closed-loop obstruction results when a single point fixes adjacent bowel loops (a proximal and distal point) (Fig. 3). Closed-loop obstruction is predisposed to ischemic strangulation of the incarcerated segment

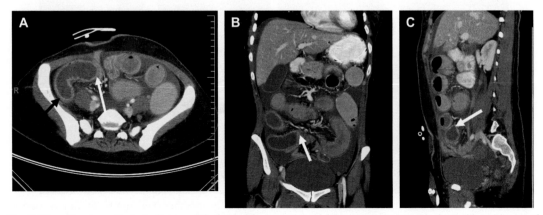

Fig. 9. Stenotic-phase Crohn's disease. (*A*) Axial, (*B*) coronal, and (*C*) sagittal CT images show dilated loops of small bowel with air-fluid levels, diffuse ascites, areas of distal ileal wall thickening (*black arrows*) and a discrete transition zone (*white arrows*). Adhesions and nonspecific ulceration were found at pathology.

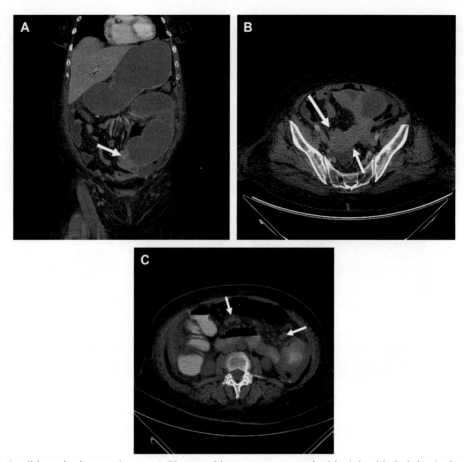

Fig. 10. Small bowel adenocarcinoma. A 73 year old women presented with right-sided abdominal pain and vomiting. (*A*) Coronal CT image shows high grade SBO due to an enhancing mass at the transition point (*arrow*). (*B*) Axial CT image shows the largest transverse dimensions of the mass (*arrows*). (*C*) Axial CT image showing mesenteric nodal metastases (*arrows*).

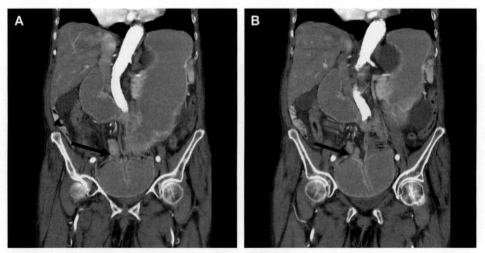

Fig. 11. (*A, B*) Small bowel adenocarcinoma. Consecutive coronal CT images show high-grade SBO causing gastric, duodenal, and jejunal dilatation to a discrete transition point (*arrow*). On CT, the transition point has the appearance of collapsed bowel, however–a 3 cm adenocarcinoma with invasion to the visceral surface causing high grade SBO was found at surgery.

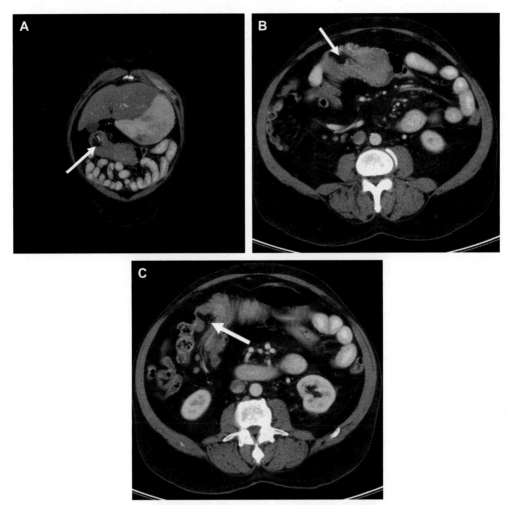

Fig. 12. Ileocecal intussusception. (*A*) Coronal and (*B, C*) contiguous axial CT images show mesenteric fat and vessels telescoping into the lumen of transverse colon (*white arrows*) consistent with intussusception. There is small bowel wall thickening proximally but no significant dilatation. On pathology, a fungating tubulovillous adenoma was in the cecum (not seen on CT).

of bowel. The risk of strangulation increases with further delay of surgery, making recognition of this entity important in early surgical management. Mortality for simple SBO is around 3% to 8%, whereas mortality is 20% to 37% once strangulation has occurred [8,9]. This mortality escalates from around 8% in the first 36 hours to 25% or more beyond 36 hours after onset of symptoms [8]. Therefore closed-loop obstruction should be considered a surgical emergency, despite the potential for reversibility with nonoperative management.

When ischemia accompanies a mechanical obstruction, it indicates that strangulation has occurred. Typically, a closed-loop obstruction rotates about the fixation point, resulting in obstruction to venous outflow. The MDCT findings of the bowel and mesentery reflect the pathophysiology of twisting and congestion. Whirling of mesenteric vessels,

mesenteric fat or fluid near involved loops, edema of the bowel wall, relative lack of wall enhancement, and, when advanced, pneumatosis may be seen. (Fig. 4 shows some of these findings.) These findings are all associated with a high morbidity and mortality; therefore, early surgical intervention may be warranted. Fig. 5 illustrates a case showing mild wall thickening and free fluid. Surgery was delayed, and bowel wall necrosis was found at surgery.

MDCT findings have been shown to correlate with pathologic tissue damage. Bowel wall hyperdensity results from compensatory vasodilation in early ischemia. Absence of wall enhancement corresponds to vasoconstriction related to overdistension of bowel wall and secondary compression of the capillary bed. Wall thickening is caused by increased capillary permeability leading to submucosal edema. Dilatation is from lack of peristalsis, which results from the edema. Pneumatosis occurs in the presence of mucosal cellular necrosis [10]. Isolated findings are not always specific for ischemia, and the absence of ischemic findings does not exclude strangulation.

Extrinsic processes

Entities causing SBO are divided broadly into those intrinsic and extrinsic to the bowel lumen. Adhesions are the main cause of SBO in the Western world, ranging from 50% to 80% of cases [3,8,11,12]. Almost all adhesions are postoperative; a minority is secondary to peritonitis or other rare entities. Although the adhesive band itself is not visualized, identification of a transition point without other obvious cause usually is attributed to adhesions in the operated patient (Fig. 6).

Hernias are the second most common cause of SBO, comprising some 10% of cases [8,11]. Hernias as a cause of SBO have diminished because of the increasing use of routine elective repair of inguinal hernias, which are the type most commonly involved in SBO. In the developing world, hernia

continues to be the leading cause of SBO [12]. In some tertiary institutions, such as The University of Chicago, incisional and peristomal hernias are very common (Fig. 7).

Hernias are defined by anatomic site and are categorized broadly as internal and external varieties. An external hernia is a defect in the abdominopelvic wall, whereas an internal hernia is through a defect in peritoneum, omentum, or mesentery [8]. MDCT is particularly useful in the minority of cases in which external hernias are not palpable or visible. Occult external hernias may become more common in the United States because of the epidemic of obesity. Internal hernias are far less common than external hernias. The diagnosis of internal hernias is almost exclusively radiographic.

Neoplasms may produce SBO in a variety of different ways. Peritoneal carcinomatosis is the most common and is suggested when extrinsic serosal disease involving the small bowel wall is seen associated with a transition zone [8]. Mesenteric metastatic carcinoid, with surrounding desmoplastic reaction, can result in retraction of surrounding loops of small bowel [13]. Although primary small

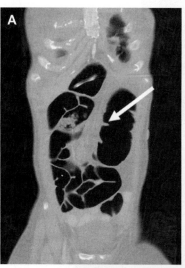
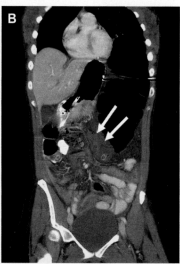
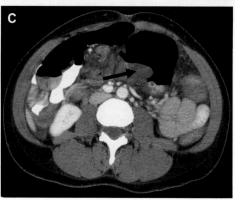

Fig. 13. Cecal volvulus. (*A*) Coronal CT image in lung windows shows dilated small bowel loops but the large loop in the left upper quadrant is colonic as indicated by the haustra (*white arrow*). (*B*) Coronal CT image shown in soft tissue windows more posteriorly shows distended cecum in the left upper quadrant. Note thickening of bowel wall possibly of adjacent loops (*white arrows*). (*C*) Axial CT image demonstrates the ileocecal valve (*arrow*) indicating that this process was a cecal volvulus, as was proven at surgery. Pathology showed a segment of ischemia and focal transmural necrosis. Distal terminal ileum was resected but was normal.

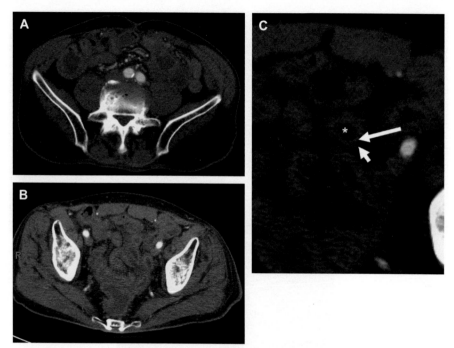

Fig. 14. (*A–C*) Shock bowel. Two axial CT images through the pelvis show diffusely thickened loops of small bowel and descending colon. This patient had shock bowel after a hypotensive episode and was not obstructed. Note three layers of small bowel in this setting: edematous bowel wall (*short arrow*), enhancing mucosa (*long arrow*), and low density intraluminal fluid (*asterisk*).

bowel lymphoma is an intrinsic process, extrinsic nodal metastases can cause obstruction by compression. Primary lymphoma of the small bowel, even when extensive or annular, is soft and generally does not cause obstruction [13]. Intraluminal small bowel neoplasms are discussed later.

Inflammatory processes, particularly appendicitis and diverticulitis, uncommonly result in SBO by secondary involvement of nearby loops of small bowel (Fig. 8). This entity must be differentiated from dilated bowel in the setting of an inflammatory process, which also may be caused by ileus.

Additional causes of extrinsic SBO include endometriosis, abscess, mycobacterial disease, desmoid tumors, aneurysm, and hematomas [8].

Intrinsic and intraluminal processes

The use of CT in the evaluation of inflammatory bowel disease is well established, but the enhanced resolution provided by thinner slices of MDCT improves the evaluation of mucosal and submucosal detail [2].

SBO in patients who have Crohn's disease can represent three common clinical situations: the initial presentation of acute disease, chronic disease in a stenotic phase, or, in patients who have undergone prior surgery, adhesions, or postoperative

stricture. Therefore, in postoperative patients, disease exacerbation versus adhesive obstruction is an important clinical distinction for which CT can aid in diagnosis. As in SBO not associated with Crohn's disease, CT is important in determining the presence of ischemia. Recognition of this entity (often using CT) is critical, because SBO in this setting is likely to subside without surgical intervention [12]. Fig. 9 shows SBO resulting from adhesions in the setting of Crohn's disease.

Subtypes of Crohn's disease have been identified to guide management in terms of medical, surgical, or no treatment [14]. A retrospective review of 14 patients who had SBO and Crohn's disease with pathologic correlation found a lack of correlation between CT findings and need for surgical treatment, however. The mainstay of management continued to be clinical judgment [15].

Intrinsic small bowel neoplasms constitute less than 2% of gastrointestinal malignancies. Although they usually present with nonspecific symptoms, they do occasionally manifest with SBO, which may be low grade and not result in significant dilatation. MDCT enterography may be useful in these cases, as discussed later [16]. When presenting with detectable SBO on MDCT, a small bowel adenocarcinoma usually is advanced and shows mural thickening at the transition zone (Fig. 10). A subtler example (not suspected prospectively) is seen in

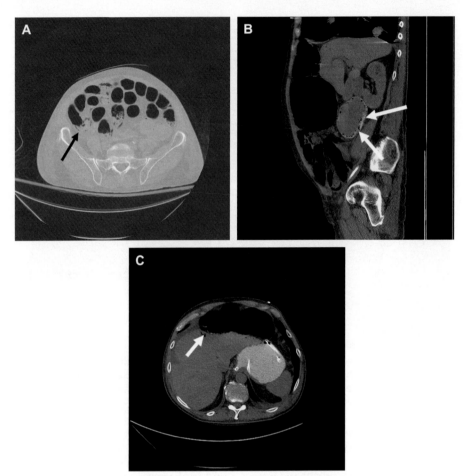

Fig. 15. Ischemic bowel. This patient, with a recent history of pulmonary embolism and COPD, presented with abdominal distension. (*A*) Axial CT image through upper pelvis in lung windows demonstrates pneumatosis intestinalis in multiple small bowel loops (*arrow*). (*B*) Sagittal CT image also shows pneumatosis (*white arrows*). Autopsy confirmed scattered areas of mucosal and transmural necrosis involving 20% of the mid to distal small bowel and a patent foramen ovale as the likely source of paradoxical embolus. (*C*) Axial CT image through the liver shows portal venous gas (*arrow*).

Fig. 11. Adenocarcinoma occurs more commonly in the duodenum and jejunum than in the ileum [13].

Many intraluminal processes can cause SBO and are divided broadly into neoplastic, inflammatory or infectious, vascular, and infiltrative (eg, hemorrhage, and others). Intraluminal lesions may obstruct the lumen mechanically or serve as lead points of intussusception (Fig. 12). In adults, unlike pediatric patients, intussusceptions are very likely to have a leading mass.

Miscellaneous intrinsic or intraluminal small bowel lesions that may lead to obstruction include gallstones (gallstone ileus), foreign bodies, bezoars, tuberculosis (especially ileocecal), radiation enteropathy, and intramural hemorrhage [8,13]. Many patients have multiple risk factors. For example, patients who have Crohn's disease often have had surgery; therefore, associated small bowel stricture or adhesions may be responsible for the obstruction.

Similarly, patients who have had prior surgery or radiation therapy for intra-abdominal neoplasm may have obstruction caused by recurrent tumor, adhesions, and/or fibrosis.

Conditions mimicking small bowel obstruction

Any condition resulting in small bowel dilatation or abdominal distension can be confused with SBO before clinical and radiographic investigations are completed and integrated. Ileus typically results in distension that may include the colon in addition to small bowel and stomach. A concurrent inflammatory process, recent surgery, gastrointestinal infection, and electrolyte disturbances are predisposing factors for ileus, and appreciation of these comorbidities is important in scan interpretation.

Cecal volvulus causes more proximal colonic obstruction and typically secondary small bowel dilatation as well. Recognition of the distended cecum is the key to differentiating volvulus from an isolated SBO (Fig. 13).

Shock bowel can present with dilated loops of small bowel, but involvement of the colon and history should help differentiate the MDCT findings from SBO (Fig. 14). Frank ischemia also can cause marked small bowel distension and simulate the appearance of obstruction (Fig. 15). Ancillary findings of bowel wall thickening, segmental bowel perfusion abnormalities, and evidence for arterial atherosclerotic disease provide evidence for an ischemic cause of the dilatation, however.

Although Crohn's disease may cause SBO because of stricture formation, stenotic-phase disease, or superimposed acute disease, it also may result in areas of dilatation and narrowing without a true obstruction (Fig. 16).

Special techniques and future modalities

CT is faster, less invasive, and more comprehensive than barium enema or CT enteroclysis. The deficiencies in CT for SBO are primarily in the setting of low-grade, partial obstruction. CT enteroclysis challenges the bowel lumen with a load of contrast that may uncover subtle adhesions and strictures and that may overcome the limitations of conventional CT in low-grade SBO [3].

Use of low-density oral contrast agents in CT enteroclysis is particularly helpful in the context of small bowel neoplasms and helps in the differentiation of extraluminal, intramural, and intraluminal

lesions [16]. As MDCT continues to advance, enteroclysis may play an increasing role in the evaluation of small bowel disease.

Although MDCT has added to diagnostic certainty, speed of diagnosis, location of possible transition points, and the presence of ischemia, fundamentals of surgical management have not altered significantly. Specifically, the surgical literature points to the inability to detect reversible ischemia, which can progress to irreversible ischemia when surgery is delayed. Progress in the detection of early, reversible strangulation will affect management more significantly [17].

Contrast-enhanced ultrasound is an emerging modality that may aid in the detection of bowel ischemia. Whereas conventional Doppler ultrasound is limited in its ability to detect slow and low-volume flow in the mucosal layer of bowel, signal from the destruction of microbubbles can be used to detect microperfusion without dependence on flow velocity to create strong color signals. Hata and colleagues [18] showed promising preliminary results in contrast-enhanced assessment of dilated bowel for the presence of ischemia. They acknowledged many limitations to their study, including subjective assessment of color signal, no analysis of intraobserver variability, and exclusion of patients with who had congestive heart failure or disseminated intravascular coagulopathy. Despite its limitations, the noninvasiveness of the test and favorable results make contrast-enhanced ultrasound a strong possibility for assessment of bowel ischemia in the future.

Ultrasound without Doppler or contrast enhancement also can provide dynamic, noninvasive

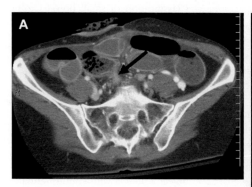
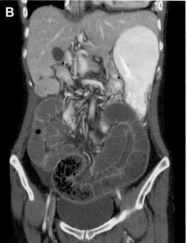

Fig. 16. A patient with known Crohn's disease and high output from an ileostomy. The patient had a total colectomy in the distant past. (*A*) Axial and (*B*) coronal CT images show dilated small bowel and a feces sign in the distal remaining ileum. In this case, the feces sign is due to the distal ileum adapting as a reservoir for stool; the patient was not clinically obstructed. A low-grade stricture (*arrow*) is likely present.

evaluation of bowel wall thickness in patients who have SBO and may aid in detection of patients initially managed with conservative measures who ultimately need surgery. A study evaluating this parameter divided obstructed patients into two groups based on the presence or absence of bowel wall thickening, as detected by ultrasound, at presentation. They were examined again 24 hours later. The decision for surgery was based on clinical toxic signs or failure of nonoperative management. Forty of 49 patients who had initial bowel wall thickening were successfully managed conservatively, compared with 68 of 72 patients who did not have initial bowel wall thickening. All 12 patients who underwent progressive wall thickening underwent surgery. Progressive increase of bowel wall thickness was determined to have a sensitivity of 92.3% and a specificity of 100% as an indication for surgery [19]. The 40 patients who had initial bowel wall thickening that did not require surgery are perhaps more interesting and probably represent the population referred to previously which may have elements of reversible ischemia. The use of an initial measurement of 3 mm as constituting "thickening" may have set low specificity for those at risk of ischemia at presentation.

Summary

SBO is a common cause of hospital admissions and emergency room visits. With an increasing tendency for conservative management, CT plays a critical role in determining which cases need early surgical treatment. MDCT has improved the ability to detect SBO, determine if SBO is complete or partial, suggest the presence of closed-loop obstruction and strangulation, and provide alternative explanations for the patient's symptoms. Multiplanar reformation and 3D capabilities improve diagnostic confidence and ultimately may improve the sensitivity and specificity of MDCT for the purposes described previously. Emerging modalities may be supplemental in determining whether ischemia is present; however, the amount of information that can be obtained in a short time from readily available CT is indispensable.

References

[1] Section XI. Splanchnology: Section 2g. The small intestine. In: Gray's anatomy of the human body. Bartleby.com edition. Available at: http://bartleby.com/107/248.html. Accessed August 25, 2006.

[2] Horton KM, Fishman EK. The current status of multidetector row CT and three-dimensional imaging of the small bowel. Radiol Clin North Am 2003;41:199–212.

[3] Maglinte D, Heitkamp DE, Howard TJ, et al. Current concepts in imaging of small bowel obstruction. Radiol Clin North Am 2003;41:263–83.

[4] Shrake PD, Rex DK, Lappas JC, et al. Radiographic evaluation of suspected small-bowel obstruction. Am J Gastroenterol 1991;86:175–8.

[5] Mallo RD, Salem L, Flum DR. Computed tomography diagnosis of ischemia and complete obstruction in small bowel obstruction: a systematic review. J Gastrointest Surg 2005;9(5):690–4.

[6] Scaglione M, Grassi R, Pinto A, et al. [Positive predictive value and negative predictive value of spiral CT in the diagnosis of closed loop obstruction complicated by intestinal ischemia]. Radiol Med (Torino) 2004;107:69–77 [in Italian].

[7] Jaffe TA, Martin LC, Thomas J, et al. Small-bowel obstruction: coronal reformations from isotropic voxels at 16 section multi-detector row CT. Radiology 2005;238:135–42.

[8] Furukawa A, Yamasaki M, Furuichi K, et al. Helical CT in the diagnosis of small bowel obstruction. Radiographics 2001;21:341–55.

[9] Ellis H. The clinical significance of adhesions: focus on intestinal obstruction. Eur J Surg 1997;577:5–9.

[10] Angelelli G, Scardapane A, Memeo M, et al. Acute bowel ischemia: CT findings. Eur J Radiol 2004; 50:37–47.

[11] Scaglione M, Romano S, Pinto F, et al. Helical CT diagnosis of small bowel obstruction in the acute clinical setting. Eur J Radiol 2004;50:15–22.

[12] Miller G, Boman J, Shrier I, et al. Etiology of small bowel obstruction. Am J Surg 2000;180:33–6.

[13] Boudiaf M, Soyer P, Terem C, et al. CT evaluation of small bowel obstruction. Radiographics 2001; 21:613–24.

[14] Maglinte DD, Gourtsoyiannis N, Rex D, et al. Classification of small bowel Crohn's subtypes based on multimodality imaging. Radiol Clin North Am 2003;41:285–303.

[15] Zissin R, Hertz M, Paran H, et al. Small bowel obstruction secondary to Crohn disease: CT findings. Abdom Imaging 2004;29:320–5.

[16] Schmidt S, Felley C, Meuwly JY, et al. CT enteroclysis: technique and clinical applications. Eur Radiol 2006;16:648–60.

[17] Hayanga AJ, Bass-Wilkins K, Bulkley GB. Current management of small-bowel obstruction. Adv Surg 2005;39:1–33.

[18] Hata J, Kamada T, Haruma K, et al. Evaluation of bowel ischemia with contrast-enhanced US: initial experience. Radiology 2005;236:712–5.

[19] Chen SC, Lee CC, Hsu CY, et al. Progressive increase of bowel wall thickness is a reliable indicator for surgery in patients with adhesive small bowel obstruction. Dis Colon Rectum 2005;48:1764–71.

ELSEVIER
SAUNDERS

RADIOLOGIC
CLINICS
OF NORTH AMERICA

Radiol Clin N Am 45 (2007) 513–524

Upper Extremity Venous Doppler Ultrasound

Therese M. Weber, MD*, Mark E. Lockhart, MD, MPH,
Michelle L. Robbin, MD

Sonography plays a major role in evaluating the upper extremity venous system. The most widely used applications include evaluation for thrombus and vessel patency, localization during venous access procedures, preoperative venous mapping for hemodialysis arteriovenous fistula (AVF) and graft placement, and postoperative hemodialysis AVF and graft assessment. Knowledge of anatomy, scanning technique, and attention to detail are important to the success of demonstrating abnormalities in the upper extremity venous system. Sonographic evaluation of the upper extremity venous system is more challenging than evaluation of the lower extremity venous system.

This article presents methods that allow easy identification of the sometimes complex anatomy and the avoidance of pitfalls that can lead to common and uncommon errors.

Normal anatomy

The venous anatomy of the neck and arm is illustrated in Fig. 1.

Deep venous system

The more clinically important aspect of the venous system of the upper extremity is the deep system, especially the proximal aspect of the venous system including the internal jugular vein, the subclavian vein, and the brachiocephalic vein. One easy way to tell if a vein is superficial or deep is to assess whether it has an artery running with it. In the upper extremity only deep veins have arteries running with them. The radial and ulnar veins in the forearm, which usually are paired, unite caudal to the level of the elbow to form the brachial veins. The brachial veins in the upper arm join with the basilic vein at a variable location, typically at the level of the teres

Department of Radiology, University of Alabama at Birmingham, 619 19th Street, South, JT N312, Birmingham, AL 35249-6830, USA
* Corresponding author.
E-mail address: tweber@uabmc.edu (T.M. Weber).

0033-8389/07/$ – see front matter © 2007 Published by Elsevier Inc.
radiologic.theclinics.com

doi:10.1016/j.rcl.2007.04.005

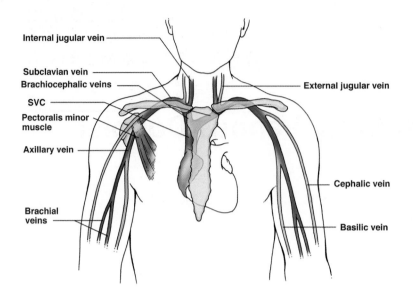

Internal jugular vein

Subclavian vein
Brachiocephalic veins
SVC
Pectoralis minor muscle
Axillary vein
Brachial veins

External jugular vein

Cephalic vein

Basilic vein

Fig. 1. Normal venous anatomy. The deep veins of the arm (*dark blue*) include the brachial vein and axillary vein. The brachiocephalic vein is formed by the internal jugular and subclavian veins. The two brachiocephalic veins join to become the superior vena cava. Superficial veins (*light blue*) include the cephalic vein, basilic vein, and external jugular vein.

major muscle. The confluence of the brachial and basilic veins continues as the axillary vein, which passes through the axilla from the teres major muscle to the first rib. As the axillary vein crosses the first rib, it becomes the lateral portion of the subclavian vein. The medial portion of the subclavian vein receives the smaller external jugular vein and the larger internal jugular vein to form the brachiocephalic (innominate) vein. Bilateral brachiocephalic veins join to form the superior vena cava.

The authors define the central veins as the brachiocephalic veins and superior vena cava, which usually cannot be demonstrated sonographically. Some angiographers include the subclavian vein when they discuss central veins. Therefore, it is important to be very specific about the vein segment examined in describing sonographic findings. The presence or absence of significant central stenosis or thrombosis needs to be inferred by evaluating the transmitted cardiac pulsatility and respiratory phasicity in the medial subclavian vein and caudal internal jugular vein, as discussed later.

Superficial venous system

The superficial venous system of the upper extremity comprises the cephalic vein located more laterally and the basilic vein located more medially. The basilic and cephalic veins typically have a variably larger vein connecting them caudally near the elbow, the median antecubital vein.

Normal arterial anatomy

The brachial artery begins in the upper arm at the lower margin of the teres major muscle tendon and usually ends about 1 cm below the elbow where is divides into the radial and ulnar arteries. Anatomic variants of the radial artery include a high take-off or high bifurcating radial artery. In some cases, the radial artery may take off from the cranial aspect of the brachial artery in the upper arm. One way to distinguish a high take-off of the radial artery from a large elbow branch artery is to follow it into the forearm down to the radial artery region at the wrist. A large arterial branch to the elbow traverses toward the elbow and does not extend into the forearm. Rarely, the ulnar artery may be absent.

Sonographic examination technique

Sonographic evaluation of the upper extremity venous system is more technically challenging than evaluation of the lower extremity venous system. These technical challenges include the inability to compress the subclavian vein because of the overlying clavicle and the need to differentiate large venous collaterals from normal veins in cases of venous obstruction.

The patient is scanned in a supine position with the examined arm abducted from the chest and with the patient's head turned slightly away from the examined arm. Real-time B-mode imaging with spectral and color flow analysis is performed using the highest frequency linear transducer that still gives adequate penetration. Typically the examination is best performed using a 5- to 10-MHz linear-array transducer moving to a higher frequency in the upper arm and forearm if possible. A curved-array transducer or sector transducer may be useful in larger individuals, especially in the axillary area, because of the increased depth of penetration and larger field of view.

All veins are examined with compression every 1 to 2 cm in the transverse plane. Gray-scale transverse images with and without compression or cine clips during compression are obtained from the cranial aspect of the internal jugular vein in the neck near the mandible to the thoracic inlet caudally. Longitudinal color and spectral images are performed also. The subclavian vein is evaluated from its medial to lateral aspect with longitudinal color and spectral images, demonstrating transmitted respiratory variability, cardiac pulsatility, and color fill-in. An inferiorly angled, supraclavicular approach with color Doppler is necessary to demonstrate the superior brachiocephalic vein and the medial portion of the subclavian vein. Use of a small-footprint sector probe in or near the suprasternal notch may facilitate visualization of the brachiocephalic veins and the cranial aspect of the superior vena cava. The midportion of the subclavian vein, located deep to the clavicle, frequently is imaged incompletely. An infraclavicular, superiorly angled approach is used to demonstrate the lateral aspect of the subclavian vein. Frequently, the subclavian vein can be compressed.

Spectral waveform evaluation is critical to upper extremity venous evaluation. Documentation of normal flow features in the medial subclavian vein is extremely important, because it confirms patency of the brachiocephalic vein and superior vena cava, which cannot be examined directly. Each spectral image is evaluated for spontaneous, phasic, and nonpulsatile flow. These samples are obtained in the longitudinal plane of the vessel with angle of insonation maintained at less than 60° (Fig. 2). Spectral analysis of the caudal internal jugular vein and medial subclavian vein is mandatory to evaluate for the presence of transmitted cardiac pulsatility and respiratory phasicity. Loss of this pulsatility may be caused by a more central venous stenosis or obstruction (Fig. 3) [1]. A normal spectral tracing should return to baseline.

Spectral tracings from the medial subclavian vein should be compared with tracings from the lateral subclavian vein. A change between the two tracings suggests subclavian vein stenosis in the midportion of the subclavian vein. Response to a brisk inspiratory sniff or Valsalva's maneuver may assist in evaluating venous patency. With a sniff, the internal jugular vein or subclavian vein normally decreases in diameter or collapses completely. Patients who have significant stenosis or obstruction of the central brachiocephalic vein or superior vena cava lose this response [1].

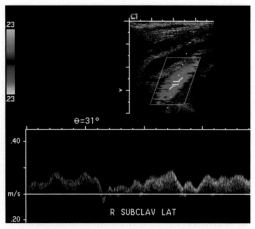

Fig. 2. Normal subclavian vein. Longitudinal color and spectral Doppler of the subclavian vein shows normal filling of the vessel with color. There is normal transmitted respiratory phasicity and cardiac pulsatility with transient reversal of flow below baseline.

Peripheral deep venous system

The remainder of the examination includes compression every 1 to 2 cm of the axillary vein, the cranial, midportion, and caudal aspect of the brachial veins, and the basilic and cephalic veins in the upper arm. Evaluation of the axilla may be limited by body habitus with subsequent limitation in seeing the vessels sonographically. Typically, the upper extremity is imaged to the antecubital fossa. If the patient has focal pain or swelling or a palpable mass in the forearm, the symptomatic area is assessed sonographically. Vessels in the forearm usually are assessed only as part of a focused evaluation of a painful or swollen area or a palpable cord.

Potential pitfalls

Pitfalls to avoid include [2–4]

1. Axillary versus cephalic vein: The axillary vein can be traced through its anatomic course into the subclavian vein. In addition, the cephalic vein, a superficial vein, does not have an adjacent artery running along its course. It may be necessary to abduct the arm further, bend the elbow, and place the hand near the patient's head to access the axilla adequately. Excessive abduction, however, can cause alteration in the venous waveform that falsely suggests a more proximal venous stenosis or occlusion. This alteration resolves with a change in position.
2. Caudal occlusion of the internal jugular vein: It is imperative to follow the caudal aspect of the internal jugular vein into the junction with the medial subclavian vein as it forms the

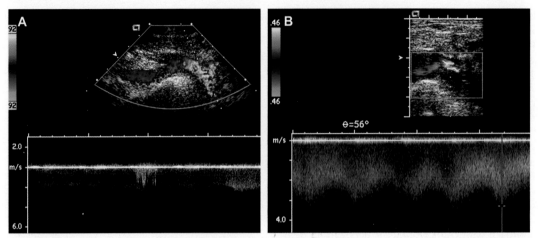

Fig. 3. Central venous occlusion. (*A*) Longitudinal Doppler demonstrates abnormal monophasic flow in the right brachiocephalic vein (Doppler gate). (*B*) Extremely high-velocity flow (329 cm/s) in the vein suggests high-grade stenosis at this level.

brachiocephalic vein. The internal jugular vein usually is in close proximity to the carotid artery. A vein located further away probably represents a collateral vessel. An additional pitfall is that normal respiratory phasicity may be seen in well-developed collaterals. The collaterals usually follow the course of the occluded vein. Collaterals frequently are multiple, somewhat serpiginous veins, rather than the normal single vein following the associated artery.

3. Mirror-image artifact: Because of reflection from the lung apex or clavicle, mirror-image artifact may give the appearance of two subclavian veins in the supraclavicular region

Imaging protocol

Training, skill, and experience are extremely important in performing all vascular ultrasound examinations, including upper extremity venous Doppler ultrasound. Participation in one of the vascular accreditation programs, such as the American College of Radiology or the Intersocietal Commission for the Accreditation of Vascular Laboratories, is strongly recommended.

The upper extremity venous imaging protocol includes the following images for each deep venous segment:

1. Transverse gray-scale image at rest and with compression or a cine clip of the compression maneuver
2. Longitudinal color Doppler with spectral waveform demonstrating transmitted cardiac and respiratory variability
   A. Internal jugular vein—cranial and caudal portions

B. Subclavian vein—mid, medial, lateral
C. Axillary vein
D. Brachial vein—cranial, mid, caudal
E. Basilic vein—upper arm
F. Cephalic vein—upper arm

Clinical diagnosis

Undiagnosed and untreated deep venous thrombosis (DVT) can result in the fatal outcome of pulmonary embolism. In 12% to 16% of pulmonary embolism cases, the source of thrombus is the upper extremities [5,6]. Fatal pulmonary embolism caused by DVT of the upper extremity has been reported [7].

Wells and colleagues [8] previously demonstrated that the use of a clinical model allows the physician to determine accurately the probability that a patient has DVT before diagnostic tests are performed. Clinical factors associated with increased probability of DVT include active cancer, immobility, localized tenderness along the distribution of the deep venous system, swollen entire extremity, pitting edema confined to the symptomatic extremity, collateral superficial veins, and previously documented DVT. The D-dimer assay has a high negative predictive value, and D-dimer is a sensitive but nonspecific marker for DVT [9–11]. Wells and colleagues [12] concluded that DVT can be ruled out in a patient who is judged clinically unlikely to have DVT and who has a negative D-dimer test and that ultrasound evaluation can be omitted safely in these patients. A problem may arise when a D-dimer is obtained without first evaluating the clinical model. D-dimer may be positive in patients who have had recent surgery or trauma, infection, atherosclerosis, congestive heart failure, or disseminated intravascular coagulation and in pregnant, puerperal, or elderly individuals. This work addressed lower extremity DVT and did not address central lines, a frequent cause of upper extremity DVT (UEDVT).

Upper extremity venous thrombosis

The most common indication for venous Doppler ultrasound of the upper extremity is to identify DVT. Indications for upper extremity venous Doppler ultrasound, as listed in the 2006 American College of Radiology practice guideline for the performance of peripheral venous ultrasound examination, include but are not limited to [13]

1. Evaluation of possible venous obstruction or thrombus in symptomatic or high-risk asymptomatic individuals
2. Assessment of dialysis access grafts
3. Venous mapping before harvest for arterial bypass or reconstructive surgery
4. Evaluation of veins before venous access
5. Evaluation for DVT in patients suspected of having pulmonary embolism
6. Follow-up for patients who have known venous thrombosis

Other causes include pain and or swelling at the site of prior phlebotomy or intravenous access site and, uncommonly, effort-related thrombosis. The pathogenesis of effort-related thrombosis is related to an anatomic constriction of the vein by the clavicle and first rib complex associated with repetitive trauma to the vein and resultant changes in the vein wall itself [14]. Radiation therapy, effort-induced thrombosis, and malignant obstructions from compression or direct venous invasion by adjacent tumor or metastatic nodal disease are more common causes of venous obstruction in the chest and arm than in the lower extremities.

Unlike the lower extremity, most cases of UEDVT are related to the presence of a central venous catheter or electrode leads from an implanted cardiac device. Thirty-five percent to 75% of patients who have upper extremity venous catheters develop thrombosis, approximately 75% of which are asymptomatic [15–17]. The complication rate varies greatly, depending on whether the catheter access site is the subclavian or the internal jugular vein. Examining only patients who had symptomatic UEDVT, Trerotola and colleagues [18] found a greater incidence of DVT in patients who had subclavian venous access than in those who had internal jugular access. Thirteen percent of the patients who had subclavian venous catheters had DVT, compared with only 3% of patients who had internal jugular vein catheters. Thus, the placement of

large-bore catheters into the subclavian vein is to be discouraged, especially in patients who have end-stage renal disease for whom dialysis access is being considered. The development of subclavian vein stenosis or thrombosis would limit dialysis access possibilities for that upper extremity.

Only 12% to 16% of patients who have UEDVT develop pulmonary embolism [6,19]. Most acute pulmonary emboli in patients who have UEDVT occur in untreated patients [5,20]. The risk of pulmonary embolism is greater in catheter-related UEDVT than in UEDVT from other causes [21]. Associated complications such as venous stasis and insufficiency caused by venous thrombosis are less common and less severe in the upper extremity than in the leg. Physiologic factors that exist in the leg, such as exposure of the deep venous system to high hydrostatic pressure, do not exist in the arm. The tendency toward development of extensive collateral venous pathways in the arm and chest after venous thrombosis or obstruction contributes to these differences.

Acute deep venous thrombosis

Current literature shows the sensitivity of venous Doppler ultrasound for UEDVT to range from 78% to 100% and its specificity to range from 82% to 100% [22–27]. The acute deep vein thrombus is seen as an enlarged, tubular structure filled with thrombus showing variable echogenicity and absence of color Doppler flow (Fig. 4). Nonocclusive thrombus may show flow outlining the thrombus, with a variable appearance depending on whether the nonocclusive thrombus is acute or

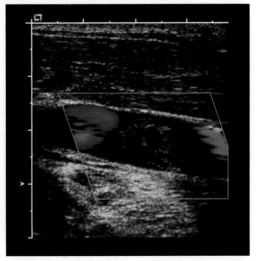

Fig. 4. Occlusive deep venous thrombosis. On longitudinal color Doppler of internal jugular vein, no flow is present around the heterogeneous clot.

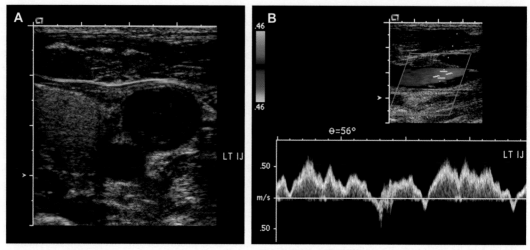

Fig. 5. Nonocclusive deep venous thrombosis. (*A*) Transverse gray-scale image shows hypoechoic thrombus that does not completely fill the internal jugular vein. (*B*) On longitudinal color and spectral Doppler, flow is present in the vein alongside the clot, and normal respiratory phasicity is present.

chronic. Nonocclusive thrombus usually does not result in enlargement of the vein (Fig. 5). When obstruction is incomplete, monophasic flow is demonstrated when the luminal narrowing is significant enough to affect the transmitted cardiac pulsatility and respiratory phasicity from the thorax. As with lower extremity venous Doppler ultrasound, attention to detail is important in areas of duplicated veins to avoid overlooking thrombus in one of the paired veins (Fig. 6).

Spectral analysis can assist in the evaluation of central thromboses. The presence of a nonpulsatile waveform (similar to portal venous flow) strongly suggests central venous disease such as thrombosis, stenosis, or extrinsic compression from an adjacent mass [22]. It is important to compare the suspicious waveform with the contralateral side to confirm its presence on only the symptomatic side. Patel and colleagues [28] found that absent or reduced cardiac pulsatility was a more sensitive parameter in patients who had unilateral venous thrombosis, even though respiratory phasicity often was asymmetric. In bilateral subclavian vein or superior vena cava occlusions the process is bilateral, and

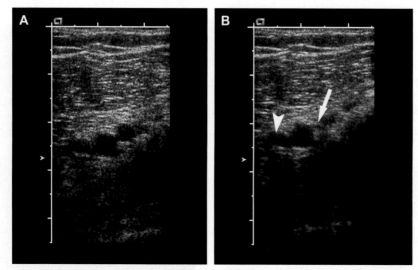

Fig. 6. Deep venous thrombosis in one paired brachial vein. (*A*) On transverse gray-scale image of brachial veins, paired veins are visible without compression. (*B*) A potential pitfall in detecting deep vein thrombosis is shown as one of the two paired brachial veins compresses normally (*arrow*). The other does not compress because of occlusive clot (*arrowhead*).

a high level of suspicion must be maintained to detect central thrombus or stenosis. Also, because of high-volume flow, there may be absence of phasicity without stenosis in the central veins if a hemodialysis graft is present in the upper arm (Fig. 7).

Chronic deep venous thrombosis

As in the lower extremity, diagnosis of chronic venous disease may be more difficult than the diagnosis of acute venous disease. Suggestive findings include frozen valve leaflets, synechia, recanalized veins with internal channels of flow, and small-caliber veins with noncompressible, thickened walls (Fig. 8) [22]. In some cases of chronic venous thrombosis, the vein may be collapsed, fibrosed, and not visible sonographically in the expected anatomic location. For example, if only one brachial vein is demonstrated, chronic scarring from prior DVT of the other brachial vein should be suggested.

Flow direction and collateral pathways should be noted also. In rare cases of brachiocephalic thrombosis, drainage may occur in a retrograde fashion through the internal jugular vein to collateral vessels (Fig. 9). In cases of occluded veins, the development of large venous collaterals may be mistaken for the thrombosed vessel. Collateral veins are tortuous venous structures that are not in the normal venous location, adjacent to the artery (Fig. 10). These collateral veins may show normal respiratory phasicity because they communicate with veins that are subject to changes in intrathoracic pressure.

The presence of a chronic thrombus in a symptomatic patient without evidence for new acute

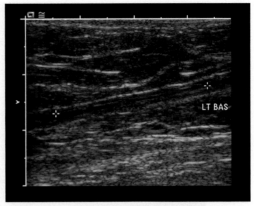

Fig. 8. Chronic superficial venous thrombosis. On longitudinal gray-scale image, thickening of the basilic vein (*cursors*) is present at site of previous catheter placement. The basilic vein is a superficial vein and usually does not require anticoagulation if a thrombus is present.

thrombus suggests postthrombotic syndrome. Postthrombotic syndrome is the most common late complication of DVT. Signs and symptoms include pain, edema, hyperpigmentation, and skin ulceration. Without the presence of acute thrombus, anticoagulant therapy is not indicated [29]. Therefore, it is important in patient management to differentiate acute from chronic changes whenever possible. Rubin and colleagues [30,31] demonstrated that sonographic elasticity imaging, a technique that measures tissue hardness, can discriminate between acute and chronic thrombi and can perform at least as well as thrombus echogenicity. Although this technique currently is not available commercially, it may play a future diagnostic role.

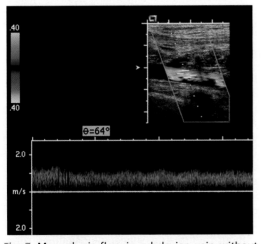

Fig. 7. Monophasic flow in subclavian vein without stenosis. Longitudinal color and spectral Doppler show monophasic waveforms due to high flow volumes from an upper arm hemodialysis graft. There was no central stenosis present on angiography.

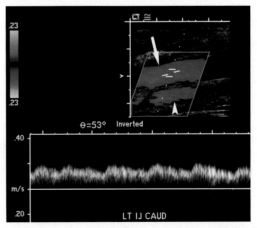

Fig. 9. Brachiocephalic vein occlusion. Reversal of flow is present on color Doppler of the internal jugular vein (*arrow*). Note the internal jugular vein and carotid artery (*arrowhead*) both demonstrate cranial flow.

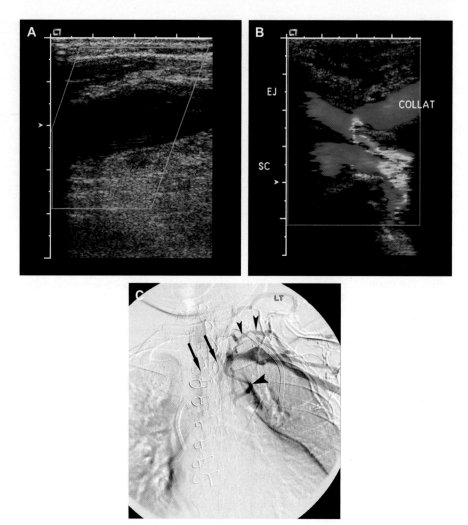

Fig. 10. Occlusive deep venous thrombosis with collaterals. (*A*) Color Doppler of internal jugular vein shows thrombus without visible flow. (*B*) A large collateral vessel is visible communicating with the external jugular vein as it bypasses the level of internal jugular vein obstruction, confirming the chronic component of the obstruction. (*C*) Catheter venogram in another patient shows absence of contrast in the left brachiocephalic vein (*arrows*) and presence of collateral vessels (*arrowheads*).

Areas of stenosis related to prior thrombosis or line placement can be demonstrated with gray-scale and color Doppler examination. A segment of vein may be narrowed significantly relative to the adjacent segments. Thickening or irregularity of the vein wall may be present. Turbulence with aliasing on color Doppler or high-velocity flow on spectral analysis may be demonstrated in these areas. Flow in the narrowed segment is not normal and may show increased pulsatility as compared with dampened, nonphasic flow in the more peripheral waveform (Fig. 11) [22].

Other vascular entities, such as a carotid artery to internal jugular fistula, may be associated with upper extremity swelling and mimic DVT (Fig. 12). Additional factors may alter venous hemodynamics. Pain and colleagues [32] demonstrated significant alteration of axillary venous flow patterns in patients who had axillary lymph node dissection and breast cancer–related lymphedema. The etiology of breast cancer–related edema is multifactorial, and abnormalities of venous drainage are a contributory factor. Further investigation is needed.

When Doppler findings are indeterminate, especially regarding central thrombosis or stenosis, or when there is high clinical suspicion for UEDVT without confirmatory sonographic findings, correlation with MR venography or catheter venography may be needed. In the authors' experience, the most frequent indications for MR venography are suspected central thrombosis and stenosis with

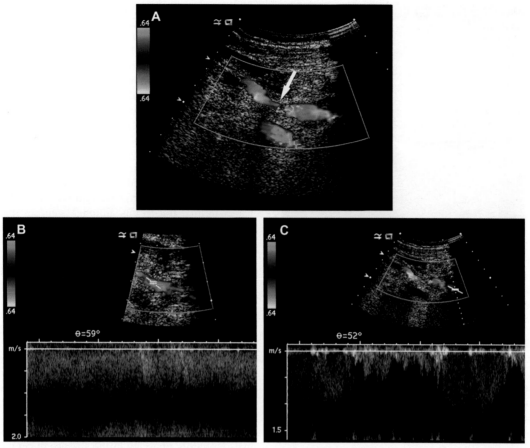

Fig. 11. Stenosis of cephalic vein. (*A*) Longitudinal color Doppler of the cephalic vein demonstrates focal narrowing (*arrow*) of the vessel with aliasing. (*B*) Spectral Doppler shows a waveform that is abnormally monophasic. (*C*) Medial to the area of stenosis, spectral Doppler shows normal venous phasicity.

unilateral or bilateral abnormal respiratory phasicity in the medial subclavian vein and internal jugular vein.

Venous access procedures

In patients who need venous access or catheterization, upper extremity venous Doppler ultrasound can identify an appropriate vessel for access. This access vessel should be screened for the possibility of central stenosis or occlusion. Ultrasound also can demonstrate the target vessel during the procedure to improve the accuracy of venipuncture, decrease potential complications, and reduce procedure time. The variability in location of vascular structures relative to external landmarks is a strong reason to use ultrasound. Povoski and Zaman [33] recommend the use of preoperative ultrasound in patients who have had previous central venous access associated with deep venous thrombosis to assess for central stenosis or occlusion. In addition,

they recommend intraprocedural venography when there is difficulty advancing the guidewire or catheter centrally or when preoperative ultrasound is negative despite previous central venous access with DVT. In an existent catheter that has been in place for a prolonged time, upper extremity ultrasound can demonstrate thrombus or fibrin sheath around a catheter (Fig. 13).

Sonographic evaluation before and after placement of hemodialysis access

Preoperative mapping

Ultrasound vascular mapping before hemodialysis access placement now is an established procedure. Robbin and colleagues [34] demonstrated that preoperative sonographic mapping before placement of hemodialysis access can change surgical management, with an increased number of AVFs placed and an improved likelihood of selecting the most functional vessels. Superficial and deep veins of the

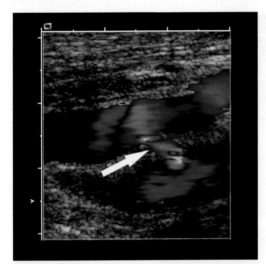

Fig. 12. Carotid-jugular fistula. Color Doppler shows direct communication (*arrow*) between the carotid artery and internal jugular vein. Arterialized flow was present in the internal jugular vein (not shown).

forearm and upper arm, as well as arteries, are evaluated for their suitability for graft or fistula placement. Criteria such as the diameter of the vein and the depth of the superficial vein from the skin are used to determine whether a fistula or a graft is recommended [35].

Arteriovenous fistula maturity assessment

Ultrasound also has a role after access placement. Upper extremity venous Doppler ultrasound can play a key role in addressing the two primary goals

of the Vascular Access Work Group of the National Kidney Foundation, to increase the prevalence and use of native AVFs and to detect access dysfunction before occlusion [36]. Ultrasound evaluation will play an increasingly important role in determining the maturity of a hemodialysis AVF [37,38]. Using color duplex ultrasound surveillance, Grogan and colleagues [38] found an unexpectedly high prevalence of critical stenoses in patent AVFs before initiation of hemodialysis and concluded that stenoses seem to develop rapidly after arterialization of the upper extremity superficial veins. They postulated that turbulent flow conditions in AVFs might play a role in inducing progressive vein wall and valve leaflet intimal thickening, although stenoses may be caused by venous abnormalities that predate AVF placement. Detection of stenosis, graft degeneration, or pseudoaneurysm formation may be important in triaging the patient toward appropriate care [39]. Ultrasound may prove useful in triaging patients toward the appropriate therapy for an immature AVF. When an AVF has low-volume flow, and one or more accessory or competing veins that may be sumping flow from the AVF are detected, ligation of accessory vein branches may be useful [40].

Because of the large amounts of arterialized flow in the hemodialysis access, there may be changes in the spectral venous flow characteristics of the draining vein. Specifically, there may be loss of the normal respiratory phasicity in the absence of central stenosis or occlusion. This loss of phasicity occurs more commonly in patients who have upper extremity hemodialysis grafts than in those who have fistulas.

Summary

It is important to understand thoroughly the normal anatomy and common variations of the upper extremity veins and arteries to avoid misdiagnosis. This understanding is particularly important because the incidence of upper extremity venous disease is increasing. The widespread use of central venous catheters, percutaneous interventional procedures performed with access through the upper extremity venous system, and implanted cardiac devices is increasing the number of patients who have upper extremity thrombosis. Ultrasound plays an important role in evaluating the upper extremity venous system and is the initial imaging modality of choice. When sonographic findings are equivocal or nondiagnostic, especially regarding central thrombosis, correlation using MR venography or catheter venography may be helpful. Ultrasound can provide an accurate, rapid, low-cost, portable, noninvasive method for screening,

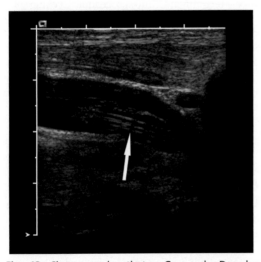

Fig. 13. Clot around catheter. Gray-scale Doppler shows occlusive clot surrounding an existing jugular venous catheter (*arrow*), a common complication of venous catheter placement.

mapping, and surveillance of the upper extremity venous system.

Acknowledgments

The authors thank Trish Thurman for her assistance in manuscript preparation.

References

[1] Gooding GA, Hightower DR, Moore EH, et al. Obstruction of the superior vena cava or subclavian veins: sonographic diagnosis. Radiology 1986;159(3):663–5.

[2] Kremkau FW, Taylor KJ. Artifacts in ultrasound imaging. J Ultrasound Med 1986;5(4):227–37.

[3] Reading CC, Charboneau JW, Allison JW, et al. Color and spectral Doppler mirror-image artifact of the subclavian artery. Radiology 1990;174(1):41–2.

[4] Pozniak MA, Zagzebski JA, Scanlan KA. Spectral and color Doppler artifacts. Radiographics 1992;12(1):35–44.

[5] Horattas MC, Wright DJ, Fenton AH, et al. Changing concepts of deep venous thrombosis of the upper extremity–report of a series and review of the literature. Surgery 1988;104(3):561–7.

[6] Monreal M, Lafoz E, Ruiz J, et al. Upper-extremity deep venous thrombosis and pulmonary embolism–a prospective study. Chest 1991;99(2):280–3.

[7] Campbell CB, Chandler JG, Tegtmeyer CJ, et al. Axillary, subclavian, brachiocephalic vein obstruction. Surgery 1977;82(6):816–26.

[8] Wells PS, Anderson DR, Bormanis J, et al. Value of assessment of pretest probability of deep-vein thrombosis in clinical management. Lancet 1997;350(9094):1795–8.

[9] Wells PS, Brill-Edwards P, Stevens P, et al. A novel and rapid whole-blood assay for D-dimer in patients with clinically suspected deep vein thrombosis. Circulation 1995;91(8):2184–7.

[10] Freyburger G, Trillaud H, Labrouche S, et al. D-dimer strategy in thrombosis exclusion–a gold standard study in 100 patients suspected of deep venous thrombosis or pulmonary embolism: 8 DD methods compared. Thromb Haemost 1998;79(1):32–7.

[11] Brill-Edwards P, Lee A. D-dimer testing in the diagnosis of acute venous thromboembolism. Thromb Haemost 1999;82(2):688–94.

[12] Wells PS, Anderson DR, Rodger M, et al. Evaluation of D-dimer in the diagnosis of suspected deep-vein thrombosis. N Engl J Med 2003;349(13):1227–35.

[13] ACR practice guideline for the performance of peripheral venous ultrasound examination. In: Practical guidelines and technical standards. Reston (VA): American College of Radiology; 2006. p. 863–6.

[14] Aziz S, Straehley CJ, Whelan TJ Jr. Effort-related axillosubclavian vein thrombosis. A new theory of pathogenesis and a plea for direct surgical intervention. Am J Surg 1986;152(1):57–61.

[15] Bonnet F, Loriferne JF, Texier JP, et al. Evaluation of Doppler examination for diagnosis of catheter-related deep vein thrombosis. Intensive Care Med 1989;15(4):238–40.

[16] McDonough JJ, Altemeier WA. Subclavian venous thrombosis secondary to indwelling catheters. Surg Gynecol Obstet 1971;133(3):397–400.

[17] Luciani A, Clement O, Halimi P, et al. Catheter-related upper extremity deep venous thrombosis in cancer patients: a prospective study based on Doppler US. Radiology 2001;220(3):655–60.

[18] Trerotola SO, Kuhn-Fulton J, Johnson MS, et al. Tunneled infusion catheters: increased incidence of symptomatic venous thrombosis after subclavian versus internal jugular venous access. Radiology 2000;217(1):89–93.

[19] Becker DM, Philbrick JT, Walker FB IV. Axillary and subclavian venous thrombosis. Prognosis and treatment. Arch Intern Med 1991;151(10):1934–43.

[20] Mustafa S, Stein PD, Patel KC, et al. Upper extremity deep venous thrombosis. Chest 2003;123(6):1953–6.

[21] Kooij JD, van der Zant FM, van Beek EJ, et al. Pulmonary embolism in deep venous thrombosis of the upper extremity: more often in catheter-related thrombosis. Neth J Med 1997;50(6):238–42.

[22] Chin EE, Zimmerman PT, Grant EG. Sonographic evaluation of upper extremity deep venous thrombosis. J Ultrasound Med 2005;24(6):829–38.

[23] Baarslag HJ, van Beek EJ, Koopman MM, et al. Prospective study of color duplex ultrasonography compared with contrast venography in patients suspected of having deep venous thrombosis of the upper extremities. Ann Intern Med 2002;136(12):865–72.

[24] Knudson GJ, Wiedmeyer DA, Erickson SJ, et al. Color Doppler sonographic imaging in the assessment of upper-extremity deep venous thrombosis. Am J Roentgenol 1990;154(2):399–403.

[25] Baxter GM, Kincaid W, Jeffrey RF, et al. Comparison of colour Doppler ultrasound with venography in the diagnosis of axillary and subclavian vein thrombosis. Br J Radiol 1991;64(765):777–81.

[26] Bernardi E, Piccioli A, Marchiori A, et al. Upper extremity deep vein thrombosis: risk factors, diagnosis, and management. SeminVasc Med 2001;1(1):105–10.

[27] Fraser JD, Anderson DR. Venous protocols, techniques, and interpretations of the upper and lower extremities. Radiol Clin North Am 2004;42(2):279–96.

[28] Patel MC, Berman LH, Moss HA, et al. Subclavian and internal jugular veins at Doppler US: abnormal cardiac pulsatility and respiratory phasicity as a predictor of complete central occlusion. Radiology 1999;211(2):579–83.

[29] Buller HR, Agnelli G, Hull RD, et al. Antithrombotic therapy for venous thromboembolic disease: the Seventh ACCP Conference on Antithrombotic and Thrombolytic Therapy. Chest 2004;126(3 Suppl):401S–28S.

[30] Rubin JM, Xie H, Kim K, et al. Sonographic elasticity imaging of acute and chronic deep venous thrombosis in humans. J Ultrasound Med 2006; 25(9):1179–86.

[31] Rubin JM, Aglyamov SR, Wakefield TW, et al. Clinical application of sonographic elasticity imaging for aging of deep venous thrombosis: preliminary findings. J Ultrasound Med 2003; 22(5):443–8.

[32] Pain SJ, Vowler S, Purushotham AD. Axillary vein abnormalities contribute to development of lymphoedema after surgery for breast cancer. Br J Surg 2005;92(3):311–5.

[33] Povoski SP, Zaman SA. Selective use of preoperative venous duplex ultrasound and intraoperative venography for central venous access device placement in cancer patients. Ann Surg Oncol 2002;9(5):493–9.

[34] Robbin ML, Gallichio MH, Deierhoi MH, et al. US vascular mapping before hemodialysis access placement. Radiology 2000;217(1):83–8.

[35] Allon M, Lockhart ME, Lilly RZ, et al. Effect of preoperative sonographic mapping on vascular access outcomes in hemodialysis patients. Kidney Int 2001;60(5):2013–20.

[36] National Kidney Foundation. K/DOQI clinical practice guidelines for vascular access, 2000. Am J Kidney Dis 2001;37(Suppl 1):S7–64.

[37] Robbin ML, Chamberlain NE, Lockhart ME, et al. Hemodialysis arteriovenous fistula maturity: US evaluation. Radiology 2002;225(1):59–64.

[38] Grogan J, Castilla M, Lozanski L, et al. Frequency of critical stenosis in primary arteriovenous fistulae before hemodialysis access: should duplex ultrasound surveillance be the standard of care? J Vasc Surg 2005;41(6):1000–6.

[39] Lockhart ME, Robbin ML. Hemodialysis access ultrasound. Ultrasound Q 2001;17(3):157–67.

[40] Beathard GA, Arnold P, Jackson J, et al. Physician operators forum of RMS lifeline. Aggressive treatment of early fistula failure. Kidney Int 2003;64(4):1487–94.

RADIOLOGIC
CLINICS
OF NORTH AMERICA

Radiol Clin N Am 45 (2007) 525–547

Ultrasound Evaluation of the Lower Extremity Veins

Ulrike M. Hamper, MD, MBA[a],*, M. Robert DeJong, RDMS, RVT, RCDS[a],
Leslie M. Scoutt, MD[b]

- Clinical presentation and differential diagnosis
- Examination technique and normal sonographic anatomy
- Controversial issues vis-à-vis the examination technique
- Sonography of acute deep venous thrombosis
- Pitfalls and limitations of diagnosis of acute deep vein thrombosis
- Sonography of chronic deep venous thrombosis
- Chronic venous insufficiency
  Pathophysiology
  Venous anatomy of the superficial veins of the lower extremity
  Method of examination
- Summary
- References

Over the past 2 decades venous ultrasonography (US) has become the standard primary imaging technique for the initial evaluation of patients for whom there is clinical suspicion of deep venous thrombosis (DVT) of the lower extremity veins. It has replaced the venogram and other diagnostic studies such as impedance plethysmography, various radionuclide studies, and conventional CT because of its noninvasive nature, the ease with which it can be performed in skilled hands, and its proven efficacy. Compression US first was described as a means of diagnosing DVT in 1986 by Raghavendra and colleagues [1] and was introduced into clinical practice in 1987 by Cronan and colleagues [2–7] from the United States and Appleman and colleagues [8] from the Netherlands. In the ensuing years multiple articles were published establishing venous US as the examination of choice for the diagnosis of venous thrombosis, further refining the US technique and diagnostic criteria with gray-scale imaging, and also incorporating the newly developed technique of Doppler US.

This article addresses the role of duplex US and color Doppler US (CDUS) in today's clinical practice for the evaluation of patients suspected of harboring a thrombus in their lower extremity veins. Clinical presentation and differential diagnoses, technique, and diagnostic criteria for both acute and chronic DVT are reviewed. In addition, sonographic evaluation of venous insufficiency is addressed.

Clinical presentation and differential diagnosis

Acute DVT is a significant health problem affecting approximately 2 million people in the United States

[a] Department of Radiology and Radiological Science, Johns Hopkins University, School of Medicine, 600 N Wolfe Street, Baltimore, MD 21287, USA
[b] Yale University, School of Medicine, 20 York Street, 2-272WP New Haven, CT 06504, USA
* Corresponding author.
E-mail address: umhamper@jhu.edu (U.M. Hamper).

doi:10.1016/j.rcl.2007.04.013

per year. Pulmonary embolism (PE) is the most dreaded complication of an untreated DVT and is reported to occur in about 50% to 60% of untreated cases with a 25% to 30% mortality rate [4,9–12]. Predisposing factors for DVT include prolonged bed rest, congestive heart failure, prior DVT, pelvic and lower extremity surgery, coagulopathies, immobilization, trauma, pregnancy, malignancies, indwelling catheters, intravenous drug abuse, dehydration, travel (probably because of prolonged immobility), and endothelial injury. In addition, oral contraceptive use, obesity, and systemic diseases such as systemic lupus erythematosus, lupus anticoagulant, nephritic syndrome, Behçet's disease, nocturnal hemoglobinuria, polycythemia vera, and hyperviscosity syndromes may predispose a patient to thromboembolism formation.

The signs and symptoms of DVT often are nonspecific, and thus the clinical diagnostic accuracy is poor. Extremity swelling, pain, and edema place the patient at risk for DVT. Significant thrombus can be present in asymptomatic patients, however. The clinical accuracy for the diagnosis of acute DVT has been reported to be about 50% in symptomatic patients [13–16]. Localized pain and calf tenderness are reported in approximately 50% of cases, but pain on forced dorsiflexion of the toes, the so-called "Homan's sign," is an unreliable diagnostic criterion and is present in only 8% to 30% of symptomatic patients harboring a DVT. Furthermore, the Homan's sign can be elicited in nearly

50% of symptomatic patients who do not have a DVT as a cause of their symptoms [4,17]. A palpable cord caused by a thrombosed superficial vessel can be present with or without involvement of the deep venous system [4]. US examination is highly sensitive and specific for the diagnosis of DVT: several series have reported sensitivities and specificities approaching 95% to 100% for the diagnosis of DVT in the proximal lower extremity. The most common causes for false-negative examinations are venous duplication, infrapopliteal thrombus, and nonocclusive focal or segmental DVT. Therefore, expeditious sonographic evaluation of patients suspected of having DVT may aid in rapid initiation of therapeutic measures to decrease the potential for developing complications such as PE or postthrombotic venous insufficiency. The limitations of US in accurately diagnosing calf vein thrombosis and DVT in obese patients is addressed later.

Examination technique and normal sonographic anatomy

The choice of transducer for evaluating the lower extremity veins depends on the patient's body habitus and the depth of the vessel to be studied. The examination is preferentially performed with a high-resolution 5- to 7.5-MHz linear array transducer. For very superficial veins (ie, the greater or small saphenous veins), a 10-MHz transducer may

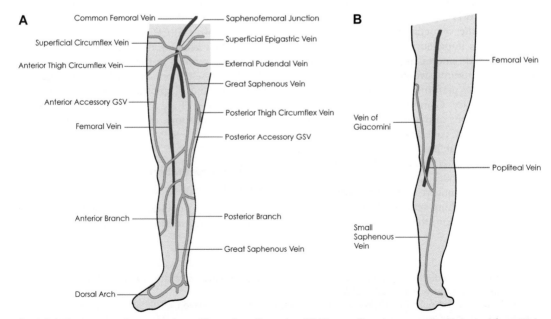

Fig. 1. (*A*) The great saphenous vein and its major tributaries. (*B*) The small saphenous vein. (*Adapted from* Weiss RA, Feied CF, Weiss MA. Vein diagnosis and treatment. New York: McGraw-Hill; 2001.)

be optimal. For large patients a lower-frequency (2.5- or 3.5-MHz) curvilinear transducer may be necessary. In general, the transducer with the highest frequency allowing adequate penetration provides the best spatial resolution. Appropriate gain settings must be applied to ensure that the vessels are free of artifactual internal echoes and that thrombus is not mistaken for echoes caused by slow-flowing blood. In addition, CDUS imaging parameters must be optimized for sensitivity to slow, low-volume flow.

The lower extremity venous system consists of a superficial system, the saphenous veins and their tributaries, and a deep system. A more detailed description of the superficial venous plexus is presented later in the section discussing venous insufficiency. Briefly, the great saphenous vein (GSV) joins the common femoral vein (CFV) just superior to its bifurcation. It travels medially in the thigh and calf extending inferiorly to the level

of the foot (Fig. 1A). It measures about 3 to 5 mm in diameter at the level of the saphenofemoral junction, tapering to about 1 to 3 mm in diameter at the level of the ankle (see Fig. 1A). Measurement of the GSV is important before harvesting for autologous vein grafting. The small saphenous vein (SSV) (formerly called the "lesser saphenous vein") extends from the ankle along the posterior aspect of the calf to insert at variable levels into the posterior proximal or mid popliteal vein (PV) (Fig. 1B). The diameter of the SSV tapers from 2 to 4 mm proximally to about 1 to 2 mm distally. Both the GSV and SSV may become enlarged and varicose in patients who have venous insufficiency or congestive heart failure. Thrombosis of these vessels may occur with ensuing superficial thrombophlebitis (Fig. 2).

The deep venous system includes the CFV, the deep femoral or profunda femoris vein, the femoral vein (FV) (previously called the "superficial femoral

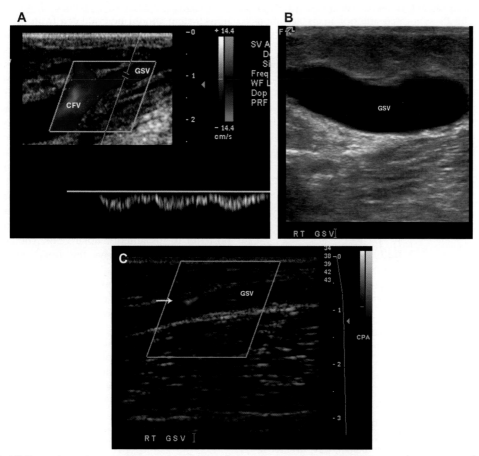

Fig. 2. (*A*) Normal greater saphenous vein/common femoral vein junction—Doppler gate in greater saphenous vein. (*B*) Large greater saphenous vein in a patient who has congestive heart failure. (*C*) Sagittal US of thrombosed greater saphenous vein with only a trickle of peripheral flow (*arrow*).

vein"), and the PV as well as the paired anterior and posterior tibial veins and the peroneal veins (Fig. 3). The CFV is the continuation of the external iliac vein and extends from the level of the inguinal ligament to the level of the bifurcation into the FV and profunda femoris vein. The profunda femoris vein lies medial to the accompanying artery and can be evaluated only in its most proximal portion. The CFV lies medial to the accompanying artery. The FV travels medial to the femoral artery through the adductor canal in the distal thigh. To avoid confusion among clinicians, the term "femoral vein" (FV) should be used instead of the previously designated term "superficial femoral vein" to describe that part of the deep venous system caudal to the bifurcation of the CFV. (In a survey performed by Bundens and colleagues [18], more than 70% of surveyed internists regarded the "superficial femoral vein" as part of the superficial and not the deep venous system and thus were under the assumption that superficial femoral vein thrombosis did not require treatment.) The PV is the continuation of the FV after its exit from the adductor canal in the posterior distal thigh. The PV is located anterior to its accompanying artery and courses through the popliteal space into the proximal calf. In general, the deep veins in the thigh are wider in diameter

than the accompanying artery unless the veins are duplicated. Duplication of the FV or PV can be seen in 20% to 35% of patients. Duplication of the FV can be segmental. It is important to mention these anatomic variants so that thrombosis in one of the duplicated limbs is not missed (Fig. 4). The paired anterior tibial veins are accompanied by their corresponding artery and arise from the popliteal vein traversing the anterior calf compartment along the interosseous membrane to the dorsum of the foot. The tibioperoneal trunk originates from the PV slightly distal to the anterior tibial veins and bifurcates into the paired posterior tibial veins and peroneal veins , both of which are accompanied by their respective arteries. The peroneal veins course medial to the posterior aspect of the fibula, whereas the posterior tibial veins course through the posterior calf muscles posterior to the tibia and along the medial malleolus. In addition, the muscles of the calf are drained by gastrocnemius and soleus veins, which do not have accompanying arteries.

In a patient suspected of having DVT, the deep venous system should be evaluated from just above the inguinal ligament to the trifurcation of the popliteal vein in the upper calf, every 2 to 3 cm, with compression. In addition, evaluation of the external iliac veins and calf veins, including anterior and posterior tibial veins and peroneal veins, can be performed. The iliac vein, CFV, and FV are best evaluated with the patient in a supine position (Fig. 5A). The popliteal veins can be studied with the patient supine and the leg flexed 20° to 30° and externally rotated or in a decubitus position with the study side up (Fig. 5B). The anterior tibial veins are best identified initially at the posterior medial ankle. When followed up the leg, the peroneal veins, which originate from the lateral ankle, are posterior to the anterior tibial veins. The anterior tibial veins run between the tibia and fibula anteriorly.

According to the American College of Radiology practice guidelines and technical standards, lower extremity Duplex sonography should include compression, color, and spectral Doppler sonography with assessment of phasicity and venous flow augmentation [19]. A complete examination includes evaluation of the full length of the CFV and saphenofemoral junction, the proximal portion of the deep femoral vein, the FV, and the PV. These veins are imaged in the transverse plane with and without compression with mild transducer pressure every 2 to 3 cm from the level of the CFV to the distal FV in the adductor canal and the PV to the popliteal trifurcation. In obese patients compression in the adductor canal may be difficult. Sometimes a

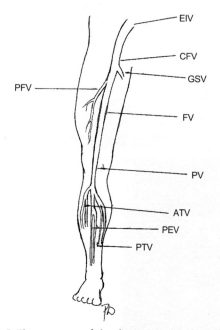

Fig. 3. The anatomy of the deep venous system. ATV, anterior tibial veins; CFV, common femoral vein; EIV, external iliac vein; FV, femoral vein; GSV, greater saphenous vein; PEV, peroneal veins; PFV, profunda femoris vein; PTV, posterior tibial veins; PV, popliteal veins.

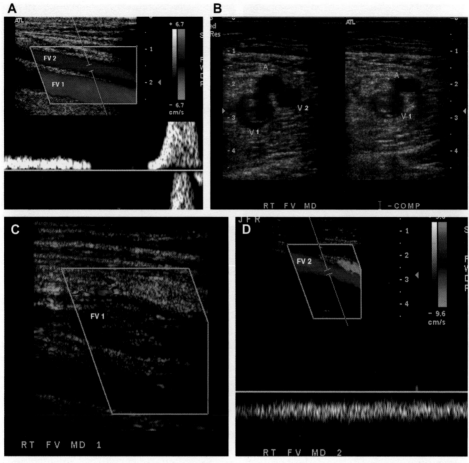

Fig. 4. (*A*) Sagittal color Doppler US of duplicated femoral vein (*FV*). (*B*) Transverse US of duplicated femoral vein demonstrating noncompressibility of thrombosed limb (*V1*). (*C*) Sagittal color Doppler US limb of a duplicated femoral vein (*FV1*). (*D*) Sagittal color Doppler US of normal flow in duplicated femoral vein (*FV2*).

two-hand technique, pushing the leg into the transducer with the free hand from behind, may help achieve adequate compression (Fig. 5C). A normal pulse of color flow Doppler signal in a suboptimally compressed or poorly visualized segment is reassuring of at least partial patency and excludes the possibility of occlusive thrombus. Compression of a normal vein completely collapses the venous lumen (Figs. 6 and 7), whereas the presence of DVT prevents coaptation of the vein walls (see Figs. 6 and 7). In the authors' laboratory, color flow Doppler US is used routinely because it speeds the identification of the vessels and facilitates identification of deeply located vessel segments. Color should fill the entire lumen of normal veins, but color flow is diminished or absent in partially or completely thrombosed veins (Fig. 8). Sometimes, particularly in veins with slow flow, squeezing the calf will augment venous flow, resulting in complete color filling of a vessel. Doppler spectral analysis is

performed to assess phasicity and augmentation responses following squeezing of the calf or plantar flexion of the foot and is helpful as a secondary means of assessing patency of the more proximal veins, particularly the iliac veins (see Fig. 8E, F). If a thrombus is identified in any segment of the veins, augmentation is not performed to avoid detaching the clot and thereby causing a PE. Because of the risk of superficial thrombophlebitis extending into the deep venous system, the authors also routinely study the GSV at its junction with the CFV (see Fig. 8F–H). Because of its increased sensitivity to low-velocity, low-volume flow, pwer Doppler US sometimes is useful in identifying early recanalization of thrombosed veins or in detecting minimal flow in nearly occluded venous segments, deep vessels, or the smaller calf veins. Power Doppler, however, does not indicate directionality of flow and is affected adversely by patient motion or calcifications.

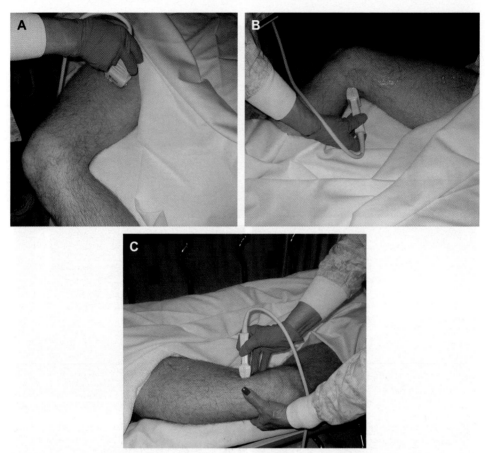

Fig. 5. (A) Transverse scan demonstrating the imaging technique of the femoral vein with the patient in a supine position. (B) Transverse scan demonstrating the imaging technique of the popliteal vein with the leg flexed and externally rotated. (C) "Two-hand technique" to visualize the femoral vein (FV) in the adductor canal.

The normal veins are easily compressible by slight transducer pressure (see Figs. 6 and 7). If one cannot compress the veins because of swelling or pain, one can attempt indirect evaluation using a Valsalva maneuver, observation of the presence or absence of respiratory phasicity, and augmentation techniques. Following a Valsalva maneuver, a normal vein expands to more than 50% of its diameter from baseline. The Valsalva maneuver has the most pronounced effect on the veins near the inguinal ligament. Proximal pelvic DVT or external compression of the pelvic veins blunts the normal dilatation of the CFV following a Valsalva maneuver. Evaluation of respiratory phasicity and augmentation also can provide indirect assessment of adjacent vein segments. Proximal (cephalic) obstruction caused by pelvic venous thrombosis or external compression of the pelvic veins by ascites, pelvic mass, or hematoma dampens respiratory phasicity in the CFV (Fig. 9). Distal (caudal) DVT blunts the normal augmentation of venous flow achieved by squeezing the leg inferior to the point of insonation. Valsalva maneuvers also can be used to evaluate venous insufficiency. With the patient supine, a temporary reversal of flow occurs if the valves are incompetent. (This phenomenon is discussed in more detail at the end of the article). Likewise changes in the venous spectral tracing can indicate more proximal cardiovascular disease. For example, in patients who have elevated right atrial pressure caused by congestive heart failure or tricuspid insufficiency, the spectral venous waveform can be quite pulsatile, mimicking a waveform more typical of the hepatic veins or inferior vena cava (Fig. 10) [20].

Controversial issues vis-à-vis the examination technique

US evaluation of the calf veins remains controversial because of its unproven clinical value and cost effectiveness, and the American College of Radiology practice guidelines do not require their evaluation. It has been shown that isolated calf vein

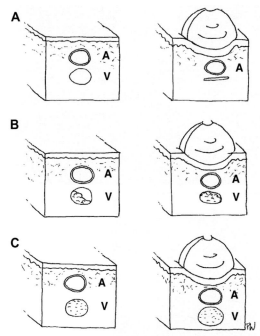

Fig. 6. Transverse compression of normal and thrombosed veins. (*A*) Compression of a normal vein completely collapses the venous lumen. (*B*) Compression of a nonocclusive, thrombosed vein partially collapses the venous lumen. (*C*) Compression of a completely thrombosed vein prevents venous coaptation.

thrombosis rarely causes significant pulmonary emboli and thus is assumed to be a benign, self-limiting disease [21]. Hence, patients who have isolated calf DVT rarely receive anticoagulation therapy in clinical practice because the risk of bleeding from the anticoagulation therapy is considered to be higher than the risk of PE even though several studies have shown that approximately 20% of calf DVTs ultimately extend into the more superior deep venous system in the thigh [21]. In addition, US evaluation of the calf veins is less accurate than evaluation of veins in the thigh because the veins in the calf are much smaller; therefore it is difficult to be certain that all of the calf vessels, some of which are duplicated, are free of thrombus. Other studies stress the clinical importance of calf vein thrombosis and argue that the 4% to 10% risk of potential bleeding with anticoagulation therapy is safer than the 20% to 30% risk of propagation and potential 5% risk for development of PE [22,23]. In a study by Badgett and colleagues [24], a complete venous examination including calf veins altered clinical management in about 30% of patients. The practice in the authors' laboratory is to evaluate the calf veins only in patients who have focal, persistent, or worsening calf symptoms.

Another controversy in the radiologic and surgical literature centers around the necessity of routinely performing bilateral lower extremity venous US examinations versus the appropriateness of performing a unilateral examination if symptoms are limited to one leg. Some studies recommend routine performance of bilateral venous US studies of the lower extremities because thrombus can occur in either leg in up to 23% of patients who have bilateral symptoms [25]. A study by Cronan [3] concluded that the likelihood of finding DVT in patients who have bilateral lower extremity symptoms is related to their predisposing risk factors, and that bilateral lower extremity sonography is indicated only in patients who have a risk factor for DVT, not in those who are at risk only for cardiac disease.

Other studies suggest that examination of an asymptomatic leg is unnecessary because, although thrombosis may occur in the asymptomatic leg in up to 14% of patients, these patients typically have DVT in the symptomatic leg as well [25–28].

An additional concern centers on the issue of performing limited examinations. Some authors have suggested a limited compression examination of the FV and PV because of the low rate of reported isolated FV thrombosis. Several studies, however, have shown that omitting the FV and evaluating only the CFVs and PVs would lead to a decrease in sensitivity because isolated thrombosis of the FV occurs in 4% to 6% of cases [26,29]. Another issue concerns the usefulness of performing augmentation in all patients being evaluated for DVT. A study by Lockhart and colleagues [30] questions the usefulness of performing venous flow augmentation maneuvers with duplex sonography because of its lack of clinical benefit and the added discomfort for the patient who has swollen and painful legs. The authors recommend using augmentation as an adjunct only in uncertain cases rather than as a routine diagnostic component of the lower extremity DVT examination.

Finally, the recent development of multislice and/or multidetector techniques in CT has led to a reconsideration of the role of CT in the diagnosis of DVT when included as part of a pulmonary angiography study. A study by Kim and colleagues [31] demonstrated that multislice helical CT detected DVT that had been missed by venous sonography in five patients, but US detected DVT that was missed by CT in one patient. On the other hand, Kim and colleagues reported [31] that indirect multidetector CT is as accurate as sonography in the detection of femoropopliteal DVT and has the advantage over sonography of being able to evaluate the pelvic veins and inferior vena cava. Particularly in a patient undergoing

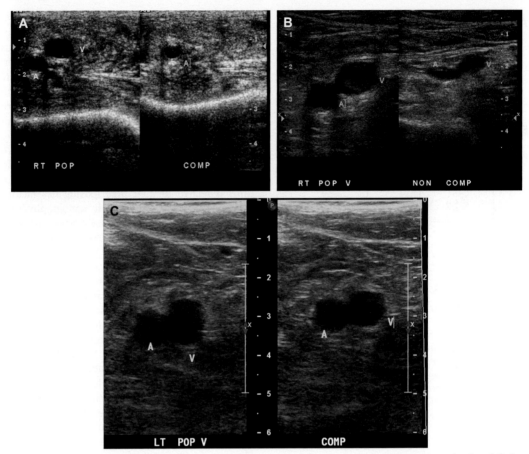

Fig. 7. Transverse sonograms demonstrating compression response of normal and thrombosed veins. (*A*) Compression of a normal popliteal vein completely collapses the venous lumen. Only the popliteal artery (*A*) remains on compression view. (*B*) Compression of a nonocclusive thrombosed popliteal vein partially collapses the venous lumen (*V*). (*C*) Compression of a completely thrombosed popliteal vein prevents venous coaptation.

CT pulmonary angiography in the ICU, the use of indirect CT venography of the lower extremities may be a reasonable alternative to sonography [32]. One must, however, consider carefully the increased radiation dose from multidetector CT when considering the use of this imaging approach to diagnose DVT.

Sonography of acute deep venous thrombosis

The hallmark gray-scale findings of acute DVT include noncompressibility of the vessel as well as direct visualization of the thrombus (see Fig. 6; Figs. 11 and 12). Thrombus may be anechoic or hypo- or hyperechoic. Anechoic or hypoechoic thrombi are thought to be more recent, although the distinction is not precise. Clot echogenicity alone cannot be used to assess the age of a clot [33]. In addition, very slowly flowing blood may be sufficiently echogenic to mimic the appearance of clot (Fig. 13A) [34]. In this instance, however, the compression US is normal (Fig. 13B). Changes in vein caliber with respiration or Valsalva maneuver are lost also when thrombus is present. Thrombi may occlude the lumen completely or partially, and they may be adherent to the wall or free floating (Fig. 14). On CDUS a filling defect can be seen indicating nonocclusive thrombus, or there may be complete absence of flow (Fig. 15).

In a large, pooled series of DVT studies, the accuracy of compression US for DVT has been shown to reach 95% with 98% specificity [4]. In other series sensitivities and specificities range from 88% to 100% and from 92% to 100%, respectively. Additional studies report a sensitivity of 95%, specificity of 99%, and accuracy of 98% for color Doppler flow imaging [35,36]. Sensitivities for isolated calf vein thrombosis are lower, ranging from 60% to 80% [4,37,38]. Protocols and techniques

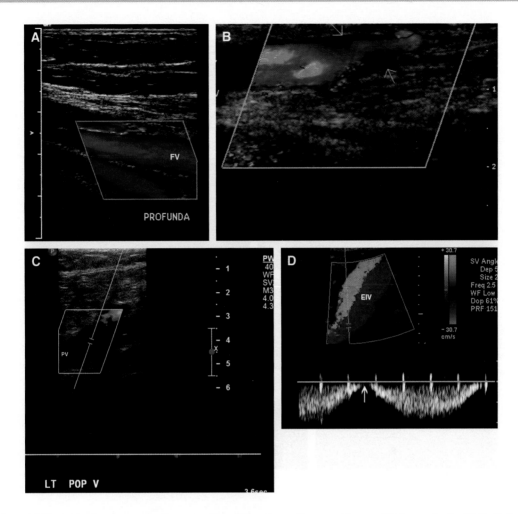

Fig. 8. (*A*) Normal veins demonstrating color flow filling the entire vessel lumen. FV, femoral vein. (*B*) Partial venous thrombosis demonstrating focal absence of color flow (*arrows*). (*C*) Occlusive venous thrombosis demonstrating complete absence of color flow in the popliteal vein. Also note absence of venous waveform on duplex spectrum. (*D*) Normal respiratory phasicity of the right iliac vein. Note return of flow to baseline during inspiration (*arrow*). (*E*) Augmentation maneuver demonstrates surge of flow in right popliteal vein when squeezing the calf (*arrow*). (*F*) Normal color flow Doppler appearance of the junction of the greater saphenous vein (*GSV*) and the common femoral vein (*CFV*). (*G*) Thrombosis of the left greater saphenou vein (*GSV*) near the junction with the common femoral vein (*arrow*). (*H*) Six days later the greater saphenous vein thrombosis has extended into the common femoral vein (*V*) as demonstrated on the transverse compression images.

for evaluation of the calf veins have not been established definitively.

Pitfalls and limitations of diagnosis of acute deep vein thrombosis

The classic clinical signs of DVT cannot be trusted because a variety of abnormalities can mimic the signs and symptoms of acute DVT. Cronan and colleagues [6] showed that in approximately 10% of patients studied for acute DVT, ancillary findings were diagnosed by sonography along with a normal

deep venous examination. US can readily distinguish those entities from venous pathology.

A variety of conditions that may cause clinical signs and symptoms indistinguishable from DVT may be caused by other underlying pathology such as adenopathy (groin swelling), arterial aneurysms, or stenoses/occlusions (Fig. 16), soft tissue tumors, hematomas or abscesses, muscle tears, and diffuse soft tissue edema (Fig. 17). Proximal obstruction by an extrinsic mass, such as adenopathy, pseudoaneurysm, or hematoma, may limit the compressibility of veins and produce the same clinical signs of DVT (see Fig. 9B; Fig. 18). Simple

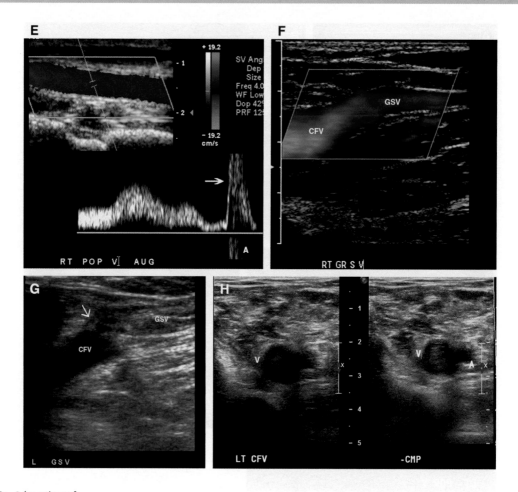

Fig. 8 (continued)

popliteal synovial cysts or cysts that communicate with the posterior bursa around the knee (Baker's cysts) can, when ruptured, cause mass effect and simulate the pain and swelling associated with popliteal DVT (Fig. 19). Popliteal artery aneurysm may cause calf pain and swelling (Fig. 20). Congestive heart failure or tricuspid insufficiency with secondary venous distension and leg swelling and edema may cause a clinically false-positive result. Often in these patients a very pulsatile venous waveform is observed (see Fig. 10) [20]. A patent SSV filled with thrombus may be mistaken for a thrombosed PV (Fig. 21). Acute or chronic clot may be difficult to differentiate, as discussed later.

False-negative US studies can occur in obese patients or in patients who have very edematous extremities. The FV in the adductor canal region may be difficult to evaluate. Small nonocclusive thrombi in the profunda femoris vein may be missed. Thrombosis of a duplicated FV (see Fig. 4B) may go undetected, and more proximal iliac vein thrombosis often is difficult to demonstrate.

Loss of phasicity in the CFV or distal iliac vein should be noted as a secondary sign indicating a more proximal thrombosis or compression by masses or collections (see Figs. 16 and 18).

It is important to recognize these pitfalls and limitations to lessen the chance of potentially severe consequences of an erroneous or missed diagnosis of DVT. False-negative imaging results may deprive the patient of appropriate anticoagulation therapy and potentially result in clot propagation, PE, and death, whereas a false-positive result may result in unnecessary anticoagulation with the associated risk of bleeding.

Sonography of chronic deep venous thrombosis

The differentiation of acute or chronic DVT by imaging methods and clinical parameters often is difficult. In about one fourth of patients, the DVT resolves completely after adequate treatment regimens. Serial studies, however, have shown

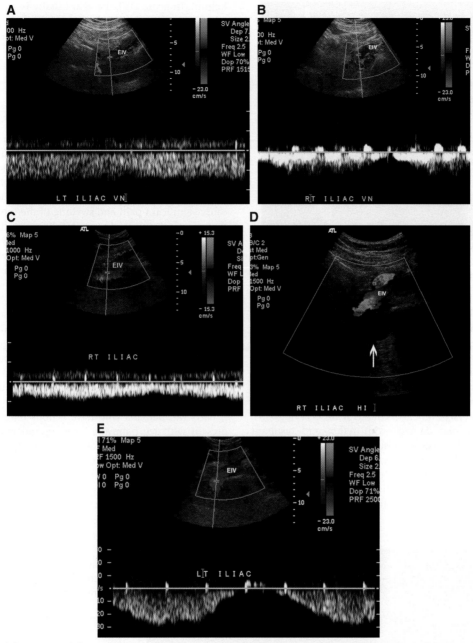

Fig. 9. (*A*) Dampened flow in left external iliac vein (*EIV*) caused by more proximal thrombosis. (*B*) Normal respiratory phasicity flow in right external iliac vein (*EIV*). (*C*) Dampened flow in right external iliac vein (*EIV*) caused by compression by fluid collection with loss of respiratory phasicity. (*D*) Right groin fluid collection (*arrow*). (*E*) Normal respiratory phasicity in left external iliac vein (*EIV*).

persistent abnormal findings on compression US 6 to 24 months later in 54% of patients who had acute DVT [4]. Without an US evaluation showing resolution of the acute DVT, recurrent DVT may be indistinguishable from chronic disease. On compression US both acute and chronic DVT may show noncompressibility of the vessel. In chronic DVT, the vessel walls often are thickened with decreased compliance (Fig. 22A). Veins may recanalize to a certain extent after an acute DVT (Fig. 22B). Residual clot, however, may manifest as organized echogenic material along the vein walls and mimic the sonographic appearance of acute clot. Because noncompressibility of a vein is a sonographic sign of

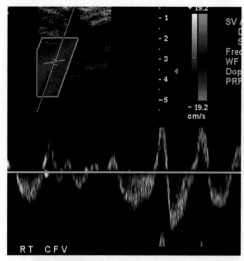

Fig. 10. Pulsatile spectral waveform in right common femoral vein (*CFV*) caused by tricuspid insufficiency.

both chronic and acute DVT, care must be taken to differentiate the two entities so that patients do not receive unnecessary anticoagulation therapy for a chronic condition. Some US findings that may help distinguish acute from chronic DVT are atretic segments (inability to identify a normal vein next to the artery), echogenic weblike filling defects within the vein (see Fig. 22B), collateral vessels (Fig. 23B), and valvular damage with reflux and resultant chronic deep venous insufficiency. Chronic thrombus usually is more echogenic and may calcify (Fig. 23A). Chronic thrombi may demonstrate thickened vein walls with a reduced venous diameter (see Fig. 22A). In addition, the size of the vein is

helpful. In acute DVT the vein usually is enlarged, whereas in chronic DVT it is normal, small, or diminutive. Recent studies demonstrating the contribution of in vitro US elasticity imaging to assess clot age may be promising for clinical use in the future [39].

Chronic venous insufficiency

Venous insufficiency is a common but often undiagnosed condition with a prevalence estimated at 25% in women and 15% in men [40–43]. The clinical significance of varicose veins is not merely cosmetic, because chronic venous insufficiency may cause significant pain and swelling of the lower extremities and ultimately may result in debilitating skin changes ranging from discoloration and induration to cutaneous and soft tissue breakdown (ie, venous stasis ulcers). Treatment costs are estimated to be as high as 3 billion dollars per year in the United States [44] and to comprise up to 1% to 3% of the total health care budget in developed countries [45–47]. Recently developed minimally invasive catheter techniques have revolutionized treatment options for patients who have varicose veins. Hence, it is important that radiologists become familiar with the US technique for evaluation of venous reflux.

Early on, patients who have venous reflux may present with leg pain and swelling and may not have obvious visible varicosities. Such patients often are referred for lower extremity venous US examinations to rule out DVT, and both clinician and radiologist may overlook the diagnosis of venous insufficiency. Hence, venous insufficiency is

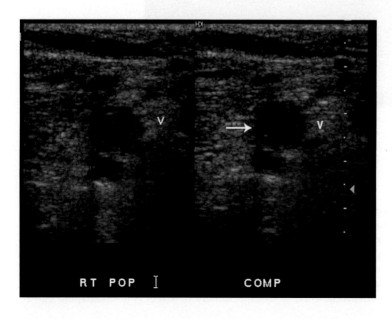

Fig. 11. Complete venous thrombosis. Transverse views of the right popliteal vein demonstrate noncompressible vein caused by acute thrombus (*arrow*).

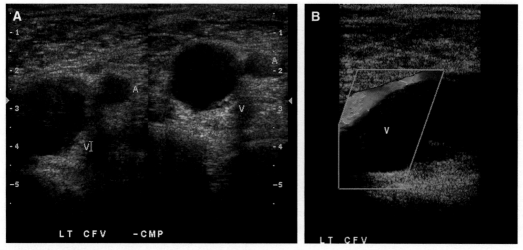

Fig. 12. (*A*) Transverse and (*B*) sagittal views of the left common femoral vein (*V*) demonstrate hypoechoic thrombus and expansion of the venous lumen.

a diagnosis that should be considered in the patient presenting with leg pain or swelling and a negative DVT US examination, particularly in someone who has persistent or recurrent symptoms. Patients who have venous reflux also may complain of leg soreness, burning, aching, throbbing, cramping, and/or muscle fatigue. Symptoms are typically exacerbated by standing or warm weather. The severity of a patient's symptoms is not necessarily related to the size or number of the varicosities or even to the amount of reflux, and significant symptoms may occur even before varicosities are clinically apparent. Over time, patients may develop chronic skin or soft tissue changes ranging from swelling and discoloration to inflammatory dermatitis and, ultimately, chronic, nonhealing leg ulcers.

Pathophysiology

Normally, venous blood flow is directed from the superficial venous system of the lower extremities through the GSV, SSV, and perforators toward the deep venous system and the heart by a series of competent, one-way valves as well as by contraction of the foot and calf muscles [48]. Valve failure is the primary cause of venous insufficiency. An incompetent valve results in retrograde flow of blood and venous pooling, which in turn dilates the more caudal veins, resulting in a cascading effect of sequential failure of more and more valves. The precise pattern of varicosities that develop depends on exactly which valves fail. Because the tributaries of the GSV and SSV are not protected by a fascial layer, they are more prone to dilate. Primary pump failure

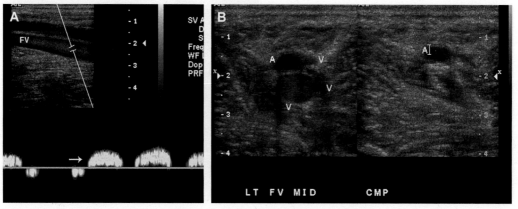

Fig. 13. Slow-flowing blood mimicking acute thrombosis. (*A*) Sagittal view of the left femoral vein demonstrates echogenic material in the venous lumen. Note venous waveform on duplex spectrum, however. (*B*) With transverse compression the venous lumen (*V*) collapses completely.

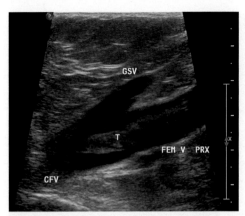

Fig. 14. Free-floating thrombus (*T*) in the left femoral vein (*FV*) extending into the common femoral vein (*CFV*).

of the calf muscles, venous obstruction from DVT, and extrinsic venous compression are much less common causes of venous insufficiency.

Risk factors for the development of venous insufficiency include any condition that distorts and/or weakens the venous valves or results in venous dilation or volume overload or increases hydrostatic pressure. Hence, risk factors include genetic predisposition, prior DVT, pregnancy, age, obesity, and occupations or activities that require prolonged standing, running, or lifting [49]. The incidence of varicose veins is nearly twice as high in women as in men [50], probably because of multiple factors including cyclic hormonal changes. Venous insufficiency also is more common in industrialized

Western countries; the increased incidence is postulated to be largely secondary to either genetic predisposition and/or diet [51].

Venous anatomy of the superficial veins of the lower extremity

The anatomy of the deep venous system in the lower extremity has been described earlier in this article. One should note here, however, several features that help discriminate the deep venous system from the superficial venous system. The veins of the deep venous system in the thigh and calf are surrounded by muscles and a deep fascial layer that help propel blood back toward the heart by means of the primary muscle pump and also help prevent reflux by limiting dilatation of the deep veins. The deep veins also always accompany an artery. The superficial veins, on the other hand, are found in the subcutaneous tissues and do not accompany an artery. A thin superficial fascial layer surrounds the saphenous trunks but not their tributaries. Thus, major branches of the saphenous system are more prone to dilate and develop reflux.

There are three major subdivisions of the superficial venous system in the lower extremity: the GSV, the SSV, and the lateral subdermic venous systems. There is substantial variability in the anatomy of the superficial venous system and in the distribution of the communicating veins (perforators) between the deep and superficial venous system.

As mentioned previously, the GSV originates medially on the foot, courses anteromedially around the medial malleolus at the ankle, and ascends anteromedially up the calf and thigh in a relatively

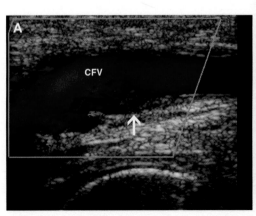

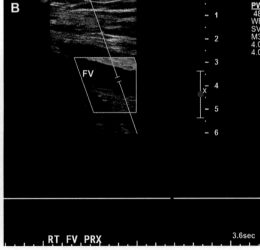

Fig. 15. (*A*) Color Doppler filling defect in the common femoral vein (*CFV*) caused by mural thrombus (*arrow*). (*B*) Absence of color flow and spectral waveform in completely thrombosed right femoral vein. Note color flow in adjacent femoral artery.

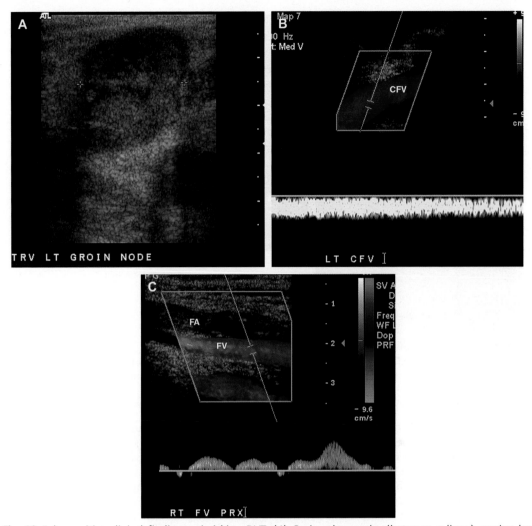

Fig. 16. False-positive clinical findings mimicking DVT. (*A*) Groin adenopathy (*between calipers*) causing leg swelling and pain. (*B*) Dampening of flow in adjacent patent left common femoral vein (*CFV*). (*C*) Right femoral artery thrombosis (*FA*) causing pain. Note normal flow in adjacent femoral vein (*FV*).

straight line, joining the CFV medially near the groin (see Fig. 1A). There always is a terminal valve at the saphenofemoral junction and usually one or two subterminal valves within 1 to 2 cm of the terminal valve. The GSV is typically 3 to 4 mm in diameter in the upper thigh and is contained in an oval fascial envelope resulting in a characteristic appearance in cross-section that has been compared with an "Egyptian eye" (Fig. 24) [52]. The most important branches of the GSV in the thigh are the posteromedial and anteromedial thigh veins, which arise in the upper to mid thigh. The lateral and medial cutaneous femoral branches, the external circumflex iliac vein, the superficial epigastric vein, and the external pudendal vein are all found near the saphenofemoral junction and terminal valves; the later three branches course superiorly (see

Figs. 1A and 24). These branches, although they may be large, are contained by the oval echogenic fascial envelope. It is estimated that 60% of patients who have varicosities have reflux in the GSV system.

The SSV originates laterally on the dorsum of the foot, passes posterior to the lateral malleolus at the ankle, and ascends the calf posteriorly, like the seam in an old-fashioned stocking (see Fig. 1B). The exact point of termination of the SSV into the deep system is quite variable. In most people, the SSV terminates directly into the PV near the popliteal crease, but the SSV may join the GSV in the lower thigh through the vein of Giacomini or even may empty directly into the FV in the thigh. The SSV also is surrounded by a fascial layer in the upper calf and typically is not wider than 3 mm in diameter. The SSV runs close to the tibial and sural

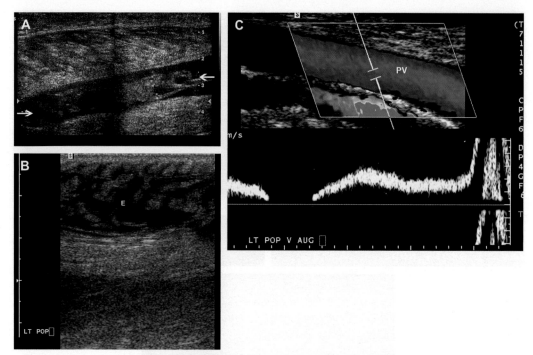

Fig. 17. False-positive clinical findings mimicking DVT. (A) Large calf hematoma (between arrows) secondary to a muscular tear. (B) Diffuse soft tissue edema (E) of the lower extremity. (C) The underlying popliteal vein (PV) was patent.

nerves, which may explain the pain associated with varicosities arising from the SSV.

The lateral subdermic venous system consists of a group of small veins found laterally above and below the knee. These veins have variable communications with the deep system. Reflux in the lateral subdermic venous system typically results in a fine telangiectasic web of superficial varicosities posterolaterally above or below the knee. Such spider-vein varicosities often occur in younger women (probably resulting from a genetic predisposition) and typically are not associated with truncal varicosities or significant pain and swelling.

Numerous short, perforating veins direct flow from the superficial to the deep system. The exact number and location of these perforators is quite variable. In general these veins are short, straight, and run perpendicular or at a slight angle from the GSV or SSV toward the deep venous system. The most common named groups are the Hunterian perforators (near the medial aspect of the upper adductor canal); Dodd's perforators (in the lower

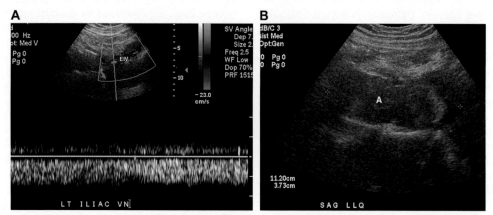

Fig. 18. Clinically false-positive results for DVT caused by groin adenopathy. (A) Dampened flow in the left external iliac vein (EIV) caused by (B) large groin adenopathy (A) from prostate cancer (between calipers).

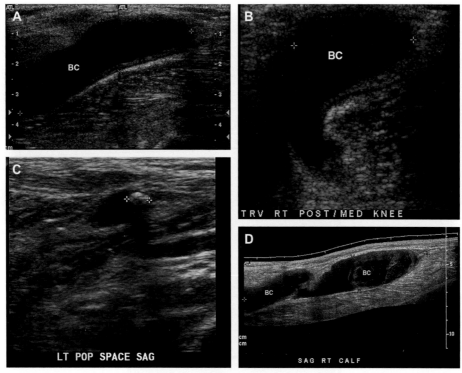

Fig. 19. Baker's cysts. (*A*) Sagittal and (*B*) transverse images of a simple Baker's cyst (*BC*). (*C*) Sagittal view of a complex Baker's cyst (*BC*) with calcifications (between calipers). (*D*) Sagittal view of a ruptured Baker's cyst (*BC*) extending into the lower calf (between calipers).

medial thigh); Boyd's perforators (in the mid calf); and Crockett's perforators (in the lower posteromedial calf) (Fig. 25). When incompetent, these perforators dilate focally and may cause "blow outs," point tenderness, or even ulceration where they join the superficial system.

Method of examination

Designing a treatment plan for a patient who has varicose veins requires identification of the highest as well as the lowest point of reflux. In addition, the source of reflux must be identified for every

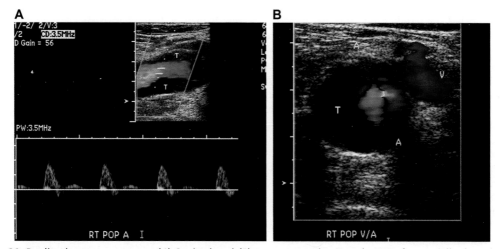

Fig. 20. Popliteal artery aneurysm. (*A*) Sagittal and (*B*) transverse color Doppler US of a partially thrombosed popliteal artery aneurysm (*A*) causing pain and calf swelling. Note absence of flow in the thrombosed portion (*T*).

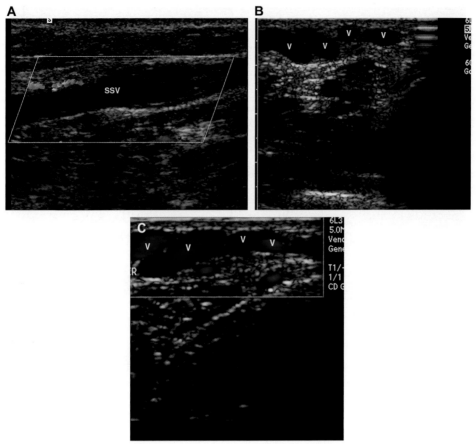

Fig. 21. (*A*) Sagittal view of a thrombosed small saphenous vein (*SSV*) mistaken for popliteal vein thrombosis. Note the very superficial location of the small saphenous vein and absence of an accompany artery. (*B*) Gray-scale image and (*C*) color Doppler US of superficial varicosities (*V*) causing pain and swelling, thus clinically mimicking DVT.

varicosity. This identification is accomplished by a combination of visual inspection and Doppler US. US examination can be quite lengthy in a patient who has numerous varicosities because patterns of reflux are highly variable and often are quite complex, with multiple sources of reflux.

The Doppler US examination for reflux begins with a standard US examination of the deep system performed with the patient in the supine position to exclude DVT. The patient then stands, and the legs are inspected visually to identify all varicose veins, because the examination should be tailored to address all varicosities in question. In general, reflux in the GSV tends to involve the medial (inner) thigh, whereas reflux in the SSV causes varicosities in the posterior calf. Telangiectastic varices developing laterally around the knee typically are secondary to reflux in the lateral subdermic venous system. Because not all symptomatic varicosities are visible, the examiner should remember to ask the patient where it hurts.

Doppler assessment of reflux always should be performed with the patient in the standing position. Because the examination can be time consuming, it may be helpful to have a walker, table, or counter to help support the patient as well as a stool for the examiner. Either color or pulse Doppler can be used, and three different maneuvers can be attempted to elicit reflux:

1. Augmentation: The leg is squeezed from below, directing flow toward the heart. If blood flows back toward the feet for more than 0.5 seconds following augmentation, the examination is positive for reflux (Fig. 26), although some examiners require a full second of reflux before considering the examination to be positive. Transient retrograde flow is normal and serves to push back the valve leaflets, causing them to close.

2. Valsalva maneuver: Reflux can be assessed in the thigh after the Valsalva maneuver because the resultant increased intra-abdominal pressure causes retrograde flow through incompetent

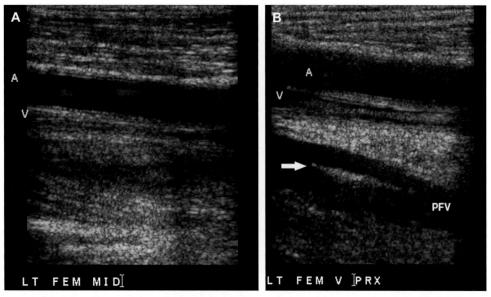

Fig. 22. DVT. (*A*) Thickened irregular vessel walls in a patient who has chronic DVT (*V*). (*B*) Linear fibrin strand in left profunda femoris vein (*PFV*), a sequela from prior DVT (*arrow*).

valves (Fig. 27). Although this technique is sensitive, it works well only in the upper thigh. If the terminal and/or subterminal valves in the GSV are competent, the Valsalva maneuver will not detect more distal points of reflux.

3. Direct or retrograde compression: Direct compression above the point of Doppler interrogation propels blood toward the feet in the setting of an incompetent valve. Although it is easiest to assess for reflux in the longitudinal plane using color or pulse Doppler interrogation, with experience the examination can be performed more efficiently in the transverse plane with color Doppler while angling the transducer toward the head or feet (Fig. 28).

In addition to Doppler interrogation, gray-scale imaging can be helpful. Often the valves themselves can be visualized directly in the GSV. If the valve leaflets are scarred, thickened, or retracted and do not meet in the midline, reflux is likely. Similarly, if the GSV measures more than 6 mm in diameter, reflux is also likely.

The standard or minimum US examination should assess for reflux in the deep venous system at the levels of the CFV (above and below the saphenofemoral junction), FV (upper, mid, and low),

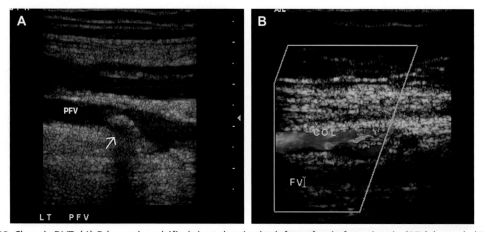

Fig. 23. Chronic DVT. (*A*) Echogenic, calcified thrombus in the left profunda femoris vein (*PFV*) (*arrow*). (*B*) Collateral vessels (*COL*) in a patient who has chronic thrombosis of the right femoral vein (*FV*).

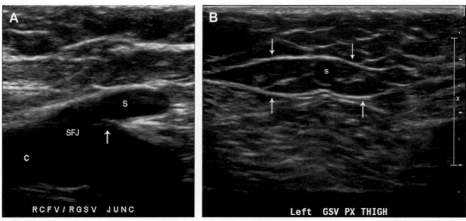

Fig. 24. Normal greater saphenous vein. (*A*) Longitudinal image at the saphenofemoral junction (*SFJ*). Note the junction of the more superficial and smaller greater saphenous vein (*S*) with the deeper and larger common femoral vein (*C*). The greater saphenous vein runs medial to the femoral vessels and joins the common femoral vein in the groin. Arrow indicates terminal valve. (*B*) Transverse image of the greater saphenous vein (*S*) within its surrounding echogenic elliptical fascial sheath creating an appearance similar to a stylized "Egyptian eye" (*arrows*). Tributaries of the greater saphenous vein pierce this fascial envelope and run more superficially in the subdermal fat and connective tissue.

and PV as well as in the GSV, from the saphenofemoral junction to the knee including the origin of the major tributaries and the PV-SSV junction. Full examination of the SSV and GSV below the knee need not be performed unless varicosities are noted in the calf. All varicosities should be traced back to the origin of reflux. In this way, reflux in major branches of the GSV or SSV or reflux originating

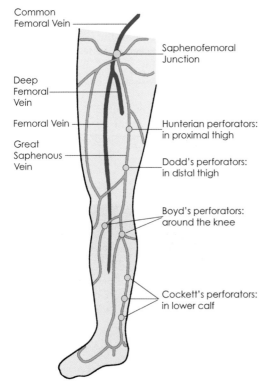

Fig. 25. Major named perforators between the superficial and deep venous system in the lower extremity. (*Adapted from* Weiss RA, Feied CF, Weiss MA. Vein diagnosis and treatment. New York: McGraw-Hill; 2001.)

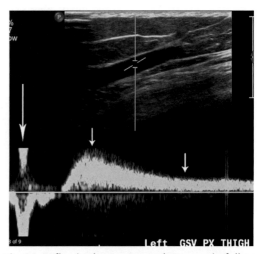

Fig. 26. Reflux in the greater saphenous vein following augmentation. Note sharp, short increase in volume and velocity of blood flow directed toward the head when the leg is squeezed from below (*long arrow*). Subsequently, there is prolonged reversed flow of blood toward the feet lasting well over several seconds (*short arrows*).

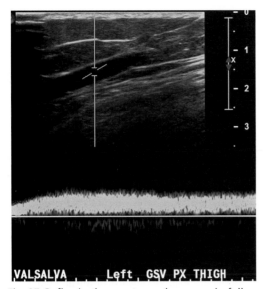

Fig. 27. Reflux in the greater saphenous vein following a Valsalva maneuver. Prolonged reflux (ie, reversed flow in the greater saphenous vein), is noted when the patient increases intra-abdominal pressure by performing a Valsalva maneuver.

from incompetent perforators may be identified even in the absence of truncal reflux in the GSV and SSV.

Summary

DVT of the lower extremities is a common clinical entity and, if left untreated, may result in chronic disability producing the postphlebitic syndrome or potentially life-threatening and devastating outcomes such as PE. Compression US now is recognized as the most appropriate primary initial imaging modality for evaluating patients at risk for a peripheral DVT, and its accuracy in diagnosing acute or chronic DVT is well established in patients who have lower extremity symptoms. The CFV, FV, and PV are examined routinely. The need for evaluation of the calf veins remains controversial, however. US also is helpful in evaluating patients who have chronic venous changes such as the postphlebitic syndrome and venous insufficiency.

The advantages of US include the noninvasiveness of the examination, lack of ionizing radiation, lack of need for intravenous nephrotoxic contrast media, relatively low cost, and portability so that even the most critically ill patients in the ICU can be

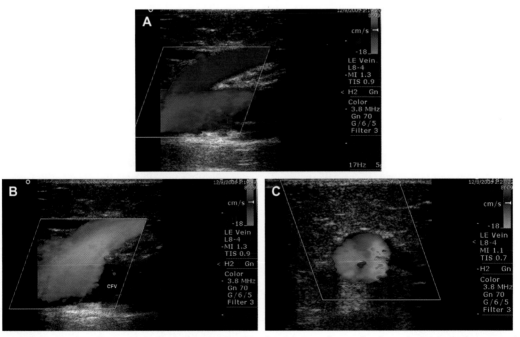

Fig. 28. (A) Color baseline examination reveals blood in the common femoral vein and greater saphenous vein heading away from the transducer toward the head (and therefore is color-coded blue). (B) Color reflux following augmentation (or the Valsalva maneuver): blood flow in the greater saphenous vein is toward the feet and away from the transducer (and therefore is color-coded red). Note no blood flow is noted in the deeper common femoral vein (*CFV*) because competent valves in the common femoral vein prevent reflux of blood toward the feet. (C) Imaging in the transverse plane with the transducer angled toward the feet demonstrates blood flowing away from the transducer (ie, refluxing toward the feet and therefore color-coded red).

examined. A thorough knowledge of regional vascular anatomy, equipment sensitivity, and scanning techniques is required. Despite its limitations in less well-visualized areas such as the iliac and calf veins, US is the most appropriate initial study to perform in patients suspected of harboring a lower extremity DVT. If US studies are nondiagnostic or equivocal, further evaluation with multidetector CT or MR venography may occasionally be necessary.

The signs and symptoms of venous insufficiency overlap with those of DVT. Hence, in a patient presenting with leg pain and swelling, the possibility of venous insufficiency may be overlooked by both clinician and the radiologist because of the overriding and more immediate concern of excluding DVT, a more serious and potentially life-threatening problem. Thus, in the acute setting, Doppler US examination of the lower extremities typically is performed solely to assess for DVT. The clinician and radiologist, however, should remember that venous insufficiency is a common cause of false-negative US examination of the lower extremities and should consider this diagnosis in patients who have leg pain and/or swelling and a negative Doppler US, particularly if symptoms are recurrent or if varicosities are visible. Consideration then should be given to referral for a more extensive Doppler evaluation of the lower extremities to evaluate for reflux.

Although more than 60% of varicosities are caused by reflux in the GSV and its major branches, other tributaries and perforators should be examined based on the patient's symptoms, visual inspection, and physical examination (focal tenderness, bulging, ulcers). If the point of origin of reflux cannot be identified by following the GSV or SSV distally, the examiner should begin at the varicosity and follow it proximally, being careful to identify the highest point of reflux. The examiner should remember that there can be complex patterns of reflux and multiple sites of origin involving tributaries and perforators with or without truncal reflux. It is important to make the diagnosis of chronic venous insufficiency, both to diagnose the cause of the patient's symptoms and because new, minimally invasive percutaneous techniques such as ambulatory phlebectomy, sclerotherapy, and endovascular thermal ablation have revolutionized treatment of this common, debilitating problem.

References

[1] Raghavendra BN, Horii SC, Hilton S, et al. Deep venous thrombosis: detection by probe compression of veins. J Ultrasound Med 1986;5:89–95.

[2] Cronan JJ. History of venous ultrasound. J Ultrasound Med 2003;22:1143–6.

[3] Cronan JJ. Deep venous thrombosis: one leg or both legs? Radiology 1996;200:429–31.

[4] Cronan JJ. Venous thromboembolic disease: the role of ultrasound. Radiology 1993;186:619–50.

[5] Cronan JJ, Leen V. Recurrent deep venous thrombosis: limitations of US. Radiology 1989;170:739–42.

[6] Cronan JJ, Dorfman GS, Grusmark J. Lower-extremity deep venous thrombosis: further experience with and refinements of US assessment. Radiology 1988;168:101–7.

[7] Cronan JJ, Dorfman GS, Scola FH, et al. Deep venous thrombosis: US assessment using vein compression. Radiology 1987;162:191–4.

[8] Appelman PT, DeJong TE, Lampmann LE. Deep venous thrombosis of the leg: US findings. Radiology 1987;163:743–6.

[9] Huisman MV, Buller HR, ten Cate JW, et al. Unexpected high prevalence of silent pulmonary embolism in patients with deep venous thrombosis. Chest 1989;95:498–502.

[10] Monreal M, Ruiz J, Olazabal A, et al. Deep venous thrombosis and the risk of pulmonary embolism. A systematic study. Chest 1992;102:677–81.

[11] Moser KM, Fedullo PF, LitteJohn JK, et al. Frequent asymptomatic pulmonary embolism in patients with deep venous thrombosis. JAMA 1994;271:223–5.

[12] Perone N, Bounameaux H, Perrier A. Comparison of four strategies for diagnosing deep vein thrombosis: a cost-effectiveness analysis. Am J Med 2001;110:33–40.

[13] Barnes RW, Wu KK, Hoak JC. Fallibility of the clinical diagnosis of venous thrombosis. JAMA 1975;234(6):605–7.

[14] Haeger K. Problems of acute deep venous thrombosis. I. The interpretation of signs and symptoms. Angiology 1969;20:219–23.

[15] Salzman EW. Venous thrombosis made easy. [editorial]. N Engl J Med 1986;314:847–8.

[16] Rosen MP, Weintraub J, Donohoe K, et al. Role of lower extremity US in patients with clinically suspected pulmonary embolism. J Vasc Interv Radiol 1995;6:439–41.

[17] Browse NR. Deep vein thrombosis. BMJ 1969;4:676–8.

[18] Bundens WP, Bergan JJ, Halasz NA, et al. The femoral vein. A potentially lethal misnomer. JAMA 1995;274:1296–8.

[19] American College of Radiology. Practical guidelines and standards for performance of the peripheral venous ultrasound examination. Reston (VA): American College of Cardiology; 2006.

[20] Abu-Yousef MM, Kakish ME, Mufid M. Pulsatile venous Doppler flow in lower limbs: highly indicative of elevated right atrium pressure. AJR Am J Roentgenol 1996;167:977–80.

[21] Gottlieb RH, Widjaja J, Mehra S, et al. Clinically important pulmonary emboli: does calf vein US alter outcomes? Radiology 1999;211:25–9.

[22] Lohr JM, Kerr TM, Lutter KS, et al. Lower extremity calf thrombosis: to treat or not to treat? J Vasc Surg 1991;14:618–23.

[23] Coon WW. Anticoagulant therapy. Am J Surg 1985;150:45–9.

[24] Badgett DK, Comerota MC, Khan MC, et al. Duplex venous imaging: role for a comprehensive lower extremity examination. Ann Vasc Surg 2000;14:73–6.

[25] Naidich JB, Torre JR, Pellerito JS, et al. Suspected deep venous thrombosis: is US of both legs necessary? Radiology 1996;200:429–31.

[26] Fard MN, Mostaan M, Zahed Pour Anaraki M. Utility of lower-extremity duplex sonography in patients with venous thromboembolism. J Clin Ultrasound 2001;29:92–8.

[27] Sheiman RG, McArdle CR. Bilateral lower extremity US in the patient with unilateral symptoms of deep venous thrombosis: assessment of need. Radiology 1995;194:171–3.

[28] Nix ML. Should bilateral venous duplex imaging be performed in a patient with unilateral leg symptoms? J Vasc Technol 1994;18:211–2.

[29] Frederick MG, Hertzberg BS, Kliewer MA, et al. Can the US examination for lower extremity deep venous thrombosis be abbreviated? A prospective study of 755 examinations. Radiology 1996;199:45–7.

[30] Lockhart ME, Sheldon HI, Robbin ML. Augmentation in lower extremity sonography for the detection of deep venous thrombosis. AJR Am J Roentgenol 2005;184:419–22.

[31] Kim T, Murakami T, Hori M, et al. Efficacy of multi-slice helical CT venography for the diagnosis of deep venous thrombosis: comparison with venous sonography. Radiat Med 2004;22:77–81.

[32] Taffoni MJ, Ravenel JG, Ackerman SJ. Prospective comparison of indirect CT venography versus venous sonography in ICU patients. AJR Am J Roentgenol 2005;185:457–62.

[33] Murphy TP, Cronan JJ. Evolution of deep venous thrombosis: a prospective evaluation with US. Radiology 1990;177:543–8.

[34] Maki DD, Kumar N, Nguyen B, et al. Distribution of thrombi in acute lower extremity deep venous thrombosis: implications for sonography and CT and MR venography. AJR Am J Roentgenol 2000;175:1299–301.

[35] Cornuz J, Pearson SD, Polak JF. Deep venous thrombosis: complete lower extremity venous US evaluation in patients without known risk factors—outcome study. Radiology 1999;211:637–41.

[36] Heijboer H, Buller HP, Lensing AWA, et al. A comparison of real-time compression ultrasonography with impedance plethysmography for the diagnosis of DVT in symptomatic outpatients. N Engl J Med 1993;329:1365–9.

[37] Yucel EK, Fisher JS, Egglin TK, et al. Isolated calf venous thrombosis: diagnosis with compression US. Radiology 1991;179:443–6.

[38] Rose SC, Zwiebel WJ, Nelson BD, et al. Symptomatic lower extremity deep venous thrombosis: accuracy, limitations, and role of color duplex flow imaging in diagnosis. Radiology 1990;175:639–44.

[39] Rubin JM, Xie H, Kim K, et al. Sonographic elasticity imaging of acute and chronic deep venous thrombosis in humans. J Ultrasound Med 2006; 9:1179–86.

[40] Callam MJ. Epidemiology of varicose veins. Br J Surg 1994;81:167–73.

[41] Brand FN, Dannenburg AL, Abbott RD, et al. The epidemiology of varicose veins: the Framingham Study. Am J Prev Med 1988;4:96–101.

[42] Beaglehole R. Epidemiology of varicose veins. World J Surg 1986;10:898–902.

[43] Evans CJ, Allan PL, Lee AJ, et al. Prevalence of venous reflux in the general population on DUS scanning: the Edinburgh vein study. J Vasc Surg 1998;28:767–76.

[44] McGuckin M, Waterman R, Brooks J, et al. Validation of venous leg ulcer guidelines in the United States and United Kingdom. Am J Surg 2002;183:132–7.

[45] Kurz X, Kahn SR, Abenhaim L, et al. Chronic venous disorders of the leg: epidemiology, outcomes, diagnosis and management. Summary of an evidence-based report of the VEINES task force. Int Angiol 1999;18:83–102.

[46] Ruckley CV. Socioeconomic impact of chronic venous insufficiency and leg ulcers. Angiology 1997;48:67–9.

[47] Van den Oever R, Hepp B, Debbaut B, et al. Socio-economic impact of chronic venous insufficiency: an underestimated public health problem. Int Angiol 1998;17:161–7.

[48] Caggiati A, Bergan JJ, Gloviczki P, et al. Nomenclature of the veins of the lower limbs: an international interdisciplinary consensus statement. J Vasc Surg 2002;36(3):416–22.

[49] Weiss RA, Feied CF, Weiss MA. Vein diagnosis and treatment. A comprehensive approach. New York: McGraw Hill Publishing; 2001. p. 4.

[50] Coon WW, Willis PW, Keller JB. Venous thromboembolism and other venous disease in the Tecumseh community health study. Circulation 1973;48:839–46.

[51] Alexander CJ. The epidemiology of varicose veins. Med J Aust 1972;1:215–8.

[52] Caggiati A. Fascial relationships of the long saphenous vein. Circulation 1999;100:2547–9.

ELSEVIER
SAUNDERS

RADIOLOGIC
CLINICS
OF NORTH AMERICA

Radiol Clin N Am 45 (2007) 549–560

Sonographic Evaluation of Ectopic Pregnancy

Shweta Bhatt, MD[a], Hamad Ghazale, MS, RDMS[b],
Vikram S. Dogra, MD[a],*

Ectopic pregnancy is a high-risk condition that occurs in 1.9% of reported pregnancies [1]. This condition is the leading cause of pregnancy-related death in the first trimester [2]. The blastocyst normally implants itself in the endometrial lining of the uterine cavity. An ectopic pregnancy results if the blastocyst implants itself elsewhere. Although the clinical triad of pain, bleeding, and amenorrhea is considered very specific for an ectopic pregnancy, ultrasound plays important role in detecting the exact location of the ectopic pregnancy and also in providing guidance for minimally invasive treatment. This article discusses the main sonographic features of ectopic pregnancy at various common and unusual locations. In addition, it provides insight into the role of hormonal markers in the diagnosis and management of ectopic pregnancy.

Clinical presentation

Ectopic pregnancy usually is an acute presentation in a woman of reproductive age presenting to the emergency department with acute pelvic or lower quadrant pain. Although the clinical triad of lower abdominal pain, vaginal bleeding, and amenorrhea is considered specific for ectopic pregnancy, women may not always present with all three symptoms. The presentation of any one of the components of the triad should prompt further investigations and tests to exclude ectopic pregnancy. Abdominal pain has been found to be the most common presenting symptom of ectopic pregnancy; abdominal tenderness is the most common physical sign [3,4]. In fact, considering the high potential mortality of this condition, any woman of reproductive age

[a] Department of Imaging Sciences, University of Rochester Medical Center, University of Rochester School of Medicine, 601 Elmwood Ave., Box 648, Rochester, NY 14642, USA
[b] Diagnostic Medical Sonography Program, Rochester Institute of Technology, 153 Lomb Memorial Drive, Rochester, NY 14623, USA
* Corresponding author.
E-mail address: vikram_dogra@urmc.rochester.edu (V.S. Dogra).

presenting to the emergency department with abdominal symptoms should have a beta-human chorionic gonadotropin (β-HCG) blood test or an ultrasound performed to exclude possibility of ectopic pregnancy. Few incidences of asymptomatic women who had ectopic pregnancy detected on routine sonographic screening have been reported [4].

Predisposing factors

Risk factors that predispose to ectopic pregnancy may not always be present, but, if present, they may be a useful adjunct in the clinical diagnosis of an ectopic pregnancy. Any factor that interferes with the normal fallopian tube function is a predisposition for an ectopic pregnancy. Gynecologic infections are a major predisposing factor in an ectopic pregnancy [5]. Other risk factors include infertility, previous ectopic pregnancy [6], previous tubal surgery (causing tubal adhesions and thus altering normal tubal function), or a history of an intrauterine contraceptive device (IUCD) [3]. Although IUCD use has been linked to ectopic pregnancy, according to Edelman and colleagues [7], no relationship exists between either current or past IUCD use or the duration of its use.

After in vitro fertilization or embryo transfer, patients also are predisposed to ectopic pregnancy, particularly those who have a prior history of tubal surgery [8]. Tubal ectopic pregnancies are predisposed by pathologic changes within the tubes, such as chronic salpingitis and follicular salpingitis [9]. Prior cesarean section is a predisposition for scar ectopic pregnancy [10]. Any congenital uterine or tubal anomalies, with or without diethylstilbestrol exposure, also can increase the risk of ectopic pregnancy. Cigarette smoking also predisposes a woman to ectopic pregnancy by causing ciliary dysfunction in the fallopian tubes. These conditions predisposing to ectopic pregnancy are summarized in Box 1.

Diagnosing ectopic pregnancy

Clinical suspicion of an ectopic pregnancy is an essential step toward diagnosis. Excluding an intrauterine pregnancy is the first step in the management of such a patient. The first-trimester screening parameters listed in Table 1 can help detect an abnormal pregnancy early. An intrauterine gestation, considerably reduces but does not exclude the possibility of an ectopic pregnancy. Heterotopic pregnancy, the simultaneous occurrence of intrauterine and extrauterine pregnancy, although rare, needs to be considered and excluded before sending the patient home. The fallopian tube is the most common location for an extrauterine pregnancy; abdominal pregnancies also have been reported, particularly in patients who have a history of assisted reproduction [11].

Endocrinology of ectopic pregnancy

HCG is a member of the glycoprotein hormone family that is composed of a common α subunit and a hormone-specific β subunit, noncovalently associated. Secretion of HCG begins very early in pregnancy and peaks at 9 to 11 weeks. Peak levels are in the range of 30 to 100 IU/L and last for only a few days; levels then decline gradually to a nadir of 5 to 10 IU/L at about 20 weeks. Transvaginal ultrasonography should be able to identify the presence of an intrauterine gestation in nearly 100% of normal pregnancies when β-HCG exceeds 2400 mIU/mL in serum [12,13]. Failure to identify an intrauterine pregnancy above this indicator of HCG is consistent with an abnormal pregnancy and may suggest either a spontaneous abortion or an ectopic pregnancy. Serial HCG values can be used to determine whether a gestation is potentially viable or spontaneously resolving. A normal pregnancy shows a doubling time of the β-HCG value of 2 days (range 1.2–2.2 days) [14]. The minimal decline of HCG in a spontaneous abortion is 21% to 35% in 2 days, depending on the initial level. A

Box 1: Conditions that predispose to ectopic pregnancy

- Tubal surgery
- Prior pelvic inflammatory disease
- Presence of an intrauterine device
- Treatment of infertility
- Previous ectopic pregnancy
- Diethylstilbestrol exposure
- Cigarette smoking

Table 1: First-trimester scanning milestones

Finding	Transabdominal ultrasound	Transvaginal ultrasound
Gestational sac	–	Present at 5 weeks (5 mm)
Yolk sac	Always present if gestational sac > 20 mm	Always present when gestational sac > 10 mm
Cardiac activity	Gestational sac > 2.5 cm	Gestational sac > 18 mm

Data from Paspulati RM, Bhatt S, Nour S. Sonographic evaluation of first-trimester bleeding. Radiol Clin North Am 2004;42:298.

slower rise or fall in serial HCG values suggests an ectopic pregnancy [15].

β-HCG is an important hormone to follow serially. A subnormal increase in serum β-HCG in early pregnancy (<66% in 48 hours) suggests that the pregnancy is not viable. An absence of this increase is suggestive of an ectopic pregnancy, although it also can be associated with early pregnancy failure. Free HCG is considered to be more specific than the other isoforms in diagnosing ectopic pregnancy. The doubling time of HCG is not constant but rather increases with increasing HCG concentration or gestational age. It has been observed, however, that there is no characteristic HCG pattern of ectopic pregnancy. The HCG levels in women who have ectopic pregnancy can simulate an intrauterine pregnancy or a completed spontaneous abortion in approximately 29% of cases [16].

Serum progesterone concentrations also may be helpful as an adjunct to β-HCG in the evaluation of ectopic pregnancy. A progesterone concentration greater than 25 ng/mL is associated with an intrauterine pregnancy in 97.5% of cases. Progesterone levels lower than 5.0 ng/mL indicate a nonviable pregnancy, regardless of location [17]. Other placental markers that can be used to diagnose an ectopic pregnancy are serum creatine kinase levels, pregnancy-specific β (1)-glycoprotein, human placental lactogen, and pregnancy-associated plasma protein-A [13].

Sonographic evaluation

Diagnosis of suspected ectopic pregnancy usually is made after a combined assessment of clinical history, hormonal markers, and sonographic features. Ultrasound usually is helpful in confirming the clinical suspicion of an ectopic pregnancy, thus enabling an early diagnosis and a considerable decrease in maternal morbidity and mortality. Morin and colleagues [18] stated that current ultrasound technology is extremely sensitive and specific in distinguishing between normal and abnormal pregnancies in the first trimester.

Ectopic pregnancy, as the name suggests, is pregnancy in an extrauterine location; this location can vary from intrapelvic to abdominal to retroperitoneal (Fig. 1). Ultrasound performed with the intent to search for ectopic pregnancy in these locations usually can lead to the correct diagnosis.

Tubal pregnancy

Ectopic pregnancy most commonly (95%) occurs in the ampullary or isthmic portions of the fallopian tube [19]. An ectopic pregnancy can be diagnosed with confidence when an adnexal mass that contains a yolk sac or viable embryo is identified

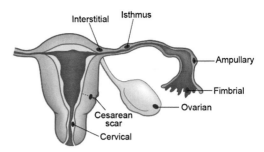

Fig. 1. The common ectopic locations of extrauterine gestation (ectopic pregnancy).

[20]. An extraovarian adnexal mass (Fig. 2), which is the most common sonographic finding in ectopic pregnancy, is seen in 89% to 100% of cases [21–23]. Independent movement of the mass and the ovary, demonstrated by the gentle probing of ultrasound transducer, is strongly associated with an ectopic pregnancy [24] and helps differentiate it from exophytic corpus luteal cyst [19].

Other adnexal findings include the tubal ring sign (the second most common sonographic finding), which is the presence of a hyperechoic ring around the gestational sac, and pelvic hemorrhage, with or without an adnexal mass. About 26% of ectopic pregnancies have normal pelvic sonograms on transvaginal ultrasound [22]. Intrauterine findings indicative of an ectopic pregnancy include the trilaminar pattern and absence of in utero pregnancy. The trilaminar pattern is considered quite specific for the diagnosis of ectopic pregnancy but has low sensitivity. The endometrial thickness tends

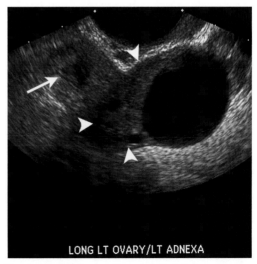

LONG LT OVARY/LT ADNEXA

Fig. 2. Surgically confirmed left tubal pregnancy. Transvaginal gray-scale ultrasound of the left adnexa demonstrates an adnexal mass with a tubal ring (*arrow*) separate from the left ovary (*arrowheads*).

to be thinner in patients who have an ectopic pregnancy [25]. Using multiple parameters in the diagnosis of ectopic pregnancy results in almost 100% sensitivity and specificity [26].

Thin-walled decidual cysts located at the junction of the endometrium and myometrium also are seen in ectopic pregnancy; however, this finding is nonspecific and also can be seen in a normal intrauterine pregnancy [21]. The thin wall of the decidual cyst helps differentiate it from the gestational sac of intrauterine pregnancy.

Pseudogestational sac is present in 10% of patients who have ectopic pregnancies. It is formed when the intrauterine fluid is surrounded by a thick decidual reaction. It is differentiated from a true sac by the absence of the two decidual layers seen in a true sac and its central location, oval shape, and a thin echogenic rim (Fig. 3) [21,22]. Color flow Doppler may assist further in differentiating between a true and a pseudo sac by demonstrating trophoblastic flow characterized by a low-resistance arterial flow pattern in a true gestational sac [22]. Sparse flow on color Doppler with low peak systolic velocities (<6 cm/s) to absent end diastolic flow suggests decidual reaction of an ectopic pregnancy [27].

Pelvic fluid within the cul-de-sac also is associated with an ectopic pregnancy. It is a nonspecific finding but may supplement the presence of other findings in making a diagnosis of an ectopic pregnancy [21]. Additionally, echogenic fluid, suggestive of hemorrhage (Fig. 4), should raise immediate concern for an ectopic pregnancy; its positive predictive value is 90%. It usually occurs following tubal rupture or tubal abortion [22]. Culdocentesis used to be the procedure of choice for diagnosing hemorrhagic fluid in the cul-de-sac, but with current ultrasound technology, transvaginal

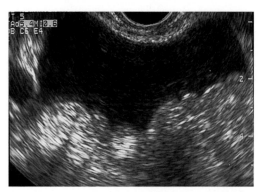

Fig. 4. Free fluid in cul de sac. Echogenic free fluid in the pelvis in a patient who has an ectopic pregnancy raises the suspicion of a ruptured ectopic pregnancy.

ultrasound is sufficient to make an accurate diagnosis. The sonographic features of ectopic pregnancy are summarized in Box 2.

Interstitial (cornual or angular) pregnancy

Interstitial gestation is a rare form of tubal pregnancy, with an incidence of about 0.7% to 4%. It results from the implantation of the gestational sac in the proximal intramural portion of the fallopian tube (within the muscular wall of the uterus). In ultrasonography, the term "interstitial pregnancy" often is used synonymously with cornual pregnancy and angular pregnancy.

Risk factors and clinical presentation are similar to those of any other ectopic pregnancy. Additionally, ipsilateral salpingectomy is a predisposing factor for interstitial pregnancy, and in vitro fertilization is a predisposing factor for heterotopic interstitial pregnancy. Contrary to previous belief,

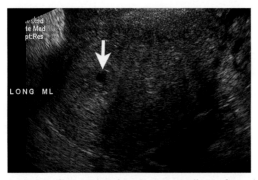

Fig. 3. Pseudogestational sac in a surgically confirmed live-twin ectopic gestation. Longitudinal gray-scale sonogram of the uterus demonstrates centrally located fluid (*arrow*) within the endometrial cavity. Please note its central location as opposed to eccentric location of intrauterine pregnancy.

Box 2: Summary of sonographic findings in ectopic pregnancy

Uterine findings
May be normal
Thick decidual cast without a gestational sac or
Pseudogestational sac

Extrauterine findings
Live embryo
Adnexal mass containing a yolk sac or non-living embryo
Tubal ring sign
Free fluid in the cul de sac
Echogenic fluid (Hemorrhagic)
Simple adnexal cyst (10% chance of ectopic pregnancy)
Complex or solid adnexal mass (no embryo, yolk sac, or tubal ring)
One third of pelvic examinations in patients who have ectopic pregnancies are normal

rupture of interstitial pregnancy occurs relatively early in pregnancy [28]. Therefore, it is necessary to diagnose this entity correctly at an early stage, before it ruptures, because rupture of an interstitial pregnancy is associated with severe hemorrhage and increased maternal morbidity and mortality.

Typical sonographic findings in an interstitial pregnancy include a gestational sac seen separate from the uterine cavity with a thin ring of myometrium surrounding the gestational sac (Fig. 5A) [29]. In an attempt to improve diagnostic accuracy, Timor-Tritsch and colleagues [30] proposed the following ultrasound criteria for the diagnosis of interstitial ectopic pregnancy: "(1) an empty uterine cavity; (2) a gestational sac located eccentrically and >1 cm from the most lateral wall of the uterine cavity; and (3) a thin (<5 mm) myometrial layer

surrounding the gestational sac." Although these criteria have a high specificity of about 90%, sensitivity for detection is as low as 40%.

The interstitial line is a useful diagnostic sonographic sign of interstitial ectopic pregnancy, with 80% sensitivity and 98% specificity for the diagnosis of interstitial pregnancy [31]. It is described as an "echogenic line that extends into the upper regions of the uterine horn and borders the margin of the intramural gestational sac" (Fig. 5B, C).

In the past few years, with technological advances in imaging and ultrasound, three-dimensional and four-dimensional multiplanar sonography has been recognized as an excellent imaging modality in the diagnosis of interstitial pregnancy [32–34]. MR imaging also plays a significant role in the diagnosis of an interstitial pregnancy, particularly

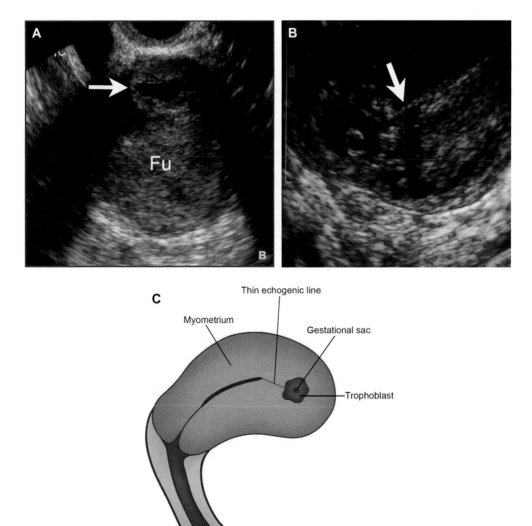

Fig. 5. Interstitial pregnancy. (*A*) Transverse gray-scale sonogram of the uterus demonstrates an eccentrically located gestational sac (*arrow*) near the fundus of the uterus (*Fu*). (*B*) Gray-scale sonogram in the same patient demonstrates the interstitial line sign (*arrow*). (*C*) The interstitial line sign in an interstitial pregnancy.

because of its increased sensitivity in detecting fresh hematoma [35].

Cervical pregnancy

Cervical pregnancy is uncommon, with an incidence of 0.1%. Predisposing risk factors include curettage, Asherman's syndrome, previous cesarean delivery, previous cervical or uterine surgery, and in vitro fertilization [36]. Delayed diagnosis of cervical ectopic pregnancy can be associated with significant morbidity and maternal death from hemorrhage.

With current ultrasound technology, cervical pregnancy can be diagnosed early in its course by identifying a gestational sac in the cervix, followed by a conservative management, thereby sparing fertility. Nearly 2 decades ago, cervical pregnancy often was misdiagnosed as an incomplete abortion and was managed with dilatation and curettage, which then resulted in severe hemorrhage. Hysterectomy was the treatment of choice to save the patient's life [37]. Today, conservative treatment, such as methotrexate therapy and uterine artery embolization, often is used for this condition, with resultant delayed spontaneous expulsion of a cervical ectopic pregnancy [38].

Kung and colleagues [39] have described criteria for diagnosis of cervical pregnancy on ultrasound including (1) identification of the gestational sac or placenta within the cervix (Fig. 6); (2) absent intrauterine pregnancy; (3) visualization of a normal endometrial stripe; (4) hourglass (figure-eight) uterus with a bulging cervical canal, as suggested by Hofmann and colleagues [40], and (5) a sac with active cardiac activity below the internal os to indicate a viable pregnancy, as suggested by Timor-Tritsch and colleagues [41].

Cervical pregnancy can be confirmed further by demonstrating the "sliding sign" by applying gentle pressure on the cervix by the probe during transvaginal scanning to exclude abortion in progression with abortus retained by a resistant external os [42].

Ovarian pregnancy

Ovarian pregnancies comprise 0.15% of all pregnancies and 0.15% to 3% of ectopic gestations, with an incidence of up to 1 in 7000 deliveries [43]. Ovarian pregnancy develops as a result of the retention of the ovum in the ovarian operculum and its continued entrapment within the ruptured ovarian follicle, which eventually is fertilized by the sperm, resulting in pregnancy. Spiegelberg [44] has described four criteria for ovarian pregnancy: "(1) intact ipsilateral tube, separate from the ovary, (2) gestational sac occupying the position of the ovary, (3) sac connected to the uterus by the ovarian ligament, and (4) histologically proven ovarian tissue located in the sac wall."

Sergent and colleagues [45] have presented additional criteria for ovarian pregnancy that, when considered along with Spiegelberg's criteria, help confirm ovarian pregnancy. These criteria include "(a) serum beta-HCG level > or = 1000 IU/L and uterine vacuity at vaginal ultrasonography, (b) ovarian implication confirmed by surgical exploration, with bleeding, (c) visualization of chorionic villi or presence of an atypical cyst on the ovary, (d) normal fallopian tubes, and (e) absence of serum beta-HCG after treatment of ovarian pregnancy."

Primary ovarian pregnancy may occur without any classical antecedent risk factors. Ultrasonography can be a useful adjunct to clinical presentation and physical examination in allowing the preoperative diagnosis of ovarian gestation [43]. Ovarian pregnancies usually appear on or within the ovary

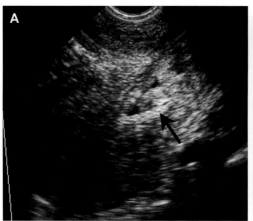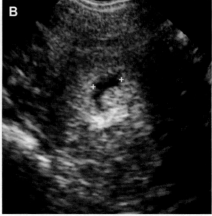

Fig. 6. Cervical pregnancy. (*A*) Longitudinal and (*B*) transverse gray-scale transvaginal ultrasound of the uterus demonstrates a gestational sac (*arrow* in panel A) in the cervix with a fetal pole within.

as a cyst with a wide echogenic outside ring. A yolk sac or embryo is seen less commonly. The appearance of the contents lags in comparison with the gestational age. Early abdominal pain is a common finding [46].

Scar pregnancy

Implantation of pregnancy within a scar of prior uterine surgery is referred to as "scar pregnancy." It often is seen in women who have a history of prior cesarean section or myomectomy who undergo in vitro fertilization. Pregnancy occurring at this unusual location can be explained by a probable implantation through a sinus tract made in the uterus during a previous uterine surgery [47]. Criteria used for diagnosis include an empty uterus and cervical canal, development of the gestational sac in the anterior part of the lower uterine segment, and thinning of myometrium between the bladder wall and the gestational sac secondary to growth of gestational sac (Fig. 7) [48]. Thinning of the myometrium caused by distension of the gestational sac predisposes the patient to uterine rupture [23].

Scar pregnancy is reported increasingly because of the growing number of uterine surgeries performed. It is important to identify it because of the high risk of rupture and severe hemorrhage and possible life-threatening sequelae [49]. Scar pregnancy can be misdiagnosed easily because spontaneous abortion is required to make a correct diagnosis; therefore a high index of suspicion and correlation of risk factors is required [50]. Although laparotomy with hysterotomy formerly was considered the definitive treatment [51], more conservative treatment choices such as local potassium chloride injections [52,53] or methotrexate (ultrasound guided injections) [54] are used now in an attempt to preserve fertility.

Abdominal pregnancy

Abdominal pregnancy is an intraperitoneal implantation exclusive of tubal, ovarian, or intraligamentous implantation. Abdominal pregnancy results from the rupture of a tubal or ovarian pregnancy with abdominal cavity implantation or direct peritoneal implantation.

The incidence of abdominal pregnancy is 1:11,000 pregnancies, and lithopedion occurs in 1.5% to 1.8% of these cases. "Lithopedion" is the name given to an extrauterine pregnancy that evolves to fetal death and calcification [55,56]. It is important to be familiar with this entity, because the majority of patients present with intra-abdominal hemorrhage, and the maternal mortality rate is estimated to be between 0.5% and 18%.

Omental pregnancy [57] and retroperitoneal pregnancy [58] are rare forms of abdominal ectopic pregnancy and usually are diagnosed only at surgical exploration. Broad ligament pregnancy also has been reported in women who have undergone salpingo-oophorectomy [59].

Heterotopic pregnancy

Heterotopic pregnancy is the simultaneous occurrence of intrauterine and extrauterine pregnancy (Fig. 8). It is particularly common in women who have had assisted conception. The incidence of heterotopic pregnancy in patients treated with infertility drugs is 1:7000, and in those who have had in vitro fertilization the incidence is approximately 1:100. Heterotopic pregnancies can be difficult to detect and often are diagnosed after the patient presents with abdominal hemorrhage. Therefore, heterotopic pregnancy must be considered in the differential diagnosis of abdominal pain in the first trimester, especially in patients who conceived by means of assisted reproductive technology.

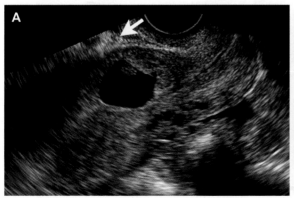
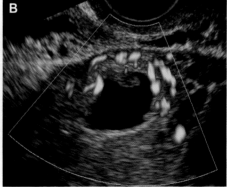

Fig. 7. Cesarean scar pregnancy. (A) Longitudinal gray-scale and (B) power Doppler sonogram of the uterus demonstrates a gestational sac with a fetal pole within in the myometrium of anterior wall of lower uterus underlying the scar (*arrow* in panel A) from prior cesarean section.

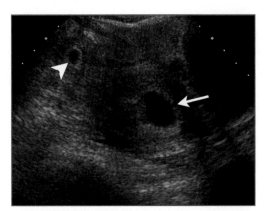

Fig. 8. Heterotopic pregnancy. Heterotopic pregnancy. Endovaginal ultrasound in this patient who had a positive pregnancy test shows presence of two true gestational sacs, one within the uterus (*arrow*) and one in the right adnexa (*arrowhead*).

Sonographic examination of the pelvis as well as the abdomen in a symptomatic woman can help detect heterotopic pregnancy at an early stage [60]. According to a comparative review of the literature by Barrenetxea and colleagues [61], heterotopic pregnancy remains a diagnostic and therapeutic challenge to practitioners.

Sonographically guided minimally invasive management of heterotopic pregnancy selectively ablates the ectopic pregnancy and permits normal continuation of the concomitant intrauterine pregnancy [52]. Good perinatal outcome can be achieved by early recognition and prompt surgical intervention for heterotopic pregnancy, directed toward preserving future fertility.

Role of color Doppler sonography

Ectopic pregnancy usually can be diagnosed easily based on the gray-scale ultrasound features described previously. Color Doppler can help confirm the diagnosis but rarely is used as the only finding for ectopic pregnancy. Ramanan and colleagues [62] described the "leash sign" on color Doppler as one of the reliable indicators of ectopic pregnancy. It is seen as a typical eccentric "leash of vessels" that has a low-resistance flow on spectral Doppler suggestive of trophoblastic tissue. This sign has a sensitivity of 100% and specificity of 99%, a positive predictive value of 95%, and a negative predictive value of 100%. Other color Doppler findings in an ectopic pregnancy include peripheral hypervascularity of the tubal ring sign, appropriately termed a "ring of fire" (Fig. 9). Although very sensitive, it has very low specificity and also can be seen around a maturing follicle or a corpus luteal cyst [63].

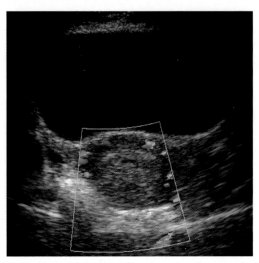

Fig. 9. Ring of fire. Color flow Doppler ultrasound of the left adnexal mass demonstrates increased peripheral vascularity that was confirmed surgically to be a tubal ectopic pregnancy.

Color Doppler also can be useful in identifying a live ectopic pregnancy. Cardiac pulsations in a live fetus can be seen on a real-time color Doppler sonogram as a pulsating color signal (Fig. 10).

Chronic ectopic pregnancy

Chronic ectopic pregnancy is an uncommon form of ectopic pregnancy manifested with minimal symptoms and a low or absent titer of HCG [64]. The term "chronic" describes only the appearance of the pelvic mass formed as a result of repeated hemorrhages (old blood clots and hematoma with surrounding adhesions) [65] and does not necessarily imply a chronic duration [66]. Its sonographic appearance may mimic pelvic inflammatory disease, endometriosis, or uterine leiomyomas [67]. Because of minimal symptoms and sonographic findings similar to many inflammatory lesions of the pelvis, preoperative diagnosis of chronic ectopic pregnancy often is not possible. A pathologist usually makes the diagnosis following surgical excision of the mass [22].

Persistent ectopic pregnancy

Failure to remove ectopic pregnancy after treatment is termed "persistent ectopic pregnancy." It may occur after surgical or nonsurgical management but is seen more commonly after conservative management of a tubal pregnancy with salpingostomy or fimbrial expression. Successful treatment of ectopic pregnancy should reduce the levels of serum HCG. The presence of elevated or plateauing serum HCG levels 1 week after management of an ectopic

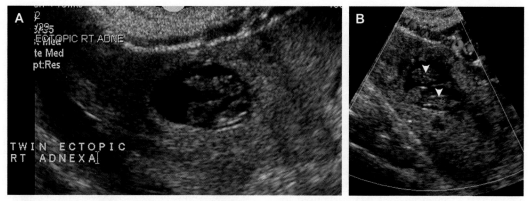

Fig. 10. Live-twin ectopic pregnancy. (*A*) Transvaginal gray-scale and (*B*) color flow Doppler sonograms of the right adnexa demonstrate two fetal poles separated by a membrane in a single gestational sac. The presence of color signals (*arrowheads*) within them on color flow Doppler suggest cardiac activity.

pregnancy is diagnosed as persistent ectopic pregnancy [68,69].

Complications

The most common complication of an ectopic pregnancy is rupture with internal bleeding that may lead to cardiovascular shock and, rarely, death. Ruptured ectopic pregnancy is the leading cause of maternal mortality in the first trimester and accounts for 10% to 15% of all maternal deaths [70]. Infertility occurs in 10% to 15% of women who have had an ectopic pregnancy. The incidence of repeat ectopic pregnancy is about 16 times greater after the first ectopic pregnancy.

Management of ectopic pregnancy

Expectant management
The dimensions of ectopic gestational tissue (<3.5 cm in its greatest dimension) and decreased or declining β-HCG values are the criteria used for expectant management. Overall, if the initial serum concentration of HCG is less than 1000 IU/L, expectant management is successful in up to 88% of patients [71,72].

Medical management
Three medications for early medical abortion have been studied and used widely: the antiprogestin mifepristone, the antimetabolite methotrexate, and the prostaglandin misoprostol. These agents cause abortion by increasing uterine contractility, either by reversing the progesterone-induced inhibition of contractions (mifepristone and methotrexate) or by stimulating the myometrium directly (misoprostol). Chemical agents that have been investigated include hyperosmolar glucose, urea, methotrexate and actinomycin, prostaglandins, and mifepristone (RU 486). When the diagnosis is certain, and an

ectopic mass is less than 3.5 cm in its greatest dimension, methotrexate therapy is an option. The time to resolution of the ectopic pregnancy is 3 to 7 weeks after methotrexate therapy. Patients treated with methotrexate should be followed with serial β-HCG levels (demonstrating serial fall) and not by ultrasound, because after methotrexate treatment the adnexal mass increases in size secondary to hemorrhage and edema and can be interpreted as failure of methotrexate therapy. Box 3 lists the requirements for methotrexate administration.

The most frequent complications of surgery are recurrence of ectopic pregnancy (5%–20%) and incomplete removal of trophoblastic tissue. It was suggested that a single dose of methotrexate should be given postoperatively as a prophylactic measure in very high-risk patients [73].

Sonographically guided treatment
Sonographically guided minimally invasive treatment of ectopic pregnancies, local intra-amniotic

---

Box 3:   Absolute and relative requirements of methotrexate administration

Absolute requirements
- Hemodynamic stability
- Ultrasound findings consistent with an ectopic pregnancy
- Willingness of the patient to adhere to close follow-up
- No contraindications to methotrexate therapy

Relative requirements
- Unruptured ectopic mass less than 3.5 cm in its greatest dimension
- No fetal cardiac motion detected
- β-subunit HCG level that does not exceed 5000 mIU/L

injections administered by percutaneous or transvaginal routes, is an effective alternative to surgical and systemic management of ectopic pregnancy. This treatment is preferred in unruptured and nonviable ectopic pregnancy and helps preserve the uterus and fallopian tubes for future pregnancies. This mode of treatment is particularly helpful in a heterotopic pregnancy, where the aim is to remove the ectopic gestation while preserving the intrauterine gestation for its normal progression [74]. In addition, intra-amniotic injection has proved useful in the treatment of unusual ectopic pregnancies such as cervical, cornual, tubal heterotopic, and cesarean scar pregnancies [52]. Materials used for intra-amniotic injection are hypertonic glucose (>50%) [75], methotrexate, RU 486 (mifepristone), and potassium chloride [76]. Methotrexate has shown better results than hypertonic glucose in the treatment of ectopic pregnancy [77].

Surgical management

Laparoscopic conservative surgery (tube-sparing salpingostomy) is the mainstay in managing ectopic pregnancy and has almost replaced the standard laparotomy and salpingectomy. Laparotomy is reserved for hemodynamically unstable patients and for a failed laparoscopic surgery.

Summary

Ectopic pregnancy is a growing problem among women of reproductive age, mostly attributed to the increasing use of assisted reproductive technologies. Early recognition of ectopic pregnancy, with the help of better ultrasound technology, has enabled a more conservative treatment of this condition, allowing patients to conceive in the future. Ultrasound also plays a role in the management of ectopic pregnancy by providing guidance for intra-amniotic injection of methotrexate or potassium chloride. The body of literature on the many possible locations of an ectopic location of pregnancy is enormous. Awareness of this possibility and a subsequent thorough ultrasound examination can lead to the detection of these ectopic pregnancies in unusual locations at a relatively early stage of gestation and thus prevent a possible catastrophe.

References

[1] Kriebs JM, Fahey JO. Ectopic pregnancy. J Midwifery Womens Health 2006;51:431–9.

[2] Lozeau AM, Potter B. Diagnosis and management of ectopic pregnancy. Am Fam Physician 2005;72:1707–14.

[3] Shah N, Khan NH. Ectopic pregnancy: presentation and risk factors. J Coll Physicians Surg Pak 2005;15:535–8.

[4] Aboud E, Chaliha C. Nine year survey of 138 ectopic pregnancies. Arch Gynecol Obstet 1998; 261:83–7.

[5] Tuomivaara LM. Ectopic pregnancy and genital infections: a case-control study. Ann Med 1990; 22:21–4.

[6] Barnhart KT, Sammel MD, Gracia CR, et al. Risk factors for ectopic pregnancy in women with symptomatic first-trimester pregnancies. Fertil Steril 2006;86:36–43.

[7] Edelman DA, Porter CW. The intrauterine device and ectopic pregnancy. Contraception 1987;36: 85–96.

[8] Zouves C, Erenus M, Gomel V. Tubal ectopic pregnancy after in vitro fertilization and embryo transfer: a role for proximal occlusion or salpingectomy after failed distal tubal surgery? Fertil Steril 1991;56:691–5.

[9] Ramirez NC, Lawrence WD, Ginsburg KA. Ectopic pregnancy. A recent five-year study and review of the last 50 years' literature. J Reprod Med 1996;41:733–40.

[10] Rotas MA, Haberman S, Levgur M. Cesarean scar ectopic pregnancies: etiology, diagnosis, and management. Obstet Gynecol 2006;107: 1373–81.

[11] Kitade M, Takeuchi H, Kikuchi I, et al. A case of simultaneous tubal-splenic pregnancy after assisted reproductive technology. Fertil Steril 2005;83: 1042.

[12] Fossum GT, Davajan V, Kletzky OA. Early detection of pregnancy with transvaginal ultrasound. Fertil Steril 1988;49:788–91.

[13] Attar E. Endocrinology of ectopic pregnancy. Obstet Gynecol Clin North Am 2004;31:779–94, x.

[14] Eyvazzadeh AD, Levine D. Imaging of pelvic pain in the first trimester of pregnancy. Radiol Clin North Am 2006;44:863–77.

[15] Seeber BE, Barnhart KT. Suspected ectopic pregnancy. Obstet Gynecol 2006;107:399–413.

[16] Silva C, Sammel MD, Zhou L, et al. Human chorionic gonadotropin profile for women with ectopic pregnancy. Obstet Gynecol 2006;107: 605–10.

[17] Dart R, Ramanujam P, Dart L. Progesterone as a predictor of ectopic pregnancy when the ultrasound is indeterminate. Am J Emerg Med 2002; 20:575–9.

[18] Morin L, Van den Hof MC. SOGC clinical practice guidelines. Ultrasound evaluation of first trimester pregnancy complications. Number 161, June 2005. Int J Gynaecol Obstet 2006;93:77–81.

[19] Webb EM, Green GE, Scoutt LM. Adnexal mass with pelvic pain. Radiol Clin North Am 2004; 42:329–48.

[20] Brown DL, Doubilet PM. Transvaginal sonography for diagnosing ectopic pregnancy: positivity criteria and performance characteristics. J Ultrasound Med 1994;13:259–66.

Sonographic Evaluation of Ectopic Pregnancy **559**

[21] Atri M, Leduc C, Gillett P, et al. Role of endovaginal sonography in the diagnosis and management of ectopic pregnancy. Radiographics 1996; 16:755–74 [discussion: 775].

[22] Dogra V, Paspulati RM, Bhatt S. First trimester bleeding evaluation. Ultrasound Q 2005;21: 69–85 [quiz: 149–50, 153–4].

[23] Dialani V, Levine D. Ectopic pregnancy: a review. Ultrasound Q 2004;20:105–17.

[24] Blaivas M, Lyon M. Reliability of adnexal mass mobility in distinguishing possible ectopic pregnancy from corpus luteum cysts. J Ultrasound Med 2005;24:599–603 [quiz: 605].

[25] Hammoud AO, Hammoud I, Bujold E, et al. The role of sonographic endometrial patterns and endometrial thickness in the differential diagnosis of ectopic pregnancy. Am J Obstet Gynecol 2005;192:1370–5.

[26] Naseem I, Bari V, Nadeem N. Multiple parameters in the diagnosis of ectopic pregnancy. J Pak Med Assoc 2005;55:74–6.

[27] Paspulati RM, Bhatt S, Nour S. Sonographic evaluation of first-trimester bleeding. Radiol Clin North Am 2004;42:297–314.

[28] Malinowski A, Bates SK. Semantics and pitfalls in the diagnosis of cornual/interstitial pregnancy. Fertil Steril 2006;86(1764):e1711–64.

[29] DeWitt C, Abbott J. Interstitial pregnancy: a potential for misdiagnosis of ectopic pregnancy with emergency department ultrasonography. Ann Emerg Med 2002;40:106–9.

[30] Timor-Tritsch IE, Monteagudo A, Matera C, et al. Sonographic evolution of cornual pregnancies treated without surgery. Obstet Gynecol 1992; 79:1044–9.

[31] Ackerman TE, Levi CS, Dashefsky SM, et al. Interstitial line: sonographic finding in interstitial (cornual) ectopic pregnancy. Radiology 1993;189:83–7.

[32] Araujo Junior E, Zanforlin Filho SM, Pires CR, et al. Three-dimensional transvaginal sonographic diagnosis of early and asymptomatic interstitial pregnancy. Arch Gynecol Obstet 2006;275(3):207–10.

[33] Chou MM, Tseng JJ, Yi YC, et al. Diagnosis of an interstitial pregnancy with 4-dimensional volume contrast imaging. Am J Obstet Gynecol 2005;193:1551–3.

[34] Izquierdo LA, Nicholas MC. Three-dimensional transvaginal sonography of interstitial pregnancy. J Clin Ultrasound 2003;31:484–7.

[35] Department of Imaging Sciences, Yoshigi J, Yashiro N, et al. Diagnosis of ectopic pregnancy with MRI: efficacy of T2*-weighted imaging. Magn Reson Med Sci 2006;5:25–32.

[36] Verma U, Maggiorotto F. Conservative management of second-trimester cervical ectopic pregnancy with placenta percreta. Fertil Steril 2006; 87(3):697, e13–6.

[37] Starita A, Di Miscia A, Evangelista S, et al. Cervical ectopic pregnancy: clinical review. Clin Exp Obstet Gynecol 2006;33:47–9.

[38] Einarsson JI, Michel S, Young AE. Delayed spontaneous expulsion of a cervical ectopic pregnancy: a case report. J Minim Invasive Gynecol 2005;12:165–7.

[39] Kung FT, Lin H, Hsu TY, et al. Differential diagnosis of suspected cervical pregnancy and conservative treatment with the combination of laparoscopy-assisted uterine artery ligation and hysteroscopic endocervical resection. Fertil Steril 2004;81:1642–9.

[40] Hofmann HM, Urdl W, Hofler H, et al. Cervical pregnancy: case reports and current concepts in diagnosis and treatment. Arch Gynecol Obstet 1987;241:63–9.

[41] Timor-Tritsch IE, Monteagudo A, Mandeville EO, et al. Successful management of viable cervical pregnancy by local injection of methotrexate guided by transvaginal ultrasonography. Am J Obstet Gynecol 1994;170:737–9.

[42] Jurkovic D, Hacket E, Campbell S. Diagnosis and treatment of early cervical pregnancy: a review and a report of two cases treated conservatively. Ultrasound Obstet Gynecol 1996;8:373–80.

[43] Nwanodi O, Khulpateea N. The preoperative diagnosis of primary ovarian pregnancy. J Natl Med Assoc 2006;98:796–8.

[44] Spiegelberg O. Zur Casuistic der Ovarialschwangerschaft. Arch Gynaekol 1878;13:73.

[45] Sergent F, Mauger-Tinlot F, Gravier A, et al. [Ovarian pregnancies: revaluation of diagnostic criteria]. J Gynecol Obstet Biol Reprod (Paris) 2002;31:741–6 [in French].

[46] Comstock C, Huston K, Lee W. The ultrasonographic appearance of ovarian ectopic pregnancies. Obstet Gynecol 2005;105:42–5.

[47] Park WI, Jeon YM, Lee JY, et al. Subserosal pregnancy in a previous myomectomy site: a variant of intramural pregnancy. J Minim Invasive Gynecol 2006;13:242–4.

[48] Li SP, Wang W, Tang XL, et al. Cesarean scar pregnancy: a case report. Chin Med J (Engl) 2004; 117:316–7.

[49] Graesslin O, Dedecker F Jr, Quereux C, et al. Conservative treatment of ectopic pregnancy in a cesarean scar. Obstet Gynecol 2005;105: 869–71.

[50] Tan G, Chong YS, Biswas A. Caesarean scar pregnancy: a diagnosis to consider carefully in patients with risk factors. Ann Acad Med Singapore 2005;34:216–9.

[51] Fylstra DL. Ectopic pregnancy within a cesarean scar: a review. Obstet Gynecol Surv 2002;57: 537–43.

[52] Doubilet PM, Benson CB, Frates MC, et al. Sonographically guided minimally invasive treatment of unusual ectopic pregnancies. J Ultrasound Med 2004;23:359–70.

[53] Seow KM, Hwang JL, Tsai YL, et al. Subsequent pregnancy outcome after conservative treatment of a previous cesarean scar pregnancy. Acta Obstet Gynecol Scand 2004;83:1167–72.

[54] Seow KM, Huang LW, Lin YH, et al. Cesarean scar pregnancy: issues in management. Ultrasound Obstet Gynecol 2004;23:247–53.

[55] Costa SD, Presley J, Bastert G. Advanced abdominal pregnancy. Obstet Gynecol Surv 1991;46: 515–25.

[56] Irick MB, Kitsos CN, O'Leary JA. Therapeutic aspects in the management of a lithopedion. Am Surg 1970;36:232–4.

[57] Onan MA, Turp AB, Saltik A, et al. Primary omental pregnancy: case report. Hum Reprod 2005;20:807–9.

[58] Lee JW, Sohn KM, Jung HS. Retroperitoneal ectopic pregnancy. AJR Am J Roentgenol 2005; 184:1600–1.

[59] Cormio G, Ceci O, Loverro G, et al. Spontaneous left broad ligament pregnancy after ipsilateral salpingo-oophorectomy. J Minim Invasive Gynecol 2006;13:84–5.

[60] Breyer MJ, Costantino TG. Heterotopic gestation: another possibility for the emergency bedside ultrasonographer to consider. J Emerg Med 2004; 26:81–4.

[61] Barrenetxea G, Barinaga-Rementeria L, Lopez de Larruzea A, et al. Heterotopic pregnancy: two cases and a comparative review. Fertil Steril 2006;87(2):417, e9–15.

[62] Ramanan RV, Gajaraj J. Ectopic pregnancy–the leash sign. A new sign on transvaginal Doppler ultrasound. Acta Radiol 2006;47:529–35.

[63] Bhatt S, Dogra VS. Doppler imaging of the uterus and adnexae. Ultrasound Clinics 2006;1:201–21.

[64] Abramov Y, Nadjari M, Shushan A, et al. Doppler findings in chronic ectopic pregnancy: case report. Ultrasound Obstet Gynecol 1997;9:344–6.

[65] Rogers WF, Shaub M, Wilson R. Chronic ectopic pregnancy: ultrasonic diagnosis. J Clin Ultrasound 1977;5:257–60.

[66] Bedi DG, Moeller D, Fagan CJ, et al. Chronic ectopic pregnancy. A comparison with acute ectopic pregnancy. Eur J Radiol 1987;7:46–8.

[67] Bedi DG, Fagan CJ, Nocera RM. Chronic ectopic pregnancy. J Ultrasound Med 1984;3:347–52.

[68] DiMarchi JM, Kosasa TS, Kobara TY, et al. Persistent ectopic pregnancy. Obstet Gynecol 1987;70: 555–8.

[69] Seifer DB, Diamond MP, DeCherney AH. Persistent ectopic pregnancy. Obstet Gynecol Clin North Am 1991;18:153–9.

[70] Tenore JL. Ectopic pregnancy. Am Fam Physician 2000;61:1080–8.

[71] Shalev E, Peleg D, Tsabari A, et al. Spontaneous resolution of ectopic tubal pregnancy: natural history. Fertil Steril 1995;63:15–9.

[72] Trio D, Strobelt N, Picciolo C, et al. Prognostic factors for successful expectant management of ectopic pregnancy. Fertil Steril 1995;63:469–72.

[73] Hajenius PJ, Engelsbel S, Mol BW, et al. Randomised trial of systemic methotrexate versus laparoscopic salpingostomy in tubal pregnancy. Lancet 1997;350:774–9.

[74] Habana A, Dokras A, Giraldo JL, et al. Cornual heterotopic pregnancy: contemporary management options. Am J Obstet Gynecol 2000;182: 1264–70.

[75] Gjelland K, Hordnes K, Tjugum J, et al. Treatment of ectopic pregnancy by local injection of hypertonic glucose: a randomized trial comparing administration guided by transvaginal ultrasound or laparoscopy. Acta Obstet Gynecol Scand 1995;74:629–34.

[76] Pansky M, Golan A, Bukovsky I, et al. Nonsurgical management of tubal pregnancy. Necessity in view of the changing clinical appearance. Am J Obstet Gynecol 1991;164:888–95.

[77] Sadan O, Ginath S, Debby A, et al. Methotrexate versus hyperosomolar glucose in the treatment of extrauterine pregnancy. Arch Gynecol Obstet 2001;265:82–4.

ELSEVIER
SAUNDERS

RADIOLOGIC
CLINICS
OF NORTH AMERICA

Radiol Clin N Am 45 (2007) 561–579

Occult Fractures of Extremities

Joong Mo Ahn, MD*, Georges Y. El-Khoury, MD

- Definition, natural history, classification, and clinical significance
- Hip
- Knee
- Wrist
- Shoulder
- Ankle and foot
- Summary
- References

It has been recognized that CT and MR imaging are useful diagnostic tools for the evaluation of patients who have experienced trauma, and these imaging modalities are frequently used before surgical interventions [1].

Multidetector row CT offers excellent spatial resolution and multiplanar reformation capabilities [2–5]. The advantages of multidetector CT include short imaging time, isotropic data sets, and the ability to reconstruct multiplanar reformatted images retrospectively in any arbitrary plane [5]. Its advantages over conventional radiology include a more precise depiction of fracture lines and depressed or distracted articular surfaces and better assessment of bone loss (Figs. 1 and 2) [6].

The multiplanar imaging capability and improved contrast resolution afforded by MR imaging make it ideal for the detection of fractures undetected by radiographs (Figs. 3 and 4) [1]. Furthermore, MR imaging is the most sensitive direct imaging technique for depicting injury to the microtrabeculae and their environs [7,8].

Occult osseous injuries may result from a direct blow to the bone, by compressive forces of adjacent bones impacting one another, or by traction forces during an avulsion injury [9]. In addition, while examining the clinical MR images of different joints for internal derangement, radiologists may encounter unsuspected fractures [10]. These fractures could be radiographically unapparent or demonstrate subtle abnormalities that are overlooked easily.

Definition, natural history, classification, and clinical significance

The term "occult fracture" is used for a fracture that is either radiographically unapparent or demonstrates subtle abnormalities that are missed at initial interpretation [10,11]. These fractures also are hidden from view at direct observation at arthroscopy [12–14]. They are termed "occult fractures" even if confirmed by other imaging tests or if the fracture is seen in retrospect [11].

Occult fractures are often referred to as "bone bruises," which are a heterogeneous group of osseous injuries ranging from diffuse trabecular involvement to localized injury contiguous with the subchondral plate or articular surface [13–17]. The terms "bone bruise" and "bone contusion" have been used synonymously and are considered to represent a spectrum of occult bone injuries of traumatic origin. Such lesions include bleeding, infarction, and edema caused by microscopic compression fractures of cancellous bone [18]. Mandalia and colleagues [19] emphasized that occult fractures involve the trabecular bone and/or

Department of Radiology, Carver College of Medicine, University of Iowa Hospitals and Clinics, 200 Hawkins Drive, Iowa City, IA 52242, USA
* Corresponding author.
E-mail address: joong-ahn@uiowa.edu (J.M. Ahn).

doi:10.1016/j.rcl.2007.04.008

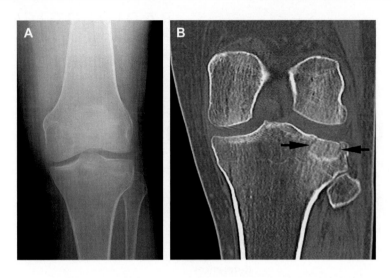

Fig. 1. A 51-year-old man who sustained a motorcycle accident. (*A*) Anteroposterior radiograph of the left knee shows no obvious fracture. (*B*) Coronal multiplanar reformatted CT image shows lateral tibial plateau fracture (*arrows*).

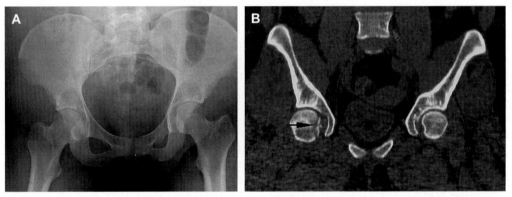

Fig. 2. A 19-year-old woman who sustained a motor vehicle accident. (*A*) Anteroposterior radiograph of the pelvis shows no obvious fracture. (*B*) Coronal multiplanar reformatted CT image shows right femoral head fracture (*arrow*).

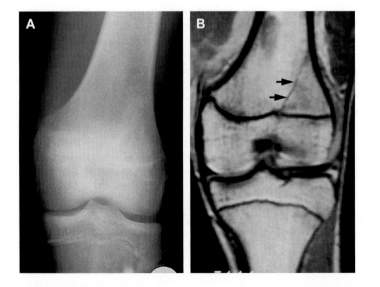

Fig. 3. A 10-year-old boy who sustained a left knee injury. (*A*) Anteroposterior radiograph of the left knee shows no obvious fracture. (*B*) T1-weighted coronal MR image of the left knee shows clearly a linear fracture line of low signal intensity (*arrows*).

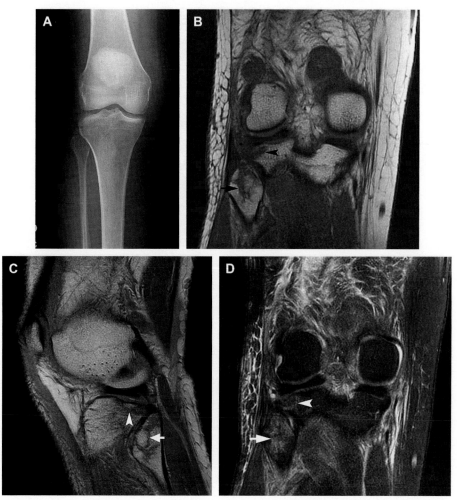

Fig. 4. A 37-year-old woman who sustained a valgus blow to her right knee. (*A*) Anteroposterior radiograph of the right knee shows no obvious fracture. (*B*) T1-weighted coronal MR image of the right knee shows subcortical compression fracture of the lateral tibial plateau (*arrowhead*) and hypointense area of geographic and nonlinear occult fracture of the proximal fibula (*arrow*). (*C*) T1-weighted sagittal MR image shows subcortical compression fracture of the lateral tibial plateau (*arrowhead*) and hypointense geographic and nonlinear occult fracture of the proximal fibula (*arrow*). (*D*) T2-weighted coronal MR image shows hyperintense area secondary to subcortical compression fracture of the lateral tibial plateau (*arrowhead*) and geographic and nonlinear occult fracture of the proximal fibula (*arrow*).

breach the adjacent cortex or osteochondral surface, whereas bone bruises or bone contusions involve only the bone marrow.

MR imaging helps in detecting nondisplaced fractures by showing a hypointense fracture line surrounded by adjacent edema (see Fig. 3; Figs. 5 and 6) [1]. In addition, the high contrast resolution afforded on MR imaging facilitates the detection of marrow edema at the site of fracture [1].

The MR imaging findings are best visualized on T1-weighted MR images as an area of amorphous low signal intensity representing an abnormal marrow signal (see Fig. 5) or as more sharply defined linear areas (see Fig. 3) of low signal intensity and

cortical irregularity that most likely represent subchondral and intraosseous fractures and cortical disruption [10].

Fluid-sensitive MR sequences may show increased signal intensity in areas of trabecular injury (see Figs. 4 and 5). It is likely that the area of low signal intensity on T1-weighted MR images and of high signal intensity on fluid-sensitive MR sequences represents intraosseous hemorrhage, edema, and microscopic compression fractures of trabecular bone, which have been suggested in histologic studies [10,12,13].

Although the reported time for the resolution of bone bruise is variable, ranging from 3 weeks to 2

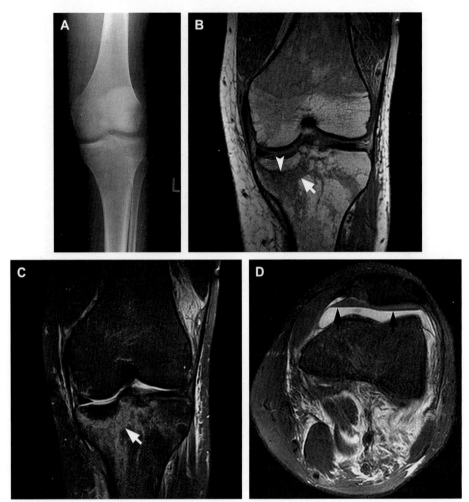

Fig. 5. An 18-year-old man who had a motorcycle crash. (*A*) Anteroposterior radiograph of the right knee shows no obvious fracture. (*B*) T1-weighted coronal MR image of the left knee shows a curvilinear fracture line (*arrowhead*) and diminished T1-signal intensity region distant from subchondral bone plate (*arrow*). (*C*) T2-weighted coronal MR image reveals bright T2-signal intensity region distant from subchondral bone plate (*arrow*). (*D*) T2-weighted axial MR image demonstrates fat–fluid level (*arrows*) indicating lipohemarthrosis.

years, follow-up MR imaging of occult fractures at 6 weeks to 3 months usually shows complete re-solution of the abnormality [12,19]. The resolution of the signal intensity is less predictable on T1-weighted MR images than on T2-weighted MR images [7]. This variation could be related to the severity and extent of the lesion [19]. Histologic evidence in the literature suggests that less severe trauma causes marrow edema without obvious injury to cellular elements, whereas more severe trauma causes microfracture and hemorrhage [19]. The severity of the trauma might influence the timing of resolution on imaging studies and the severity of clinical symptoms.

The MR imaging findings of occult fracture may be nonspecific, and the diagnosis of occult fractures depends primarily on the clinical setting. A closely related entity that could create addi-tional confusion is stress fracture of the amor-phous type [12,14,20]. The history of a single traumatic event rather than a period of unusual physical activity is useful in diagnosing an occult fracture. If the clinical history is unknown, the lo-cation of the lesion may aid in the differentiation from stress fracture [12]. Occult fractures involve large segments of the epiphysis and metaphysis (see Figs. 4 and 6), whereas stress fractures pre-dominantly involve the metaphysis [12,14]. For example, occult fractures in the leg commonly in-volve the subchondral bone within the medullary space of the epiphysis, whereas stress fractures tend to occur in the proximal tibial metaphysis

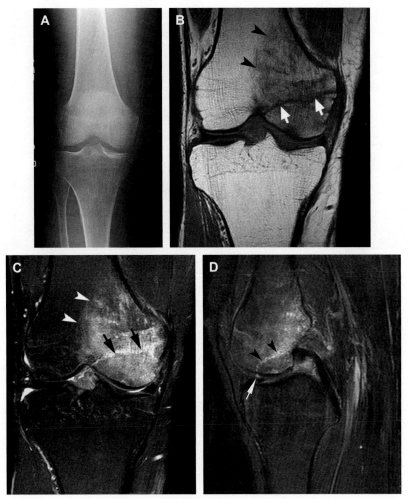

Fig. 6. A 46-year-old man who had an injury to his right knee. (*A*) Anteroposterior radiograph of the right knee shows no obvious fracture. (*B*) T1-weighted coronal MR image of the right knee reveals a hypointense fracture line (*arrows*) with area of diminished T1-signal intensity (*arrowheads*) in the medial femoral condyle of the left distal femur. (*C*) T2-weighted coronal MR image demonstrates a hyperintense fracture line (*arrows*) with bright area of bone marrow edema (*arrowheads*). (*D*) T2-weighted sagittal MR image shows a hyperintense fracture line (*arrowheads*), which extends into the articular cartilage (*arrow*).

or diaphysis but usually do not involve the epiphyses [12–14].

In the radiology literature, various classification systems for occult bone fractures have been proposed [8,14,21]. Mink and Deutsch [14] reported 66 cases of occult fractures with MR imaging and defined four categories of occult fracture in the knee: bone bruise, subchondral fracture, osteochondral fracture, and stress fracture. Bone bruise is defined as a geographic and nonlinear subchondral area of decreased signal intensity on T1-weighted images and increased signal intensity on T2-weighted images (Fig. 7). A subchondral fracture is defined as a linear or pronged area of decreased signal intensity on T1-weighted images and increased signal intensity on T2-weighted images that frequently extends vertically to reach the cortical bone and articular surface (Fig. 8). Osteochondral fracture is defined as the fracture of articular cartilage along with a small underlying bone segment (see Fig. 6). Stress fracture is defined as a linear zone of decreased signal intensity on T1- and T2-weighted images [13,14].

Vellet and colleagues [21] categorized occult fractures according to the MR imaging appearance in 120 patients and modified the classification system of Mink and Deutsch by introducing five categories: reticular fracture, geographic fracture, subcortical linear fracture, impaction fracture, and osteochondral fracture. Reticular fracture is defined as

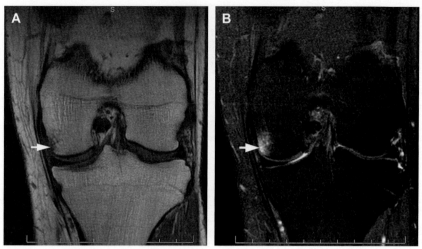

Fig. 7. A 33-year-old man who had left knee pain. (*A*) T1-weighted coronal MR image of the left knee shows an area of decreased signal intensity in the medial femoral condyle (*arrow*). (*B*) T2-weighted coronal MR image reveals increased signal intensity of the lesion in the medial femoral condyle (*arrow*).

serpiginous region of diminished T1-weighted signal intensity distant from the subchondral bone plate (see Fig. 5). The geographic fracture is defined as a discrete confluent focus of low signal intensity contiguous with the subchondral bone plate. The subcortical linear fracture is a discrete linear zone of diminished signal intensity on T1-weighted images less than 2 mm in diameter (see Figs. 6 and 8), with a sharp zone of transition into adjacent bone marrow fat. The impaction fracture is a depression of the articular surface in conjunction with

a geographic lesion. The osteochondral fracture is defined as geographic lesion with a discrete interface of low signal intensity that separates the lesion from the surrounding trabecular bone and communicates with the joint space (see Fig. 6) [13,21].

Lynch and colleagues [8] proposed a classification comprising three types. A type I lesion is a diffuse, often reticulated area of decreased signal intensity in the epiphyseal and metaphyseal regions on T1-weighted images and increased signal intensity on T2-weighted images (see Fig. 4). A type II lesion is

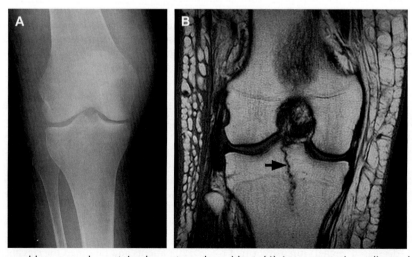

Fig. 8. A 59-year-old woman who sustained a motorcycle accident. (*A*) Anteroposterior radiograph of the right knee shows no obvious fracture. (*B*) T1-weighted coronal MR image of the right knee reveals a vertically oriented hypointense fracture line (*arrow*). (*C*) T2-weighted coronal MR image shows a vertically oriented hyperintense fracture line (*arrow*). (*D*) T1-weighted sagittal MR image shows vertically oriented fracture line (*arrows*) and associated subcutaneous hematoma (*arrowhead*).

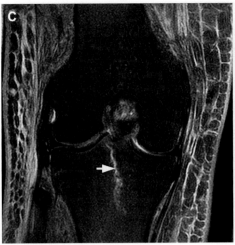

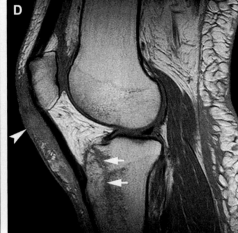

Fig. 8 (*continued*)

similar to type I lesion but is associated with an interruption in the smooth cortical line (see Fig. 6). A type III lesion is defined as an area of profound decrease of signal intensity restricted to the immediate subcortical region, seen on T1-weighted images (Figs. 9 and 10). Lynch and colleagues emphasized that even the bone bruises without cortical disruption may represent regions of bone at increased risk for the subsequent development of insufficiency fractures if the bone is not protected adequately during trabecular healing [8]. There is controversial evidence regarding the prognostic significance of the different types of bone bruise [19].

It is important to detect and diagnose occult fractures accurately for several reasons. First, they may be the only abnormalities present and can help explain the patient's symptoms without the need for surgical procedures [15]. Second, it is important for patients who have occult fractures to avoid bearing weight on the fracture to prevent compressions of bone in the areas of trabecular fractures and collapse of the damaged overlying articular cartilage that may then lead to pain or premature osteoarthritis [15,21]. Finally, associated soft tissue injuries such as ligamentous injuries are known to occur also. These ligamentous abnormalities often are of greater clinical importance than the occult fractures. Thus, detection of occult fractures may force referring physicians to pay closer attention to the ligamentous structures [15].

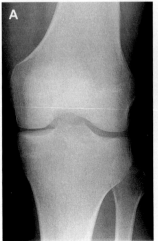

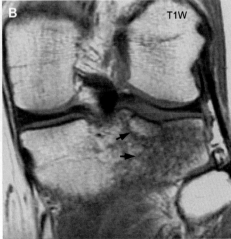

Fig. 9. A 22-year-old man who sustained a twisting injury to his left knee. (*A*) Anteroposterior radiograph of the left knee shows no obvious fracture. (*B*) T1-weighted coronal MR image of the left knee shows fracture lines (*arrows*).

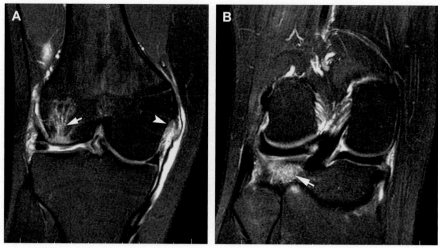

Fig. 10. A 19-year-old woman who sustained a twisting injury to her right knee. (*A*) T2-weighted coronal MR image of the right knee shows bone marrow edema in the lateral femoral condyle (*arrow*) and torn medial collateral ligament (*arrowhead*). (*B*) T2-weighted coronal MR image obtained posterior to the image in panel A reveals bone marrow edema in the lateral tibial plateau (*arrow*).

Hip

Trauma to the hip from falls or other causes is commonplace and is a major source of morbidity. Hip fracture is among the most commonly encountered orthopedic injuries in the emergency department [22]. The diagnosis of a hip fracture most frequently is made on physical examination and plain radiographs [23]. A large proportion of these fractures may be missed on plain radiography, however (Fig. 11) [24,25], particularly in osteoporotic hips or in the presence of degenerative osteophytes.

The incidence of occult hip fracture is estimated to be 2% to 10% in the patients presenting with painful hip after trauma [26–28]. Occult fractures may be secondary to trauma or secondary to stress [24].

Although displaced fractures are diagnosed readily, in many cases initial radiographs of nondisplaced fractures of the femoral neck may be normal or equivocal, resulting in uncertainty with regard to diagnosis and treatment [29]. Patients who have recognized undisplaced femoral neck fractures require acute admission and early screw

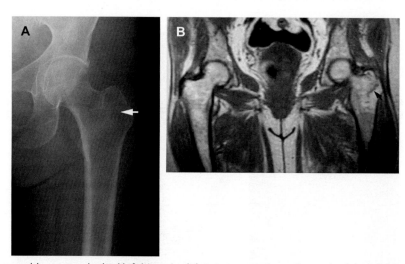

Fig. 11. A 59-year-old woman who had left hip pain. (*A*) Anteroposterior radiograph of the left hip shows a questionable lucency in the greater trochanter (*arrow*). (*B*) T1-weighted coronal MR image of the pelvis demonstrates a low signal intensity of linear fracture line (*arrow*) that does not correspond to a normal anatomic structure.

fixation [1]. Patients who have unrecognized fractures continue to bear weight as much as is tolerable following discharge until fracture fragments displace with drastic consequences such as avascular necrosis or non-union following delayed operative intervention [1,30]. Although femoral neck fractures usually are identified on plain radiographs, undisplaced fractures may remain occult before further imaging studies [1]. Undisplaced fractures may be particularly difficult to detect in elderly osteopenic patients in whom minor alterations in trabecular alignment may be harder to perceive [1].

Numerous studies have shown that MR imaging is the modality of choice for studying occult hip fractures [31]. The sensitivity and specificity of MR imaging for the detection of occult fractures of the femoral neck are better than those of bone scintigraphy [26] and have been reported to be as high as 100% [23,26,32]. Deutsch and colleagues [29] studied occult fractures of the proximal femur with MR imaging. They identified fractures in nine patients who had normal radiographs and found no false positives or false negatives. The MR imaging finding of a linear, oblique, or serpiginous low signal intensity on T1-weighted MR images that remains dark on T2-weighted images and does not correspond to a normal anatomic structure is assumed to represent a fracture line (Fig. 12) [31]. A fracture line may be distinguished from other dark abnormal intraosseous bands such as a bone infarct, avascular necrosis, or metastasis (Fig. 13). The less defined region of decreased signal intensity on T1-weighted MR images that becomes bright on

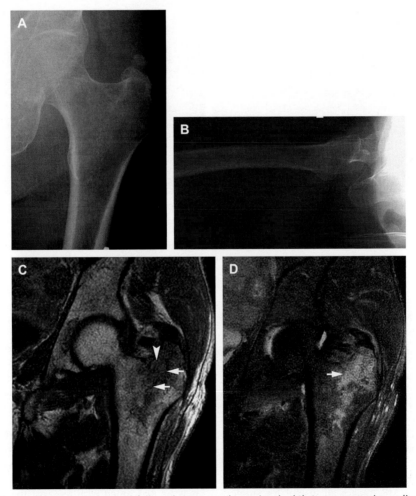

Fig. 12. A 67-year-old woman who had fallen about 1 week previously. (*A*) Anteroposterior radiograph of the left hip shows no obvious fracture. (*B*) Cross-table lateral view of the left hip is negative. (*C*) T1-weighted coronal MR image shows the low signal intensity of a serpiginous fracture line (*arrows*) in the greater trochanter and an area of decreased signal intensity in the intertrochanteric region (*arrowhead*). (*D*) T2-weighted coronal MR image shows increased signal intensity in the intertrochanteric region (*arrow*) representing bone marrow edema.

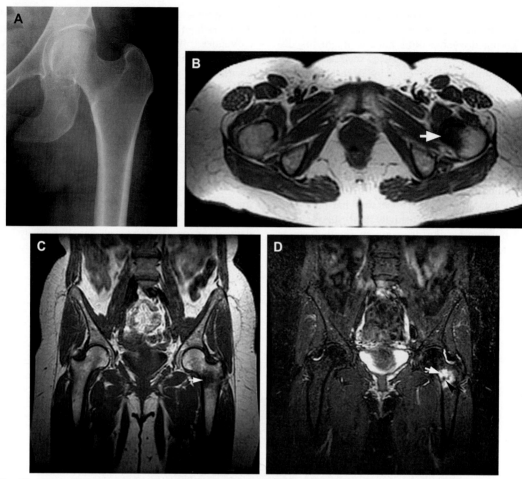

Fig. 13. A 55-year-old woman who had left hip pain. (*A*) Anteroposterior radiograph of the left hip is a negative examination. (*B*) T1-weighted axial MR image shows decreased signal intensity in the lesser trochanter (*arrow*). (*C*) T1-weighted coronal MR image demonstrates hypointense lesion in the lesser trochanter (*arrow*). (*D*) T2-weighted coronal MR image shows area of bright signal intensity (*arrow*) and serpiginous low signal intensity (*arrowhead*) representing edema and the fracture line, respectively.

T2-weighted MR images probably represents a zone of edema, intraosseous hemorrhage, or granulation tissue (see Fig. 12) [29]. The short inversion time inversion recovery (STIR) sequence demonstrates the fracture as a bright line [29].

Another advantage of MR imaging in patients who have occult fractures of the proximal femur is the ability to assess the extent of these fractures [29,33,34]. The diagnosis of incomplete intertrochanteric fractures, a subset of intertrochanteric fracture, can be established with certainty only with MR imaging (see Figs. 11–13) [34]. Furthermore, coronal MR images are useful for surgical planning (see Fig. 13) [23].

The advantages of early detection of an occult fracture of the proximal femur lie in decreasing the chances of a displacement of simple nondisplaced fracture. Early diagnosis and treatment of femoral fractures potentially can lead to a shorter hospital stay, reduced morbidity, and therefore decreased costs [31,35]. In addition to complete occult fractures that breach the cortex, several types of subtle or radiographically occult fractures can be diagnosed definitively with MR imaging [12,14,15].

Limited and rapid MR protocols that use only T1-weighted coronal MR images without other imaging sequences may be sufficient for a specific diagnosis of occult fracture of the proximal femur and may be performed with less cost than more complex protocols [23,31,35]. Some centers use a limited protocol in which T1-weighted coronal MR images are the preferred imaging modality for the detection of radiographically occult fractures [23].

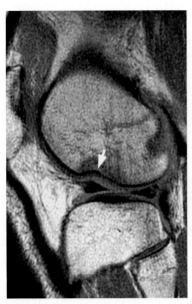

Fig. 14. Terminal sulcus on the lateral femoral condyle of the femur. Proton density-weighted sagittal MR image demonstrates the terminal sulcus, which is an anatomic sulcus on the lateral femoral condyle of the femur (*arrow*).

Haramati and colleagues [31], however, recommended that both coronal and axial T1-weighted MR images be performed.

Knee

Occult osseous injuries were first described in the knee [14,21], and focal abnormal signal intensity within the distal femoral condyles or proximal tibial plateaus is seen frequently on MR imaging of the knee (see Figs. 9 and 10) [8]. Although bone bruises in the knee do not alter management significantly, they may be a cause of pain (see Fig. 7) [36]. This pain usually is mild and resolves without therapy in a period of 4 to 8 weeks [36]. The prompt detection and correct diagnosis of occult fracture should be of particular value in patients who have knee injuries without associated meniscal or capsuloligamentous lesions and perhaps in those for whom the MR images otherwise would be interpreted as normal, despite the presence of significant clinical symptoms [10].

The preponderance of occult fractures around the knee within the lateral joint compartment is consistent with pre-existent or induced valgus forces at the time of injury, whether or not the injury is associated with rotational or deceleration forces [21]. This predominance of bone bruises in the lateral femoral condyle and the lateral tibial plateau can be explained by the usual mechanism of injury (ie, anterior subluxation of the lateral tibial plateau relative to the lateral femoral condyle during a pivot shift injury) (see Figs. 4, 9, and 10) [15,18,37]. Such factors also would account for the high prevalence of associated ligamentous injuries [21]. In addition, the presence of bone bruise is associated with more severe presenting symptoms [18].

The lateral femoral condyle and posterolateral tibial plateau are the two most common occult fractures or bone bruises associated with an acute anterior cruciate ligament tear [7,15,21]. On sagittal and coronal MR images, the occult fractures or bone bruises are located directly and invariably over the lateral femoral condyle terminal sulcus.

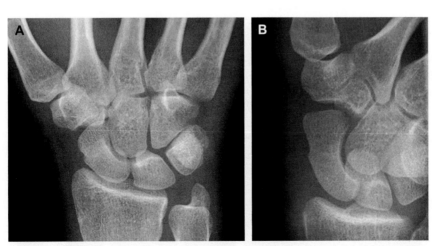

Fig. 15. A 19-year-old woman who injured her right hand. (*A*) Anteroposterior radiograph of the right wrist is negative. (*B*) Scaphoid view is essentially negative. (*C*) T1-weighted coronal MR image reveals nondisplaced fracture (*arrow*) in the waist of the scaphoid. (*D*) T2-weighted coronal MR image shows bright signal intensity of bone marrow edema (*arrow*) in the waist of the scaphoid.

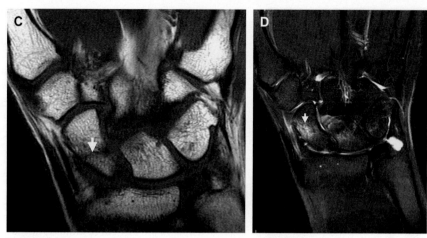

Fig. 15 (continued)

The terminal sulcus is an anatomic sulcus on the lateral femoral condyle of the femur [7]. The terminal sulcus actually represents the junction between the tibiofemoral articular surface and the patellofemoral articular surface (see Fig. 14) [7].

Occult fractures vary in size and signal intensity, but the greatest signal intensity typically is contiguous with the subchondral plate [7]. The occult osseous lesion can extend vertically but rarely crosses the physeal scar. The physeal scar seems to serve as a barrier to contain and limit the propagation of the abnormal signal intensity [7]. Axial MR images demonstrate direct continuity of the osseous lesion with the lateral femoral cortex.

The distribution of occult fractures or bone bruises around the knee is like a footprint left behind at the time of the impact, providing valuable clues about the associated soft tissue injuries occurring in the knee [9]. In many instances, the mechanism of knee injury can be determined by studying the distribution of the occult fractures and bone bruise; this information enables the radiologists to predict with accuracy the specific soft tissue abnormalities that are likely to be present.

Wrist

The scaphoid is the most commonly fractured bone of the wrist. Scaphoid fractures occur most often in young adults (age range, 15–40 years), and such fractures are known to have a high rate of complications [38]. These complications include delayed

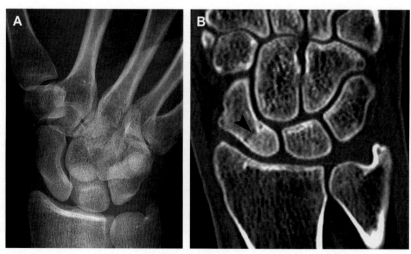

Fig. 16. A 28-year-old woman who injured dorsiflexion injury in her right hand. (*A*) Scaphoid view is essentially negative. (*B*) Coronal multiplanar reformatted CT image shows definite fracture lucency in the waist of the scaphoid (*arrowhead*).

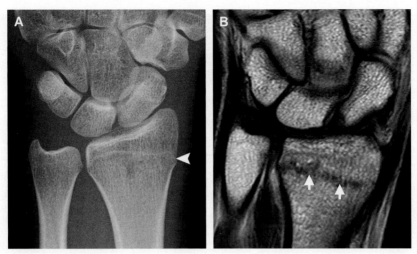

Fig. 17. A 29-year-old woman who fell on her outstretched left hand. (*A*) Anteroposterior radiograph of the left wrist shows questionable buckling in the radial cortex (*arrowhead*). (*B*) T1-weighted coronal MR image reveals nondisplaced fracture (*arrows*) in the left distal radius.

union, non-union, or avascular necrosis, especially if diagnosis is delayed. The incidence of radiographically occult scaphoid fractures is relatively high (see Figs. 15 and 16) [38].

Plain radiography is the first step in the evaluation of the scaphoid injuries, and it is effective in diagnosing most but not all scaphoid fractures. If radiography is negative, and clinical suspicion of a scaphoid fracture persists, further investigation with special radiographic views, CT scan, or MR

imaging is necessary (see Figs. 15 and 16) [38]. In many clinical settings, the diagnosis of a scaphoid fracture on the basis of radiography is delayed up to 2 weeks or more after the injury, when follow-up radiographs demonstrate the initially occult scaphoid fracture because hyperemia and bone resorption at the fracture site make the fracture line more visible [38].

Criteria for an occult fracture on multidetector row CT are the presence of a sharp lucent line

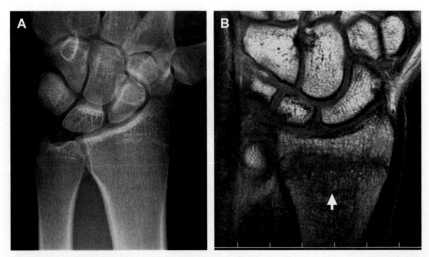

Fig. 18. An 18-year-old man who fell on his outstretched left hand. (*A*) Anteroposterior radiograph of the left wrist is negative. (*B*) T1-weighted coronal MR image reveals extensive area of decreased signal intensity representing bone marrow edema (*arrow*) in the left distal radius. (*C*) T2-weighted coronal MR image demonstrates large area of bone marrow edema (*arrow*) in the left distal radius. (*D*) T2-weighted axial MR image also shows bone marrow edema (*arrow*) in the left distal radius.

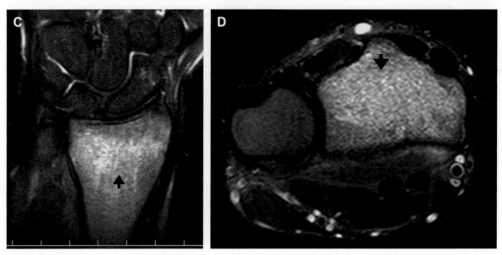

Fig. 18 (continued)

within the bone pattern, a discontinuity in the trabecular meshwork, and a break or step-off in the cortex (see Fig. 16).

Accurate diagnosis using CT or MR imaging initiates early treatment with 6-week immobilization for the wrist fracture [38]. Another advantage of CT or MR imaging is the ability to show fracture lines more clearly than plain radiography (Fig. 17). CT is more sensitive than radiography for detecting subtle or occult fractures [38,39]. CT is a rapid and comfortable method for examining the hand and wrist and is a valuable diagnostic tool in the evaluation of the patients who have suffered trauma in hand and wrist in which an explanation for the patient's symptoms cannot be found with conventional imaging studies [39]. CT also has been widely used in the follow-up of fracture healing of the scaphoid and distal radius, especially in the presence of hardware.

MR imaging is exquisitely sensitive to bone marrow abnormalities and therefore renders even nondisplaced fractures obvious (see Fig. 15; Fig. 18). A STIR sequence is sensitive in identifying cortical fracture lines in the scaphoid [38]. These findings are present immediately after the trauma.

Although CT has a high sensitivity for occult wrist fractures, MR imaging seems to be superior as an initial examination because it enables visualization of bone marrow abnormalities in nondisplaced fractures (see Figs. 15 and 18) [38].

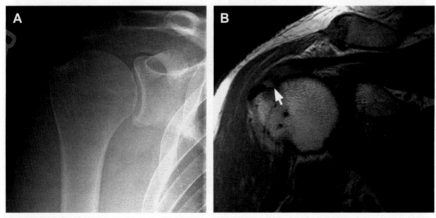

Fig. 19. A 42-year-old woman who fell from a horse. She had a limitation of her right arm elevation with pain and was referred for MR imaging of the shoulder to evaluate for rotator cuff tear. (*A*) Anteroposterior view of the right shoulder shows no fracture. (*B*) T1-weighted coronal MR image reveals hypointense band with cortical disruption in the greater tuberosity (*arrow*) representing subcortical nondisplaced fracture.

MR imaging can be cost effective in the setting of acute trauma with normal radiographs because MR imaging reduces the interval between the initial symptoms and the definitive diagnosis. Early MR imaging obviates the need for other examinations such as bone scanning or short-term follow-up radiography and therefore makes the diagnosis a simple one-step procedure.

Shoulder

Fractures of the greater tuberosity are caused by a variety of mechanisms but most commonly result from seizures, glenohumeral dislocations, or forced abduction with direct impaction of the greater tuberosity on the acromion. Most fractures of the greater tuberosity are minimally displaced and

traditionally are treated conservatively. Because clinical presentation simulates a rotator cuff tear, patients who have occult fractures often are referred for MR imaging to look for a rotator cuff tear (Fig. 19) [40].

Subtle fractures of the greater tuberosity may go undetected with plain radiography. Irregularities or defects of the curved surface of the greater tuberosity are revealed on plain radiographs only when viewed tangentially. Negative radiographic findings do not totally exclude a greater tuberosity fracture because fractures may not be visible when the X-ray beams are not tangential to the curved surface of the proximal humerus. Fluoroscopy has been used when MR imaging is not readily available. Such fractures can be diagnosed confidently on MR imaging, however, and are evaluated best on

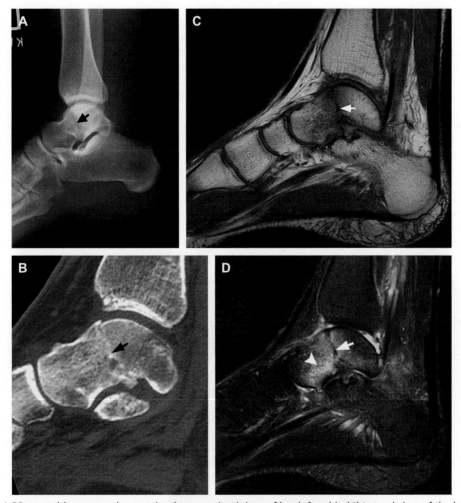

Fig. 20. A 38-year-old woman who sustained an eversion injury of her left ankle (*A*) Lateral view of the left ankle shows suspicious lucency (*arrow*) in the talar neck. (*B*) Sagittal multiplanar reformatted CT image shows fracture line in the talar neck (*arrow*). (*C*) T1-weighted sagittal MR image demonstrates low signal intensity line of talar neck fracture (*arrow*). (*D*) T2-weighted sagittal MR image demonstrates low signal intensity line of talar neck fracture (*arrow*). Note also adjacent bone marrow edema (*arrowhead*).

oblique coronal T1- and T2-weighted MR images. Fractures of the greater tuberosity present as crescentic or oblique lines of decreased signal intensity close to the surface of the bone, and they frequently are surrounded by marrow edema [40].

The degree of superior or posterior displacement of the fracture fragment is evaluated best on oblique coronal T1-weighted MR images. Because most fractures of the greater tuberosity are associated with rotator cuff abnormalities, the rotator cuff should be inspected carefully in patients who have such fractures [40].

Ankle and foot

Early detection of occult fractures in the ankle and foot helps avoid chronic disability [41]. CT and MR imaging each have particular advantages in the assessment of unexplained posttraumatic pain of the ankle and foot (Fig. 20) [41]. These modalities provide excellent sensitivity and specificity in the evaluation of ankle and foot fractures and allow visualization of soft tissue structures. CT provides optimal assessment of the bone, whereas MR imaging provides optimal assessment of ligaments, tendons, and bone marrow edema or contusions [41].

Fractures of the talus are not common injuries, and most of these injuries occur in the talar neck or talar dome [42]. Fractures of the talar neck usually are caused by forced ankle dorsiflexion (see Fig. 20) [42] and occasionally are very subtle, especially when undisplaced. CT and MR imaging are diagnostic in occult talar neck fracture.

The dome of the talus articulates with the tibia and fibula and has a key role in ankle motion and in supporting the axial load during weight bearing

[43]. Fractures of the talar dome generally result from inversion injuries of the ankle. They are located medially or laterally with equal frequency (Fig. 21) [44]. Lateral talar dome fractures are almost always associated with trauma, whereas medial talar dome lesions can be traumatic or atraumatic in origin. Although the talar dome lesions usually can be diagnosed with plain radiographs, CT or MR imaging often is required because these fractures are easily missed on plain radiographs, and the diagnosis can be challenging (see Fig. 21).

Tarsal navicular stress fractures usually occur in elite athletes including runners, gymnasts, basketball players, and football players, typically linebackers [45]. The correct diagnosis of a tarsal navicular stress fracture is often delayed, partly because the clinical onset is insidious with nonspecific signs and symptoms and also because in most cases these stress injuries are not evident on radiographs [46]. The interval between the onset of symptoms and the diagnosis often is between 7 weeks to 4 months but may be much longer in some patients. Early diagnosis in athletes is essential for initiation of conservative therapy or internal fixation. Tarsal navicular stress fractures may be incomplete or complete. Incomplete fractures usually involve the dorsal 5 mm of the navicular adjacent to the talonavicular joint, an area that is difficult to evaluate radiographically [47]. MR imaging detects the bone marrow edema associated with the osseous stress reaction, which often is present before a fracture line is visualized (Fig. 22) [48]. MR imaging is the modality of choice in patients who have early symptoms suggesting a tarsal navicular stress fracture.

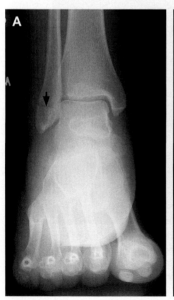 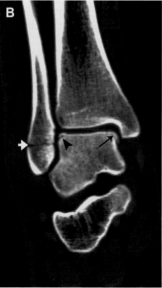

Fig. 21. A 19-year-old man who sustained a motorcycle accident. (*A*) Anteroposterior view of the right ankle shows a transverse fracture of the distal fibula (*arrow*). The talar dome appears intact. (*B*) Coronal multiplanar reformatted CT image shows transverse fracture of the distal fibula (*thick arrow*). In addition, medial (*slender arrow*) and lateral (*arrowhead*) talar dome fractures, which were not evident on plain radiography, are well visualized.

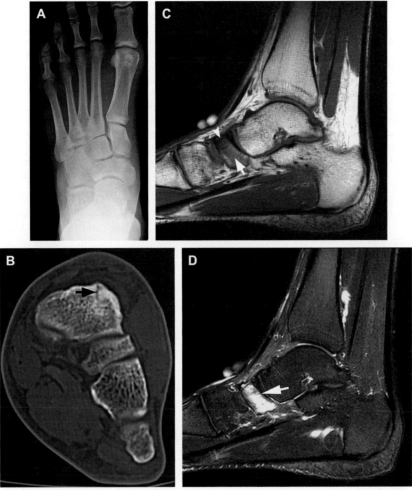

Fig. 22. A 21-year-old man who experienced left foot pain. (*A*) Anteroposterior view of the left foot is negative. (*B*) Coronal multiplanar reformatted CT image shows linear fracture line in the left tarsal navicular (*arrow*). (*C*) T1-weighted sagittal MR image demonstrates low signal intensity fracture line (*arrowhead*) and hypointense area of bone marrow edema (*arrow*) in the tarsal navicular. (*D*) T2-weighted sagittal MR image demonstrates hyperintense bone marrow edema in the left tarsal navicular (*arrow*).

Summary

CT and MR imaging have been shown to be excellent imaging techniques that superiorly display and delineate the occult fractures whenever plain radiographs are negative or indeterminate.

CT findings of occult fracture are the presence of a sharp lucent line within the trabecular bone pattern and a break in the continuity of the cortex. The typical MR imaging findings of occult fracture are intraosseous speckled or linear regions of low signal intensity on T1-weighted MR images and irregular areas of high signal intensity in corresponding areas on fluid-sensitive MR imaging sequences.

Although plain radiographs provide nearly complete evaluation of fractures in most cases, CT and MR imaging enable detection of traumatic injuries in patients who have negative plain radiographs and a high clinical suspicion of occult fracture before treatment. CT has been proved to be accurate in depicting occult fracture with cortical involvement and is used successfully for this purpose.

MR imaging has high sensitivity and specificity in detecting occult fractures and remains the reference standard for early diagnosis of occult fractures of the extremity.

References

[1] Eustace S. MR imaging of acute orthopedic trauma to the extremities. Radiol Clin North Am 1997;35(3):615–29.

[2] Memarsadeghi M, Breitenseher MJ, Schaefer-Prokop C, et al. Occult scaphoid fractures: comparison of multidetector CT and MR imaging–initial experience. Radiology 2006;240(1): 169–76.

[3] Hu H, He HD, Foley WD, et al. Four multidetector-row helical CT: image quality and volume coverage speed. Radiology 2000;215(1):55–62.

[4] Breederveld RS, Tuinebreijer WE. Investigation of computed tomographic scan concurrent criterion validity in doubtful scaphoid fracture of the wrist. J Trauma 2004;57(4):851–4.

[5] Buckwalter KA, Farber JM. Application of multidetector CT in skeletal trauma. Semin Musculoskelet Radiol 2004;8(2):147–56.

[6] Ahn JM, El-Khoury GY. Computed tomography of knee injuries. Imaging Decisions 2006;10(1): 14–23.

[7] Speer KP, Spritzer CE, Bassett FH 3rd, et al. Osseous injury associated with acute tears of the anterior cruciate ligament. Am J Sports Med 1992; 20(4):382–9.

[8] Lynch TC, Crues JV 3rd, Morgan FW, et al. Bone abnormalities of the knee: prevalence and significance at MR imaging. Radiology 1989;171(3): 761–6.

[9] Sanders TG, Medynski MA, Feller JF, et al. Bone contusion patterns of the knee at MR imaging: footprint of the mechanism of injury. Radiographics 2000;20(Spec No):S135–51.

[10] Berger PE, Ofstein RA, Jackson DW, et al. MRI demonstration of radiographically occult fractures: what have we been missing? Radiographics 1989;9(3):407–36.

[11] Weishaupt D, Schweitzer ME. MR imaging of the foot and ankle: patterns of bone marrow signal abnormalities. Eur Radiol 2002;12(2):416–26.

[12] Yao L, Lee JK. Occult intraosseous fracture: detection with MR imaging. Radiology 1988;167(3): 749–51.

[13] Boks SS, Vroegindeweij D, Koes BW, et al. Follow-up of occult bone lesions detected at MR imaging: systematic review. Radiology 2006;238(3): 853–62.

[14] Mink JH, Deutsch AL. Occult cartilage and bone injuries of the knee: detection, classification, and assessment with MR imaging. Radiology 1989; 170(3 Pt 1):823–9.

[15] Kaplan PA, Walker CW, Kilcoyne RF, et al. Occult fracture patterns of the knee associated with anterior cruciate ligament tears: assessment with MR imaging. Radiology 1992; 183(3):835–8.

[16] Wright RW, Phaneuf MA, Limbird TJ, et al. Clinical outcome of isolated subcortical trabecular fractures (bone bruise) detected on magnetic resonance imaging in knees. Am J Sports Med 2000; 28(5):663–7.

[17] Miller MD, Osborne JR, Gordon WT, et al. The natural history of bone bruises. A prospective study of magnetic resonance imaging-detected trabecular microfractures in patients with isolated medial collateral ligament injuries. Am J Sports Med 1998;26(1):15–9.

[18] Vincken PW, Ter Braak BP, van Erkel AR, et al. Clinical consequences of bone bruise around the knee. Eur Radiol 2006;16(1):97–107.

[19] Mandalia V, Fogg AJ, Chari R, et al. Bone bruising of the knee. Clin Radiol 2005;60(6): 627–36.

[20] Daffner RH. Stress fracture: current concepts. Skeletal Radiol 1978;2:221–9.

[21] Vellet AD, Marks PH, Fowler PJ, et al. Occult posttraumatic osteochondral lesions of the knee: prevalence, classification, and short-term sequelae evaluated with MR imaging. Radiology 1991;178(1):271–6.

[22] Perron AD, Miller MD, Brady WJ. Orthopedic pitfalls in the ED: radiographically occult hip fracture. Am J Emerg Med 2002;20(3): 234–7.

[23] Bogost GA, Lizerbram EK, Crues JV 3rd. MR imaging in evaluation of suspected hip fracture: frequency of unsuspected bone and soft-tissue injury. Radiology 1995;197(1):263–7.

[24] Alba E, Youngberg R. Occult fractures of the femoral neck. Am J Emerg Med 1992;10(1):64–8.

[25] Verbeeten KM, Hermann KL, Hasselqvist M, et al. The advantages of MRI in the detection of occult hip fractures. Eur Radiol 2005;15(1): 165–9.

[26] Rizzo PF, Gould ES, Lyden JP, et al. Diagnosis of occult fractures about the hip. Magnetic resonance imaging compared with bone-scanning. J Bone Joint Surg Am 1993;75(3):395–401.

[27] Lubovsky O, Liebergall M, Mattan Y, et al. Early diagnosis of occult hip fractures MRI versus CT scan. Injury 2005;36(6):788–92.

[28] Cumming RG, Nevitt MC, Cummings SR. Epidemiology of hip fractures. Epidemiol Rev 1997; 19(2):244–57.

[29] Deutsch AL, Mink JH, Waxman AD. Occult fractures of the proximal femur: MR imaging. Radiology 1989;170(1 Pt 1):113–6.

[30] Asnis SE, Gould ES, Bansal M, et al. Magnetic resonance imaging of the hip after displaced femoral neck fractures. Clin Orthop Relat Res 1994; 298:191–8.

[31] Haramati N, Staron RB, Barax C, et al. Magnetic resonance imaging of occult fractures of the proximal femur. Skeletal Radiol 1994;23(1): 19–22.

[32] Brossmann J, Biederer J, Heller M. MR imaging of musculoskeletal trauma to the pelvis and the lower limb. Eur Radiol 1999;9(2):183–91.

[33] Feldman F, Staron RB. MRI of seemingly isolated greater trochanteric fractures. AJR Am J Roentgenol 2004;183(2):323–9.

[34] Schultz E, Miller TT, Boruchov SD, et al. Incomplete intertrochanteric fractures: imaging features and clinical management. Radiology 1999; 211(1):237–40.

[35] Quinn SF, McCarthy JL. Prospective evaluation of patients with suspected hip fracture and

indeterminate radiographs: use of T1-weighted MR images. Radiology 1993;187(2):469–71.

[36] Schweitzer ME, Karasick D. MRI of the ankle and hindfoot. Semin Ultrasound CT MR 1994;15(5): 410–22.

[37] Costa-Paz M, Muscolo DL, Ayerza M, et al. Magnetic resonance imaging follow-up study of bone bruises associated with anterior cruciate ligament ruptures. Arthroscopy 2001;17(5):445–9.

[38] Breitenseher MJ, Metz VM, Gilula LA, et al. Radiographically occult scaphoid fractures: value of MR imaging in detection. Radiology 1997; 203(1):245–50.

[39] Hindman BW, Kulik WJ, Lee G, et al. Occult fractures of the carpals and metacarpals: demonstration by CT. AJR Am J Roentgenol 1989;153(3): 529–32.

[40] Mason BJ, Kier R, Bindleglass DF. Occult fractures of the greater tuberosity of the humerus: radiographic and MR imaging findings. AJR Am J Roentgenol 1999;172(2):469–73.

[41] Clark TW, Janzen DL, Ho K, et al. Detection of radiographically occult ankle fractures following

acute trauma: positive predictive value of an ankle effusion. AJR Am J Roentgenol 1995;164(5): 1185–9.

[42] Santavirta S, Seitsalo S, Kiviluoto O, et al. Fractures of the talus. J Trauma 1984;24(11):986–9.

[43] Keene JS, Lange RH. Diagnostic dilemmas in foot and ankle injuries. JAMA 1986;256(2): 247–51.

[44] Canale ST, Belding RH. Osteochondral lesions of the talus. J Bone Joint Surg Am 1980;62(1): 97–102.

[45] Torg JS, Pavlov H, Cooley LH, et al. Stress fractures of the tarsal navicular. A retrospective review of twenty-one cases. J Bone Joint Surg Am 1982;64(5):700–12.

[46] Kiss ZS, Khan KM, Fuller PJ. Stress fractures of the tarsal navicular bone: CT findings in 55 cases. AJR Am J Roentgenol 1993;160(1):111–5.

[47] Pavlov H, Torg JS, Freiberger RH. Tarsal navicular stress fractures: radiographic evaluation. Radiology 1983;148(3):641–5.

[48] Spitz DJ, Newberg AH. Imaging of stress fractures in the athlete. Radiol Clin North Am 2002;40(2):313–31.

RADIOLOGIC
CLINICS
OF NORTH AMERICA

Radiol Clin N Am 45 (2007) 581–592

ELSEVIER
SAUNDERS

Renal Trauma

Young Joon Lee, MD, Soon Nam Oh, MD, PhD,
Sung Eun Rha, MD, PhD, Jae Young Byun, MD, PhD*

Trauma is the leading cause of death in men and women under 40 years of age. Urinary tract injury occurs in 10% of all abdominal trauma patients, and the kidney is the most commonly injured organ in the urinary tract [1].

There is a broad consensus in favor of less invasive procedures and conservative management of traumatic renal injuries when a patient is stable, except in cases of severe injury such as pedicle injury or complete laceration of the ureteropelvic junction [2–4]. Therefore, it is crucial to diagnose the extent and type of renal injury accurately to assure adequate treatment.

Ultrasound, CT, and MR imaging are cross-sectional imaging modalities for renal trauma; among them, CT with contrast enhancement is the modality of choice for renal trauma because it quickly and accurately can demonstrate injury to the renal parenchyma, renal pedicles, and associated abdominal or retroperitoneal organs [5].

This article reviews the mechanism, clinical features, imaging modalities, and CT imaging findings according to the classification of the renal trauma. Trauma to underlying abnormal kidneys, iatrogenic renal injuries, and complications of renal trauma are reviewed also.

Mechanism of renal injuries

The kidneys are protected from damage posteriorly by the psoas and quadratus lumborum muscles and anteriorly by the peritoneum. Perinephric fat and the lower rib cage also protect the kidneys. Despite this protection, renal injury frequently occurs because of trauma to the back, flank, lower thorax, or upper abdomen.

It is important to distinguish between blunt and penetrating injuries. Blunt trauma accounts for 80% to 90% of all renal injury [1,6,7]. The most common cause of blunt trauma is motor vehicle accident. A direct blow to the flank or abdomen during sports activities is another common cause of blunt trauma injury. Sudden deceleration or a crash injury may result in contusion, laceration, or avulsion of the renal parenchyma. Tension in the renal pedicles may produce an intimal tear leading to thrombosis of a renal artery or vein.

Department of Diagnostic Radiology, Division of Abdominal Radiology, Kangnam St. Mary's Hospital, The Catholic University of Korea, 505 Banpo-dong Seocho-gu, Seoul 137-701, Republic of Korea
* Corresponding author.
E-mail address: jybyun@catholic.ac.kr (J.Y. Byun).

doi:10.1016/j.rcl.2007.04.004

Penetrating trauma accounts for approximately 10% of all renal injuries such as those caused by gunshot or stabbing injuries [1,6]. Iatrogenic injuries caused by renal biopsies or interventional procedures, such as percutaneous nephrostomy or renal artery angioplasty, are other causes of penetrating trauma. Penetrating injury produces direct tissue disruption of the renal parenchyma, vascular pedicles, or collecting system. A gunshot wound produces a radiating current of energy and cavitation known as the "blast effect," which may produce delayed tissue necrosis from an area that initially seemed viable [7].

Clinical features and indications for imaging

In general, hematuria is present in more than 95% of cases of renal trauma, and gross hematuria may be associated with more severe renal trauma than is microscopic hematuria [7]. Hematuria may be absent in 10% to 25% of renal injuries, however [7]. Ureteropelvic junction injuries, including renal pedicle injury, can occur without hematuria in 25% to 50% of patients, and there is no direct relationship between the degree of hematuria and the extent of renal injury [8].

In penetrating trauma, major renal vessels or the ureter may be severed despite little or no hematuria, and the majority of patients who have penetrating injuries of the kidney also have damage to other organs [9]. Therefore, renal imaging should be performed in all patients who have penetrating injury and hematuria except for those who are hemodynamic instable and require immediate surgery [10].

In blunt trauma, renal imaging is indicated if the patient has gross hematuria or microscopic hematuria with (1) shock, (2) clinical suspicion of abdominal organ injury, or (3) rapid deceleration injury, including a fall from a height [10].

Imaging modalities

Traditionally, intravenous urography (IVU) and cystography were used to assess genitourinary injuries, but the IVU findings usually were normal or nonspecific in many, large, published studies because of the lack of sensitivity and specificity for renal injuries. Nonvisualization, contour deformity, or extravasation of contrast medium on IVU indicates a major renal injury and should prompt further radiographic evaluation with CT or angiography [11]. The primary usefulness of IVU may be to indicate a normally functioning kidney on the uninjured side [10,11].

Ultrasonography has been the subject of interest for the evaluation of abdominal trauma because of its low cost, wide availability, portability, and lack of invasiveness. The sensitivity of ultrasonography for detecting free fluid was found to correlate with organ injury in the range of 80% to 90% [12–14]. Ultrasonography, however, is less sensitive for detecting solid-organ injuries, including renal parenchymal injuries, and free fluid is depicted in only 35% of the reported cases of isolated renal injuries [13,15–17]. Nevertheless, ultrasonography is a valuable screening test for children and adults who are presumed to have minor trauma because it has a high negative predictive value (approximately 98%) [18,19].

Since the mid-1980s, CT has become the best initial imaging modality for patients suspected of having renal injury. CT can assess accurately the extent of damaged tissue and perirenal hemorrhage, extravasation of urine, renal pedicle or vascular injuries, and injuries to other intra-abdominal structures such as the liver, pancreas, and spleen. The CT protocol is important for optimal evaluation of entire urinary systems including the renal vasculature and the collecting system. Both physiologic and morphologic information can be obtained by using CT with contrast enhancement. The usual contrast dose is approximately 120 to 150 mL for adults and 1.5 to 2 mL/kg for children [20]. An injection rate of 3 to 4 mL/second (ie, at least faster than 2 mL/second) is required for appropriate evaluation of vascular and parenchymal injuries [20]. Automatic bolus tracking is better than fixed scan delay for optimal vascular-phase scans. Nephrographic-phase scans must be obtained for parenchymal injuries, and late excretory-phase scans sometimes should be obtained to evaluate the possibility of urinary contrast extravasation if there is significant perinephric or periureteral fluid [20,21]. The optimal section thickness of multidetector CT for renal vascular imaging is 0.5 to 1.25 mm, because the diameter of the main renal artery is 4 to 6 mm and that of the accessory renal arteries is usually 0.5 to 3 mm. A section thickness of 2.5 to 5 mm is sufficient for evaluation of the renal parenchyma [21].

Because MR imaging offers excellent detail of the renal anatomy, combining it with gadolinium may be useful for trauma patients who have severe allergies to CT contrast. The use of MR imaging is limited in acute renal trauma, however, because of motion artifacts and the much longer scanning time than with CT.

Angiography is used less frequently for suspicious renal artery injuries because vascular extravasation can be detected more easily and more quickly on 16- or 64-channel multidetector CT. As nonsurgical management of trauma patients becomes more widely accepted, angiography with transcatheter embolization is becoming a desirable treatment for patients who have arteriovenous fistula, pseudoaneurysm, or active arterial bleeding [22–27].

Because nuclear medicine studies can evaluate the renal function of injured kidneys or repaired kidneys, they also are well suited for the follow-up evaluation of renal function [28]. They are rarely used in an acute setting, however, because they provide insufficient evaluation of the morphology of renal injuries and of other possible organ injuries.

Classification and imaging findings

Various classification systems of renal injuries have been devised, but the grading system of the American Association for the Surgery of Trauma (AAST) is now widely accepted and used (Table 1) [11,29]. This system classifies renal injury according to its depth and the involvement of vessels or the collecting system, and it is well correlated with any abnormalities detected on CT (Fig. 1) [20,29].

Table 1: **American Association for the Surgery of Trauma grading system for renal injury**

Grade[a]	Type of Injury	Description of Injury
I	Contusion	Microscopic or gross hematuria; urologic studies normal
	Hematoma	Subcapsular, nonexpanding without parenchymal laceration
II	Hematoma	Nonexpanding perirenal hematoma confined to renal retroperitoneum
	Laceration	< 1.0 cm parenchymal depth of renal cortex without urinary extravasation
III	Laceration	> 1.0 cm parenchymal depth of renal cortex without collecting system rupture or urinary extravasation
IV	Laceration	Parenchymal laceration extending through renal cortex, medulla, and collecting system
	Vascular	Main renal artery or vein injury with contained hemorrhage
V	Laceration	Completely shattered kidney
	Vascular	Avulsion of renal hilum which devascularizes kidney

[a] Advance one grade for bilateral injuries up to grade III.

Grade I injuries

Grade I injuries are the most common type of renal trauma and account for approximately 80% of all renal injuries. This grade includes hematuria with normal imaging studies, contusion, and nonexpanding subcapsular hematoma without parenchymal laceration (Fig. 2) [20]. Contusions are ill defined or, occasionally, distinct areas of decreased enhancement and excretion; they are distinguished from segmental infarctions by the presence of contrast enhancement. A renal parenchymal contusion may appear as an area of somewhat high density on precontrast scans because of the hemorrhage. In blunt trauma subcapsular hematoma is less common than perinephric hematoma [20]. A subcapsular hematoma between the renal capsule and the renal parenchyma also shows high-density fluid on precontrast scans as well as some deformity of the underlying kidney. A subcapsular hematoma is crescent or biconvex in shape. Longstanding hematoma may calcify, and older hematoma can be demonstrated only after contrast administration [30].

Grade II and grade III injuries

Grade II injuries include nonexpanding perinephric hematoma confined to the retroperitoneum and renal parenchymal lacerations less than 1 cm in depth and without urinary extravasation. Grade III injuries include renal parenchymal lacerations more than 1 cm in depth and without collecting system rupture or urinary extravasation.

Perinephric hematoma is identified readily on CT as a typically ill-defined, high-density fluid collection between the renal parenchyma and Gerota's fascia (Fig. 3). Thickening of the lateroconal fascia, compression of the colon, and displacement of the kidney by perinephric hematoma also can be seen in perinephric hematomas [31,32]. A large perinephric hematoma may cross to the opposite perirenal space along a communicating plane anterior to the lower aorta and the inferior vena cava [33]. Renal contour deformity usually does not occur even in a large perinephric hematoma, in contrast to its usual appearance in subcapsular hematoma.

Renal parenchymal laceration appears as an irregular, moderately well-defined linear or wedge-shaped defect in the renal enhancement pattern [34]. In grade III injuries, renal parenchymal laceration involves the renal cortex and the medulla while preserving the collecting system (Fig. 4) [21].

Grade IV injuries

Grade IV injuries are characterized by corticomedullary laceration involving the renal collecting system and by damage to the main renal vessels. The

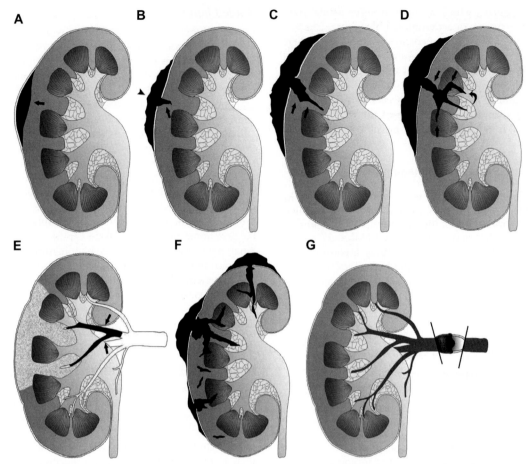

Fig. 1. The AAST grading of renal injury. (*A*) Grade I, subcapsular hematoma (*arrow*). (*B*) Grade II, cortical laceration less than 1 cm deep (*arrow*) and perinephric hematoma (*arrowhead*). (*C*) Grade III, cortical laceration more than 1 cm deep (*arrows*) and perinephric hematoma. (*D*) Grade IV, laceration extending through the renal cortex, medulla (*arrows*), and collecting system (*curved arrow*). (*E*) Grade IV, segmental infarction caused by thrombosis of segmental renal artery branches (*arrows*). (*F*) Grade V, shattered kidney. (*G*) Grade V, avulsion of renal hilum that devascularizes the kidney.

hallmark of grade IV injury on CT is extravasation of opacified urine into the perirenal space (Fig. 5) [34]. Only late excretory-phase scans occasionally demonstrate the critical extravasation of opacified urine. Therefore, late excretory-phase scanning should be obtained to evaluate urine extravasation when there are lacerations extending through the kidney, significant perinephric fluid, or fluid around the renal hilum on the nephrographic phase. Urinary extravasation alone is not an indication for surgical exploration, however, because it resolves spontaneously in approximately 80% of cases [10].

Grade IV injuries include segmental infarctions caused by thrombosis, dissection, or laceration of the segmental arteries. The CT features of segmental infarctions are well circumscribed linear or wedge-shaped nonenhancing areas extending through the renal parenchyma in a radial or segmental

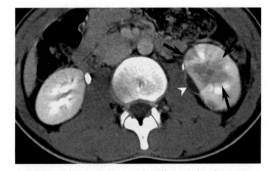

Fig. 2. Renal contusion with subcapsular hematoma (grade I) in a 16-year-old male who had sustained blunt abdominal trauma. Contrast-enhanced excretory-phase CT scan demonstrates multifocal areas of decreased enhancement in the interpolar region of the left kidney (*arrows*). A bow-shaped, low-density lesion is a liquefied subcapsular hematoma in the medial aspect of the left kidney (*arrowhead*).

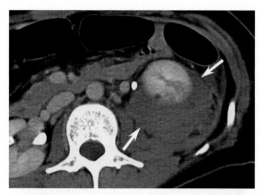

Fig. 3. Perinephric hematoma (grade II) after renal biopsy in a 37-year-old woman. Contrast-enhanced CT scan in the nephrographic phase shows large hematoma (*arrows*) in the perirenal space surrounding the lower pole of the left kidney.

orientation (Fig. 6) [20]. Segmental infarctions often resolve with conservative treatment.

Grade V injuries

Grade V injuries include shattered or devascularized kidney, ureteropelvic junction avulsion, and complete laceration or thrombosis of the main renal artery or vein. A shattered kidney is the most severe form of renal laceration, which is fractured into three or more separate segments with associated injuries to the collecting system (Fig. 7). Ureteropelvic junction avulsion occurs more commonly in children than in adults. The hallmark of ureteropelvic junction avulsion is the absence of opacification of the distal ureter, but partial ureteropelvic junction avulsion may demonstrate contrast in the distal ureter. Collections of urine medial to the renal pelvis and ureteropelvic junction are commonly noted in ureteropelvic junction avulsion or in penetrating injuries of the renal pelvis [31,35].

Renal pedicle injuries constitute up to 5% of all renal traumas and often are combined with associated injuries to other organs [36]. Hematuria may be absent, especially if there are no other associated injuries. Hematoma located between the aorta and the kidney and a laterally displacing injured kidney are suggestive of a renal pedicle injury [37].

The most common vascular pedicle injury resulting from blunt trauma is renal artery occlusion. Marked stretching of the renal artery causes an intimal tear leading to dissection, platelet aggregation, and vessel occlusion. Traumatic renal infarction also can occur at any time subsequent to and even long after the initial renal trauma [34]. Isolated intimal injury to the renal artery can be present without extensive retroperitoneal hemorrhage or hematuria. The CT findings of renal artery occlusion are characterized by the well-defined segmental or global absence of parenchymal enhancement but with preservation of the renal contour (Fig. 8) [38]. The renal vein may be opacified retrograde from the inferior vena cava, and abrupt truncation of the renal artery can be seen. Retrograde filling of the renal vein is applicable only to the right kidney, because the right renal vein is shorter than left renal vein and lacks the additional venous inflow from the adrenal, lumbar, and gonadal veins that is commonly found with the left renal vein [39–41]. The cortical rim sign caused by collateral perfusion on capsular and subcapsular enhancement may not be seen during the first few hours after infarction, because it takes a minimum of 8 hours for the cortical rim sign to be seen in trauma-induced renal infarction [42].

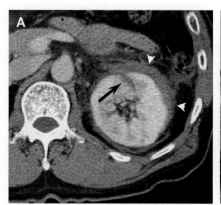
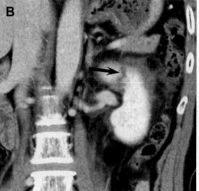

Fig. 4. Cortical laceration (grade III) in a 61-year-old man who had sustained blunt abdominal trauma. (*A*) Contrast-enhanced CT scan in the nephrographic phase shows a cortical laceration (*arrow*) more than 1 cm deep as well as perinephric hematoma (*arrowheads*). (*B*) Multiplanar reformatted image in the coronal plane shows the cortical laceration (*arrow*).

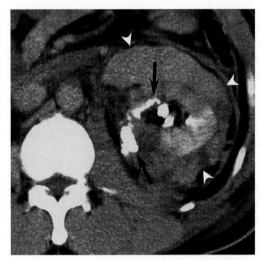

Fig. 5. Laceration of the collecting system (grade IV) in a 43-year-old woman who had sustained blunt abdominal trauma. Contrast-enhanced CT scan in the late excretory phase shows leakage of contrast material (*arrows*) caused by laceration of the collecting system as well as a hematoma in the perinephric space (*arrowheads*).

Isolated renal vein injuries are the most infrequent type of renal vascular pedicle injury [43]. Trauma-induced renal vein thrombosis almost always occurs in combination with an arterial or parenchymal injury [44]. The CT findings of renal vein thrombosis are renal enlargement, decreased early nephrogram, and prolonged corticomedullary nephrogram with diminished or absent opacification of the pelvocaliceal system [45]. Laceration of the renal vein appears on CT as a medial or circumferential subcapsular or perinephric hematoma [20].

Trauma to underlying abnormal kidneys

Pre-existing renal abnormalities predispose the kidneys to an increased risk of injury following blunt abdominal trauma [46]. It is difficult to evaluate accurately injuries to a kidney with a pre-existing congenital anomaly or acquired disease [47].

Rupture or bleeding into a renal cyst is the most common complication of renal trauma with underlying abnormality (Fig. 9). Computer models have been used to measure the force transmission and stress distribution of renal cysts in traumatized kidneys. In these models, higher hydrostatic pressures caused by liquid-filled inner compartments have led to higher stress concentrations in the model periphery [48]. Longstanding hydronephrosis caused by conditions such as a ureteropelvic junction stricture or a renal stone also can lead to elevated intrapelvic and intracystic pressures, thereby making the kidneys vulnerable to rupture. CT can distinguish ruptured simple renal cysts from hemorrhage because of the presence of near-water-density perirenal fluid.

Congenital renal anomalies may predispose an individual to blunt abdominal trauma because of the location, size, and shape of the kidneys. Horseshoe kidneys occur in approximately 0.25% of the general population and may accompany associated congenital problems such as ventricular septal defect, skeletal malformation, trisomy 18, neural tube defects, anorectal anomalies, hypospadias, undescended testes, and bicornuate uterus [49]. Horseshoe kidneys are not protected by the lower ribs and may be compressed or fractured against the lumbar vertebral column by blunt abdominal trauma. Traumatic injuries of horseshoe kidneys are easily identified on CT (see Fig. 7).

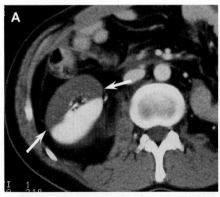
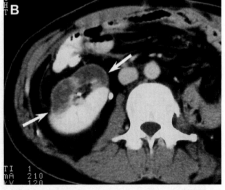

Fig. 6. Segmental infarction (grade IV) of the right kidney in a 34-year-old man who had sustained blunt abdominal trauma. (*A*) Contrast-enhanced CT scan in the nephrographic phase demonstrates a sharply demarcated, wedge-shaped area of decreased attenuation in the interpolar region of the right kidney (*arrows*). (*B*) Contrast-enhanced CT scan in the excretory phase, obtained 21 days later, shows low attenuation of the anterior segment with capsular rim nephrogram (*arrows*).

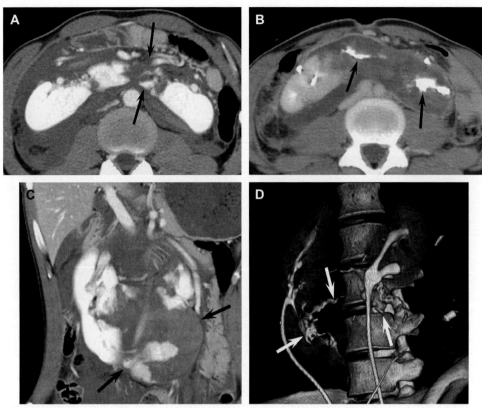

Fig. 7. Shattered kidney (grade V) with ureteropelvic junction laceration in a 30-year-old man who had an underlying horseshoe kidney. (*A*) Contrast-enhanced axial CT scan in the nephrographic phase shows multiple fragments of renal parenchyma (*arrows*) at the fused site of both kidneys and large amount of hematoma in the bilateral anterior and posterior pararenal spaces. (*B*) Contrast-enhanced axial CT scan shows extravasation of contrast media (*arrows*). (*C*) Multiplanar reformatted image in the coronal plane in the nephrographic phase shows a shattered horseshoe kidney with a large amount of hematoma in the perinephric space (*arrows*). (*D*) In a volume-rendered oblique coronal image, a large volume of contrast media extravasation (*arrows*) from the left kidney can be seen at a glance.

Compared with blunt trauma in adults, the pediatric kidney is more vulnerable to blunt trauma because of the lesser protection offered by the pliable thoracic cage, weaker abdominal musculature, and the relatively larger size of the pediatric kidneys proportionate to a child's body. In one series, 12.6% of all pediatric blunt renal trauma occurred in pathologic kidneys [50]. Underlying congenital malformations causing hydronephrosis, such as ureteropelvic junction stenosis, extrarenal pelvis, and reflux, predispose the pediatric kidney to significant injuries with only minor force (Fig. 10) [50].

Iatrogenic renal trauma

Ultrasound-guided percutaneous core-needle biopsy is a frequently used and relatively safe procedure for the diagnosis of renal parenchymal disease and to evaluate a transplanted kidney. Biopsy complications, including perirenal hematoma,

laceration of the renal arterial branch, arteriovenous fistula, and pseudoaneurysm, may occur, however. The majority of acquired renal arteriovenous fistulae resulting from renal biopsy heal spontaneously, but angiography with intervention can be performed effectively to achieve hemostasis and to maximize the preservation of renal function with persistent or symptomatic vascular injuries accompanied by deterioration of renal function, uncontrolled hypertension, or hematuria (Fig. 11) [51,52].

Renal vascular injury can occur during angiography with or without intervention. Renal artery angioplasty or a stenting procedure requires the stability of heavy-duty guidewires, because manipulation of these guidewires alone can injure the artery [53].

Extracorporeal shock-wave lithotripsy (ESWL) is an effective treatment for urolithiasis. Perirenal hematoma, rupture of the kidney, and kidney

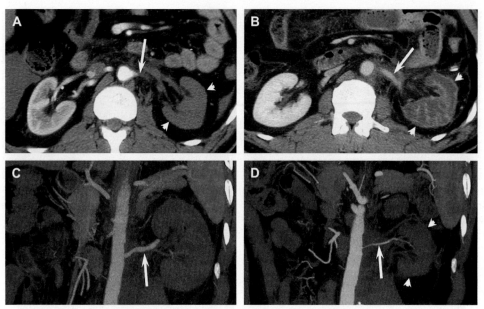

Fig. 8. Renal infarction (grade V) of the left kidney in a 49-year-old man who had sustained blunt abdominal trauma. (*A*) Contrast-enhanced CT scan in the corticomedullary phase shows an abruptly nonenhancing segment of the left main renal artery (*arrow*) and lack of enhancement of the left kidney (*arrowheads*). (*B*) Follow-up contrast-enhanced CT scan in the nephrographic phase after surgical reconstruction of the renal artery shows enhancement of the left main renal artery (*arrow*) and a diffusely swollen left kidney with capsular rim nephrogram (*arrowheads*). Most of the renal parenchyma is unenhanced, however. (*C*) Maximum intensity projection image in the coronal plane after the surgery shows a recanalized, well-enhancing left main renal artery (*arrow*) without enhancement of the renal parenchyma. (*D*) Maximum intensity projection image in the coronal plane obtained 2 months after the surgery shows diffuse thinning of the left renal artery (*arrow*) and contracted left kidney (*arrowheads*) without enhancement.

lacerations following ESWL procedure have been reported, however [54–56]. Perirenal hematoma is detected in 15% to 30% of the cases of ESWL [54]. Because some degree of renal injury is inevitable following ESWL, if a patient presents with persistent abdominal pain and a history of ESWL, adjunctive imaging surveillance should be considered for bleeding or other potential complications.

Complications of renal trauma

Complications of renal trauma occur in 3% to 33% of patients who suffer renal trauma. Complications after renal trauma include urinary extravasation, urinoma, infected urinoma, secondary hemorrhage, perinephric abscess, pseudoaneurysm, hypertension, arteriovenous fistula, and pulmonary complications [57].

Extravasation of urine is the most common complication of renal trauma (see Figs. 5 and 7) [2]. It is present in all patients who have grade IV parenchymal injury and grade V ureteropelvic junction avulsion. Urinoma is a urine collection that may be seen in 1% to 7% of all patients who have experienced renal trauma [58]. Delayed-phase CT images obtained 5 to 20 minutes after contrast enhancement

are important for the diagnosis of urinoma because iodinated urine increases the attenuation of a urinoma over time. Most urinomas reside in a subcapsular location or in the perirenal space within Gerota's

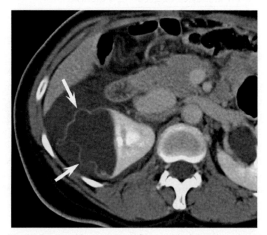

Fig. 9. Traumatic rupture of an underlying renal cyst in a 47-year-old woman who had sustained blunt abdominal trauma. Contrast-enhanced CT scan in the excretory phase shows a large cyst with undulated contour (*arrows*) in the right kidney with a fluid collection in the perirenal space and right anterior pararenal space.

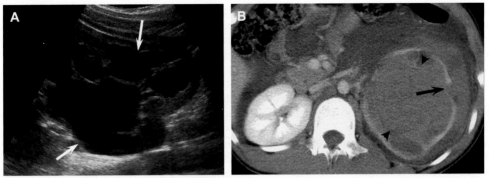

Fig. 10. Traumatic renal injury in an 11-year-old boy who had pre-existing hydronephrosis caused by ureteropelvic junction stricture. (*A*) Longitudinal renal ultrasonography obtained a year before the trauma showed marked dilatation of the renal pelvis and calyces of the left kidney (*arrows*). (*B*) Contrast-enhanced CT scan obtained on the day of blunt trauma shows focal cortical breakage (*arrow*), dilated renal pelvis, and calyces filled with high-attenuating hematoma (*arrowheads*).

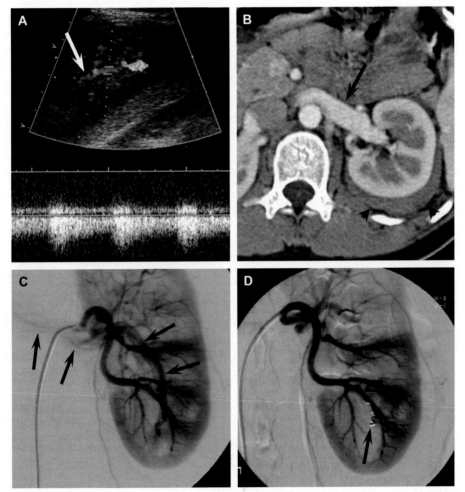

Fig. 11. Arteriovenous fistula with perinephric hematoma after renal biopsy. (*A*) Color Doppler ultrasonography shows a pulsatile flow pattern resembling artery in the inferior segmental renal vein (*arrow*). (*B*) Contrast-enhanced CT scan in the corticomedullary phase shows an engorged left renal vein (*arrow*) and perinephric hematoma (*arrowheads*) surrounding the left kidney. (*C*) Selective renal angiography demonstrates early contrast filling of the left renal vein by means of the inferior segmental renal vein (*arrows*). (*D*) After embolization of arteriovenous fistula with coils (*arrow*), early contrast filling of the renal vein during arteriography regressed.

fascia; however, a urinoma, if extensive, may cross the midline into the contralateral perirenal space. Intraperitoneal urine extravasation is usually a result of penetrating or iatrogenic injury [59].

An infected urinoma and perinephric abscess can be secondary to local or systemic bacterial seeding of a urinoma or caused by coexisting enteric or pancreatic injuries. Both entities can be managed by percutaneous catheter drainage [60].

Secondary hemorrhage is common in cases of renal injuries that are more severe than grade III or IV and especially in penetrating trauma managed conservatively. Secondary hemorrhage often is caused by a traumatic pseudoaneurysm or arteriovenous fistula. The mean interval between the injury and the onset of secondary hemorrhage is approximately 12 days [61].

Pseudoaneurysm is a well-known iatrogenic complication after procedures such as percutaneous surgery, open surgery, renal biopsy, and endoscopic renal surgery, but it can be caused penetrating or blunt renal trauma as well [62–64]. Pseudoaneurysm enhances on the arterial phase and washes out on the delayed phase of CT, and Doppler ultrasound is diagnostic with a characteristic to-and-fro swirling in an anechoic lesion [65]. Angiography is the criterion standard for the diagnosis and first-line treatment of a pseudoaneurysm that appears as a round or oval structure opacified from the main renal artery or from one of its branches.

The majority of small arteriovenous fistulas heal spontaneously, but most of those that occur after major renal trauma do not heal spontaneously and may induce compromised renal function, uncontrolled hypertension, or hematuria. On CT, an arteriovenous fistula demonstrates early enhancement of the engorged renal vein and inferior vena cava (see Fig. 11) [66,67].

"Page kidney" refers to hypertension secondary to renal compression caused by a perirenal hematoma or by fibrosis, as Engel and Page [68] first described renin-dependant hypertension based on their experiments. External compression of the kidney induces renal hypoperfusion and ischemia related to excess renin secretion resulting in water retention and hypertension [69]. A "Page kidney" shows attenuated contrast enhancement of the kidney with a surrounding fibrotic band that may be calcified [70]. Posttraumatic renovascular hypertension may occur a few weeks to decades following the injury but usually occurs within an average of 34 months later [11].

Summary

Renal imaging is indicated in patients who have penetrating trauma, gross hematuria, and blunt trauma with microscopic hematuria plus shock, all clinical signs indicating abdominal organ injury or significant deceleration injury. CT with contrast enhancement is the best initial imaging study for patients suspected of having renal injury, because it may provide accurate grading of the AAST by demonstrating the depth of injury and the involvement of vessels or the collecting system. Delayed CT scanning can provide the critical observation for diagnosing grade IV injuries and therefore may be needed also. The majority of renal injuries have been managed conservatively, but severe renal injuries greater than grade IV, especially those with coexisting other organ injuries, more often require intervention or surgery.

Acknowledgments

The authors thank Bonnie Hami, MA (USA) for her editorial assistance in preparing the manuscript and Kyung Me Lee for her editorial assistance in preparing the drawings and photographs for the manuscript.

References

[1] Baverstock R, Simons R, McLoughlin M. Severe blunt renal trauma: a 7-year retrospective review from a provincial trauma centre. Can J Urol 2001;8(5):1372–6.

[2] Matthews LA, Smith EM, Spirnak JP. Nonoperative treatment of major blunt renal lacerations with urinary extravasation. J Urol 1997;157(6): 2056–8.

[3] Moudouni SM, Hadj Slimen M, Manunta A, et al. Management of major blunt renal lacerations: is a nonoperative approach indicated? Eur Urol 2001;40(4):409–14.

[4] Traub KB, Hua V, Broman S, et al. Introduction of a genitourinary trauma database for use as a multi-institutional urologic trauma registry. J Trauma 2001;51(2):336–9.

[5] Sandler CM, Amis ES Jr, Bigongiari LR, et al. Diagnostic approach to renal trauma. American College of Radiology. ACR appropriateness criteria. Radiology 2000;215(Suppl):727–31.

[6] Miller KS, McAninch JW. Radiographic assessment of renal trauma: our 15-year experience. J Urol 1995;154:352–5.

[7] Sagalowsky AI, Peters PC. Genitourinary trauma. In: Walsh PC, Retik AB, Vaughan ED Jr, et al, editors. Campbell's urology, vol 3. 7th edition. Philadelphia: WB Saunders; 1999. p. 3085–119.

[8] Kawashima A, Sandler CM, Corl FM, et al. Imaging of renal trauma: a comprehensive review. Radiographics 2001;21(3):557–74.

[9] Cass AS. Renovascular injuries from external trauma. Diagnosis, treatment, and outcome. Urol Clin North Am 1989;16(2):213–20.

[10] Heyns CF. Renal trauma: indications for imaging and surgical exploration. BJU Int 2004;93(8): 1165–70.

[11] Santucci RA, Wessells H, Bartsch G, et al. Evaluation and management of renal injuries: consensus statement of the renal trauma subcommittee. BJU Int 2004;93(7):937–54.

[12] Boulanger BR, Brenneman FD, McLellan BA, et al. A prospective study of emergent abdominal sonography after blunt trauma. J Trauma 1995; 39(2):325–30.

[13] Bode PJ, Niezen RA, van Vugt AB, et al. Abdominal ultrasound as a reliable indicator for conclusive laparotomy in blunt abdominal trauma. J Trauma 1993;34(1):27–31.

[14] Hoffmann R, Nerlich M, Muggia-Sullam M, et al. Blunt abdominal trauma in cases of multiple trauma evaluated by ultrasonography: a prospective analysis of 291 patients. J Trauma 1992; 32(4):452–8.

[15] Tso P, Rodriguez A, Cooper C, et al. Sonography in blunt abdominal trauma: a preliminary progress report. J Trauma 1992;33(1):39–43.

[16] Rothlin MA, Naf R, Amgwerd M, et al. Ultrasound in blunt abdominal and thoracic trauma. J Trauma 1993;34(4):488–95.

[17] McGahan JP, Richards JR, Jones CD, et al. Use of ultrasonography in the patient with acute renal trauma. J Ultrasound Med 1999;18(3):15–6 [quiz: 207–13].

[18] Dolich MO, McKenney MG, Varela JE, et al. 2,576 ultrasounds for blunt abdominal trauma. J Trauma 2001;50(1):108–12.

[19] Rose JS, Levitt MA, Porter J, et al. Does the presence of ultrasound really affect computed tomographic scan use? A prospective randomized trial of ultrasound in trauma. J Trauma 2001;51(3):545–50.

[20] Smith JK, Kenney PJ. Imaging of renal trauma. Radiol Clin North Am 2003;41(5):1019–35.

[21] Park SJ, Kim JK, Kim KW, et al. MDCT Findings of renal trauma. AJR Am J Roentgenol 2006; 187(2):541–7.

[22] Chatziioannou A, Brountzos E, Primetis E, et al. Effects of superselective embolization for renal vascular injuries on renal parenchyma and function. Eur J Vasc Endovasc Surg 2004;28(2):201–6.

[23] Vignali C, Lonzi S, Bargellini I, et al. Vascular injuries after percutaneous renal procedures: treatment by transcatheter embolization. Eur Radiol 2004;14(4):723–9.

[24] Sofocleous CT, Hinrichs C, Hubbi B, et al. Angiographic findings and embolotherapy in renal arterial trauma. Cardiovasc Intervent Radiol 2005; 28(1):39–47.

[25] Cantasdemir M, Adaletli I, Cebi D, et al. Emergency endovascular embolization of traumatic intrarenal arterial pseudoaneurysms with N-butyl cyanoacrylate. Clin Radiol 2003;58(7):560–5.

[26] Miller DC, Forauer A, Faerber GJ. Successful angioembolization of renal artery pseudoaneurysms after blunt abdominal trauma. Urology 2002;59(3):444.

[27] Hagiwara A, Sakaki S, Goto H, et al. The role of interventional radiology in the management of blunt renal injury: a practical protocol. J Trauma 2001;51(3):526–31.

[28] Lang EK, Sullivan J, Frentz G. Renal trauma: radiological studies. Comparison of urography, computed tomography, angiography, and radionuclide studies. Radiology 1985;154(1):1–6.

[29] Moore EE, Shackford SR, Pachter HL, et al. Organ injury scaling: spleen, liver, and kidney. J Trauma 1989;29(12):1664–6.

[30] Amparo EG, Fagan CJ. Page kidney. J Comput Assist Tomogr 1982;6(4):839–41.

[31] Sclafani SJ, Becker JA. Radiologic diagnosis of renal trauma. Urol Radiol 1985;7(4):192–200.

[32] McCort JJ. Perirenal fat infiltration by hemorrhage: radiographic recognition and CT confirmation. Radiology 1983;149(3):665–7.

[33] Kneeland JB, Auh YH, Rubenstein WA, et al. Perirenal spaces: CT evidence for communication across the midline. Radiology 1987;164(3):657–64.

[34] Federle MP. Renal trauma. In: Pollack HM, McClennan BL, editors. Clinical urography, vol 2. 2nd edition. Philadelphia: W.B. Saunders; 2000. p. 1772–84.

[35] Kenney PJ, Panicek DM, Witanowski LS. Computed tomography of ureteral disruption. J Comput Assist Tomogr 1987;11(3):480–4.

[36] Cass AS, Susset J, Khan A, et al. Renal pedicle injury in the multiple injured patient. J Urol 1979; 122(6):728–30.

[37] Sclafani SJ, Goldstein AS, Panetta T, et al. CT diagnosis of renal pedicle injury. Urol Radiol 1985; 7(2):63–8.

[38] Lupetin AR, Mainwaring BL, Daffner RH. CT diagnosis of renal artery injury caused by blunt abdominal trauma. AJR Am J Roentgenol 1989; 153(5):1065–8.

[39] Balkan E, Kilic N, Dogruyol H. Indirect computed tomography sign of renal artery injury: retrograde filling of the renal vein. Int J Urol 2005; 12(3):311–2.

[40] McKenney MG, Martin L, Lentz K, et al. 1,000 consecutive ultrasounds for blunt abdominal trauma. J Trauma 1996;40(4):607–10.

[41] Cain MP, Matsumoto JM, Husmann DA. Retrograde filling of the renal vein on computerized tomography for blunt renal trauma: an indicator of renal artery injury. J Urol 1995;153(4): 1247–8.

[42] Kamel IR, Berkowitz JF. Assessment of the cortical rim sign in posttraumatic renal infarction. J Comput Assist Tomogr 1996;20(5):803–6.

[43] Stables DP, Thatcher GN. Traumatic renal vein thrombosis associated with renal artery occlusion. Br J Radiol 1973;46(541):64–6.

[44] Kau E, Patel R, Fiske J, et al. Isolated renal vein thrombosis after blunt trauma. Urology 2004; 64(4):807–8.

[45] Glazer GM, Francis IR, Gross BH, et al. Computed tomography of renal vein thrombosis. J Comput Assist Tomogr 1984;8(2):288–93.

[46] Leslie CL, Simon BJ, Lee KF, et al. Bilateral rupture of multicystic kidneys after blunt abdominal trauma. J Trauma 2000;48(2):336–7.

[47] Rhyner P, Federle MP, Jeffrey RB. CT of trauma to the abnormal kidney. AJR Am J Roentgenol 1984;142(4):747–50.

[48] Schmidlin FR, Schmid P, Kurtyka T, et al. Force transmission and stress distribution in a computer-simulated model of the kidney: an analysis of the injury mechanisms in renal trauma. J Trauma 1996;40(5):791–6.

[49] Glenn JF. Analysis of 51 patients with horseshoe kidney. N Engl J Med 1959;261:684–7.

[50] Chopra P, St-Vil D, Yazbeck S. Blunt renal trauma-blessing in disguise? J Pediatr Surg 2002;37(5):779–82.

[51] deSouza NM, Reidy JF, Koffman CG. Arteriovenous fistulas complicating biopsy of renal allografts: treatment of bleeding with superselective embolization. AJR Am J Roentgenol 1991;156(3):507–10.

[52] Beaujeux R, Saussine C, al-Fakir A, et al. Superselective endo-vascular treatment of renal vascular lesions. J Urol 1995;153(1):14–7.

[53] Lee-Elliott C, Khaw KT, Belli AM, et al. Iatrogenic arteriovenous fistula in a renal allograft: the result of a TAD guidewire injury. Cardiovasc Intervent Radiol 2000;23(4):306–9.

[54] Knapp PM, Kulb TB, Lingeman JE, et al. Extracorporeal shock wave lithotripsy-induced perirenal hematomas. J Urol 1988;139(4):700–3.

[55] Fukumori T, Yamamoto A, Ashida S, et al. Extracorporeal shock wave lithotripsy-induced renal laceration. Int J Urol 1997;4(4):419–21.

[56] Ozucelik DN, Karcioglu O. Kidney rupture following extracorporeal shock wave lithotripsy. Acad Emerg Med 1999;6(6):664–5.

[57] Al-Qudah HS, Santucci RA. Complications of renal trauma. Urol Clin North Am 2006;33(1): 41–53.

[58] Titton RL, Gervais DA, Hahn PF, et al. Urine leaks and urinomas: diagnosis and imaging-guided intervention. RadioGraphics 2003;23(5): 1133–47.

[59] Lang EK, Glorioso L 3rd. Management of urinomas by percutaneous drainage procedures. Radiol Clin North Am 1986;24(4):551–9.

[60] Husmann DA, Gilling PJ, Perry MO, et al. Major renal lacerations with a devitalized fragment following blunt abdominal trauma: a comparison between nonoperative (expectant) versus surgical management. J Urol 1993;150(6): 1774–7.

[61] Heyns CF, Van Vollenhoven P. Selective surgical management of renal stab wounds. Br J Urol 1992;69(4):351–7.

[62] Lee RS, Porter JR. Traumatic renal artery pseudoaneurysm: diagnosis and management techniques. J Trauma 2003;55(5):972–8.

[63] Jebara VA, El Rassi I, Achouh PE, et al. Renal artery pseudoaneurysm after blunt abdominal trauma. J Vasc Surg 1998;27(2):362–5.

[64] Swana HS, Cohn SM, Burns GA, et al. Renal artery pseudoaneurysm after blunt abdominal trauma: case report and literature review. J Trauma 1996;40(3):459–61.

[65] Vasile M, Bellin MF, Helenon O, et al. Imaging evaluation of renal trauma. Abdom Imaging 2000;25(4):424–30.

[66] Sprouse LR 2nd, Hamilton IN Jr. The endovascular treatment of a renal arteriovenous fistula: placement of a covered stent. J Vasc Surg 2002; 36(5):1066–8.

[67] Hirai S, Hamanaka Y, Mitsui N, et al. High-output heart failure caused by a huge renal arteriovenous fistula after nephrectomy: report of a case. Surg Today 2001;31(5):468–70.

[68] Engel WJ, Page IH. Hypertension due to renal compression resulting from subcapsular hematoma. J Urol 1955;73(5):735–9.

[69] McCune TR, Stone WJ, Breyer JA. Page kidney: case report and review of the literature. Am J Kidney Dis 1991;18(5):593–9.

[70] Sterns RH, Rabinowitz R, Segal AJ, et al. 'Page kidney'. Hypertension caused by chronic subcapsular hematoma. Arch Intern Med 1985;145(1): 169–71.

RADIOLOGIC
CLINICS
OF NORTH AMERICA

Radiol Clin N Am 45 (2007) 593–599

Mesenteric Ischemia

Angela D. Levy, MD, COL, MC, USA

Ischemic injury to the intestine occurs when the mesenteric blood supply fails to meet the local tissue demands so that the intestines are deprived of oxygen and nutrients necessary to maintain cellular integrity. Despite advances in clinical diagnosis and cross-sectional imaging, the diagnosis of mesenteric ischemia remains difficult because the clinical presentation often is nonspecific and the cross-sectional imaging features overlap those of with other intestinal diseases. Moreover, intestinal ischemic injury represents a continuum of pathologic changes that range from mild mural edema to infarction. Consequently, there is range in the cross-sectional imaging findings of intestinal ischemia and infarction depending on the onset, duration, origin, and extent of intestinal involvement. When mesenteric ischemia is a clinical concern, multidetector CT (MDCT) is the imaging modality of choice because of its ability to image the mesenteric vasculature and small intestine and to evaluate the abdomen for other pathologies. This article reviews the clinical, pathophysiologic, and CT features of acute and chronic mesenteric ischemia.

Acute mesenteric ischemia

Clinical features

The diagnosis of acute mesenteric ischemia requires a high index of suspicion because the clinical manifestations vary greatly depending on the severity and chronicity of the process. Acute mesenteric ischemia accounts for the majority of cases and should be considered in older patients who present with abdominal pain and have long-standing congestive heart failure, cardiac arrhythmias, recent myocardial infarction, or hypotension. Younger patients also may develop ischemia but usually have an underlying disease or condition, such as collagen vascular disease, vasculitis, hypercoagulable state, vasoactive medication, or cocaine use, that predisposes them to abnormalities in splanchnic blood flow [1].

Abdominal pain that is out of proportion to the degree of abdominal tenderness on physical examination is the hallmark of acute mesenteric ischemia [2]. Sudden, severe abdominal pain with rapid, forceful bowel evacuation is very suggestive of an arterial embolus [1]. Patients who have mesenteric venous thrombosis usually have colicky abdominal pain and have had symptoms for more than 48 hours before they seek medical care [3]. Nausea, vomiting, anorexia, and diarrhea may also be present. Stools containing occult blood are common. Massive and sometimes fatal hemorrhage may occur when infarction is present.

The initial physical examination frequently is normal. The abdomen usually is soft and

The opinions and assertions contained herein are the private views of the author and are not to be construed as official or as reflecting the view of the Department of the Army or Defense.
Department of Radiology and Radiologic Sciences, Uniformed Services University of the Health Sciences, 4301 Jones Bridge Road, Bethesda, MD 20814-4799, USA
E-mail address: adlevy@usuhs.mil

0033-8389/07/$ – see front matter. Published by Elsevier Inc.
radiologic.theclinics.com

doi:10.1016/j.rcl.2007.04.012

nontender or is minimally tender at the onset of acute ischemia. Abdominal tenderness with guarding and rebound occurs later and indicates progression toward infarction. There are no specific laboratory tests that are sensitive or specific for the diagnosis of acute mesenteric ischemia or intestinal infarction. Leukocytosis, acidosis, and elevations in serum amylase usually occur late in the course of acute mesenteric ischemia.

Etiology and pathophysiology

Ischemia frequently is classified by origin: arterial or venous. Loss of arterial blood flow is a more common cause of acute ischemia than venous occlusion. Causes of arterial ischemia include arterial emboli, nonocclusive mesenteric ischemia, and superior mesenteric artery thrombosis. Embolic occlusions account for the more than 50% of cases. Emboli usually originate from left atrial or ventricular thrombi and lodge in branch points in the middle or distal superior mesenteric artery. Nonocclusive mesenteric ischemia accounts for 20% to 30% of cases and occurs when there is hypoperfusion from low cardiac output in the settings of cardiac infarction, congestive heart failure, arrhythmia, or aortic insufficiency [4]. Less commonly, hypovolemia in the setting of shock from trauma or massive hemorrhage may cause nonocclusive mesenteric ischemia. Acute occlusion of the superior mesenteric artery typically occurs in patients who have atherosclerotic vascular disease when thrombus occludes pre-existing atherosclerotic lesions of the superior mesenteric artery. These occlusions invariably occur in the proximal portion of the vessel.

Mesenteric venous thrombosis accounts for 5% to 15% of cases of mesenteric ischemia and infarction [5]. Ninety-five percent of all mesenteric venous thrombosis involves the superior mesenteric vein [5] and most often are secondary to an underlying condition such as a hypercoagulable state, portal venous hypertension, trauma, or an inflammatory processes. Rarely, there is no underlying cause, and the thrombosis is classified as primary mesenteric venous thrombosis. Obstruction of venous return also may occur as a complication of small bowel obstruction when severe bowel dilatation, closed-loop obstruction, adhesions or bands, or intussusceptions compromise venous return.

CT features

In patients who have suspected mesenteric ischemia, MDCT protocols should be optimized for an MDCT angiographic study of the mesenteric vasculature as well as for a thorough assessment of the intestines and mesentery. Consequently, intravenous and intraluminal contrast agents are necessary.

Recent data suggest that low-attenuation intraluminal contrast agents (water, methylcellulose, or other such agents) are better than conventional high-attenuation intraluminal contrast media (barium and iodine preparations) because intestinal wall enhancement can be assessed more easily and because low-attenuation intraluminal contrast agents do not interfere with the computer algorithms that are used to manipulate three-dimensional MDCT angiography data [6].

Direct visualization of vascular occlusion such as arterial thrombus in the superior mesenteric artery or venous thrombosis of the superior mesenteric vein and its tributaries on two-dimensional or three-dimensional CT data sets is direct evidence of the underlying cause of acute mesenteric ischemia. Arterial thrombus is hypoattenuating and generally is located at the site of atherosclerotic narrowing of the involved vessel, usually in the proximal portion of the vessel. Calcification generally is adjacent to the hypoattenuating acute thrombus (Figs. 1 and 2). Emboli in the distal branches of the superior mesenteric artery are more difficult to detect directly by CT because they tend to lodge at branch points in the smaller arterial tributaries. Therefore, in patients who have embolic ischemia, the CT manifestations generally are limited to the intestine and adjacent mesenteric fat.

Thrombus within the mesenteric veins appears as focal rounded or tubular hypoattenuation in the affected vein. There is a rim of peripheral contrast enhancement if the vein is partially occluded (Fig. 3).

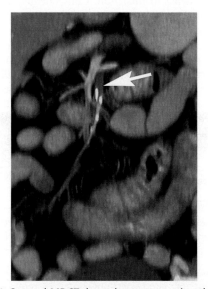

Fig. 1. Coronal MDCT shows hypoattenuating thrombus (*arrow*) in the proximal superior mesenteric artery adjacent to calcified plaque in a 50-year-old man who complained of acute abdominal pain and diarrhea.

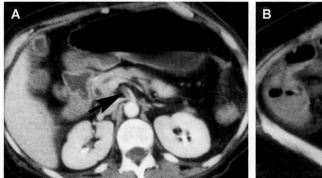
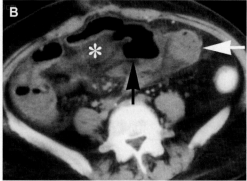

Fig. 2. Acute mesenteric ischemia with small intestinal infarction in a 65-year-old woman who complained of severe, acute abdominal pain. (*A, B*) Intravenous contrast-enhanced CT scan shows hypoattenuating thrombus occluding the origin of the superior mesenteric artery (*arrow* in panel A), mesenteric edema (*asterisk* in panel B), mural thickening (*white arrow* in panel B) and dilatation (*black arrow* in panel B) of the small intestine.

In complete thrombotic occlusion a thin rim of hyperattenuation surrounding the thrombus represents the wall of the vein (Fig. 4). Acute thrombus also may increase the size of the affected vein, and, occasionally, the outer margin of the vein may be ill defined.

In acute mesenteric ischemia the most common intestinal CT finding is mural thickening [6]. Mural thickening in ischemia typically is symmetric and circumferential and usually does not exceed 1.5 cm in thickness [7]. Mural thickening represents submucosal edema, inflammation, or hemorrhage in the bowel wall. On CT, mural thickening may be homogeneous in attenuation (Fig. 5), have a target or halo pattern of enhancement (see Fig. 4), or be heterogeneous with areas of high-attenuation hemorrhage and areas of hypoattenuation that reflect hypoperfusion [8].

Lack of mural enhancement is the only direct finding in the intestine that indicates absence of mesenteric blood flow (Fig. 6). The finding of unenhanced segments of bowel wall was shown to have a specificity of 100% for ischemia in the series reported by Zalcman and colleagues [9]. In the series by Taourel and colleagues [10], lack of mural enhancement was one of the findings, in addition to mesenteric vascular occlusion, pneumatosis, and visceral infarction, that increased the sensitivity of CT for the detection of ischemia to greater than 90%. Other authors, however, have noted that, in practice, lack of mural enhancement may be difficult to detect [11].

"Shock bowel" is a term that has been applied to the prolonged enhancement of the small bowel wall in the setting of hypovolemic shock [12]. The finding involves the small bowel diffusely with a normal-appearing colon. The small bowel may be dilated with fluid- or gas-filled segments. Typically, other signs of hypovolemic shock, such as a flattened inferior vena cava, are present. It has

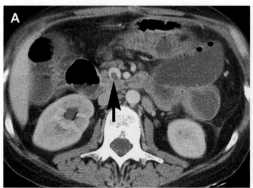
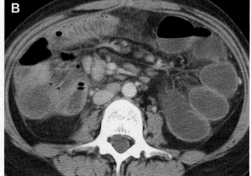

Fig. 3. Partial thrombotic occlusion of the superior mesenteric vein in a 40-year-old woman with protein S deficiency. (*A, B*) Intravenous contrast-enhanced CT scan shows nonoccluding thrombus in the superior mesenteric vein (*arrow* in panel A), dilated small intestine, and an engorged mesentery. Hydronephrosis of the right kidney is present.

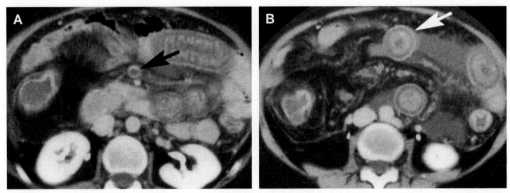

Fig. 4. Acute mesenteric ischemia with small bowel infarction in a 70-year-old man who complained of abdominal pain, nausea, and vomiting. (*A, B*) Intravenous contrast-enhanced CT scan shows hypoattenuating thrombus occluding of the superior mesenteric vein (*arrow* in panel A), an edematous small bowel mesentery, and extensive mural thickening throughout the small intestine with a target pattern of mural enhancement (*arrow* in panel B).

been suggested that prolonged enhancement of the small bowel wall occurs when there is splanchnic vasoconstriction and slowed perfusion. Patients who have shock bowel often have complete recovery with return of the small bowel to normal morphologic appearance, suggesting that the finding represents reversible ischemic changes [12].

The distribution and extent of the intestinal abnormality depends on which artery or vein is compromised. If the superior mesenteric artery or vein is thrombosed or occluded, the entire small intestine, right colon, and proximal transverse colon may be affected. The extent of involvement also is affected by the presence of collateral circulation. In the case of arterial emboli, the distribution and extent of abnormalities vary greatly depending on the caliber and number of vessels affected by emboli. Multifocal abnormalities are present in many cases of emboli ischemia.

The presence of intramural gas (pneumatosis) and portal venous gas usually indicates infarction

and has high specificity (see Fig. 5), but pneumatosis and portal venous gas also may be seen in nonischemic conditions when overdistension, trauma, or inflammatory, infectious, or neoplastic disease severely damages or ulcerates the intestinal mucosa [13]. Wiesner and colleagues [14] showed that bandlike pneumatosis and the combination of pneumatosis and portal venous gas on CT are strongly associated with intestinal infarction, whereas bubblelike pneumatosis and isolated portal venous gas were related to partial mural intestinal ischemia in one third of cases they studied.

In patients who have small bowel obstruction, ischemia is a major cause of morbidity and mortality. Strangulation and ischemia should be suspected in the setting of small bowel obstruction when there is diminished bowel wall enhancement, small bowel feces sign, ascites, diffuse mesenteric haziness, an unusual course of the mesenteric vessels, or diffuse mesenteric haziness (see Fig. 4) [8,15–17]. The sensitivity of CT for the diagnosis of

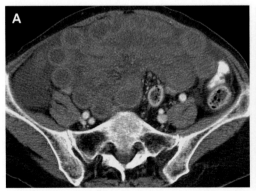
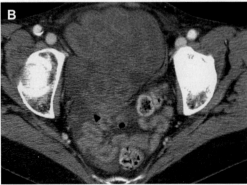

Fig. 5. Small intestinal ischemia in a 76-year-old woman who had a history of uterine prolapse, presented with nausea and vomiting, and was found to have a closed-loop small bowel obstruction. (*A, B*) Intravenous contrast-enhanced CT scans show ascites and a radial distribution of dilated small bowel consistent with a closed-loop obstruction. There is homogenous mural thickening of the involved small bowel.

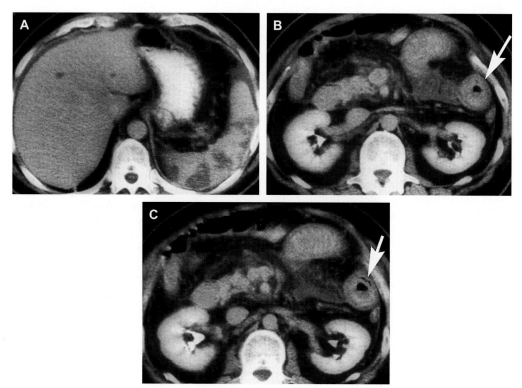

Fig. 6. Small intestinal ischemia and infarction from multiple arterial emboli in a 52-year-old man who had atrial fibrillations. (*A*, *B*, *C*) Intravenous contrast-enhanced CT scan shows multiple splenic infarctions, mesenteric edema, ascites, and mural thickening in the small intestine. Lack of mural enhancement (*arrow* in panel B) and pneumatosis (*arrow* in panel C) are present.

ischemia in small bowel obstruction ranges from 76% to 100%, and its specificity ranges from 60% to 93% [16–18]. The findings of ischemia and strangulation in small bowel obstruction overlap with the findings of uncomplicated small bowel obstruction because mural thickening, small bowel feces sign, mesenteric edema, and ascites commonly are present in cases of uncomplicated small bowel obstruction. Correlating the clinical assessment of the patient with the CT findings may be necessary in equivocal cases [8].

Other CT findings that occur in acute mesenteric ischemia include increased attenuation in the mesentery from mesenteric vascular engorgement or mesenteric fluid, small intestinal dilatation, and ascites. Although these findings are observed commonly in patients who have acute mesenteric ischemia, they generally are not diagnostically helpful because they occur in many other acute abdominal conditions such as pancreatitis, inflammatory bowel disease, peritonitis, and mechanical bowel obstruction. Arterial-phase imaging can aid in the discrimination of ischemia from other disorders because it enables the evaluation of arterial causes of ischemia and also improves bowel wall enhancement.

Chronic mesenteric ischemia

Clinical features

Chronic mesenteric ischemia accounts for less than 5% of all intestinal ischemia and almost always is associated with atherosclerosis of the mesenteric vessels. Chronic mesenteric ischemia has a more insidious presentation than acute mesenteric ischemia. Patients who have chronic mesenteric ischemia generally are elderly, have a heavy smoking history, and have diffuse atherosclerotic vascular disease. Women are affected more than men (female:male ratio, 3:1) [19]. Chronic mesenteric ischemia often is called "abdominal angina" because of the common clinical presentation of pain after eating. Typically, patients may complain postprandial abdominal pain that occurs within 30 minutes after eating that gradually increases in severity and slowly resolves over 1 to 3 hours [1]. Their symptoms generally are present for a long time, sometimes as long as a year before clinical presentation. Fear of eating (sitophobia) may occur in patients who have chronic mesenteric ischemia because they may reluctant to eat or stop eating to avoid the development of pain. As a result, weight loss is common and may be profound. Other symptoms such as nausea, diarrhea, malabsorption, and constipation may occur, but weight loss and postprandial abdominal pain are the most characteristic. On physical examination, the patient may have cachexia. The abdomen usually is soft and nontender.

Etiology and pathogenesis

Chronic mesenteric ischemia most commonly occurs in patients who have atherosclerotic plaque that narrows or occludes the celiac, superior mesenteric, and inferior mesenteric arteries. Less frequent causes include vascular obstructions in fibromuscular dysplasia and Takayasu arteritis. Tumors in the retroperitoneum and mesentery that encase or obstruct the major vessels, radiation injury, and median arcuate ligament syndrome may have similar clinical presentations. Intestinal infarction is uncommon in chronic mesenteric ischemia, because the development of atherosclerosis occurs over a long period of time, and collateral circulation develops to compensate for the loss of blood supply. Patients usually develop symptoms when adequate collateral blood supply does not exist.

CT features

The diagnosis is based on clinical symptoms and the demonstration of occlusive atherosclerotic lesions in the splanchnic arterial supply and exclusion of other gastrointestinal diseases. Occlusions or severe stenoses in at least two of the three major splanchnic vessels (celiac, superior mesenteric, and inferior mesenteric arteries) should be present to consider the diagnosis. In more than half of patients who have chronic mesenteric ischemia, all three vessels are involved [1]. Occasionally, symptoms develop when there is a single occluded vessel, and the remaining two are critically narrowed. CT may show calcified plaque in the aorta and at the origin of the celiac, superior mesenteric, and inferior mesenteric arteries as well as luminal stenoses on arterial-phase imaging. Collateral vessels may be present within the mesentery. The intestine usually is normal in appearance. It is important to exclude extrinsic causes of vascular occlusion such as tumor encasement or compression and other reasons for the patient's symptoms. Multiplanar two-dimensional and three-dimensional reconstructions with MDCT data sets provide a noninvasive alternative to traditional angiography for diagnosis and planning for interventional radiology or surgical management. The degree of stenosis and anatomic configuration of the vessel can be viewed in multiple planes with MDCT.

Summary

Acute and chronic mesenteric ischemia is a difficult clinical diagnosis to establish because the clinical and CT manifestations often are nonspecific and overlap with those of inflammatory, neoplastic, and obstructive disorders of the gastrointestinal tract. Prompt and early diagnosis of mesenteric ischemia requires a high index of suspicion and correlation of CT findings with the patient's clinical symptomatology. Mural thickening is the most common finding identified on CT, and lack of mural enhancement is the most specific finding in patients who have mesenteric ischemia. Lack of mural enhancement may be difficult to observe in practice but should be sought out carefully in patients suspected of having ischemia. MDCT is the imaging examination of choice because it enables the mesenteric vasculature, intestine, and other abdominal structures to be evaluated in a single examination.

References

[1] Brandt LJ. In: Feldman M, Friedman LS, Brandt LJ, editors. Sleisenger and Fordtran's gastrointestinal and liver disease. 8th edition, Intestinal ischemia, Vol 2. Philadelphia: Saunders; 2006. p. 2563–85.

[2] Brunicardi FC, Schwartz SI. Schwartz's principles of surgery. 8th edition. New York: McGraw-Hill, Health Pub. Division; 2005.

[3] Kumar S, Sarr MG, Kamath PS. Mesenteric venous thrombosis. N Engl J Med 2001;345(23): 1683–8.

[4] Trompeter M, Brazda T, Remy CT, et al. Non-occlusive mesenteric ischemia: etiology, diagnosis, and interventional therapy. Eur Radiol 2002; 12(5):1179–87.

[5] Fenoglio-Preiser CM. Gastrointestinal pathology: an atlas and text. 2nd edition. New York: Lippincott-Raven; 1999.

[6] Horton KM, Fishman EK. Multi-detector row CT of mesenteric ischemia: can it be done? Radiographics 2001;21(6):1463–73.

[7] Segatto E, Mortele KJ, Ji H, et al. Acute small bowel ischemia: CT imaging findings. Semin Ultrasound CT MR 2003;24(5):364–76.

[8] Rha SE, Ha HK, Lee SH, et al. CT and MR imaging findings of bowel ischemia from various primary causes. Radiographics 2000;20(1):29–42.

[9] Zalcman M, Sy M, Donckier V, et al. Helical CT signs in the diagnosis of intestinal ischemia in small-bowel obstruction. AJR Am J Roentgenol 2000;175(6):1601–7.

[10] Taourel PG, Deneuville M, Pradel JA, et al. Acute mesenteric ischemia: diagnosis with contrast-enhanced CT. Radiology 1996;199(3):632–6.

[11] Macari M, Balthazar EJ. CT of bowel wall thickening: significance and pitfalls of

interpretation. AJR Am J Roentgenol 2001; 176(5):1105–16.

[12] Mirvis SE, Shanmuganathan K, Erb R. Diffuse small-bowel ischemia in hypotensive adults after blunt trauma (shock bowel): CT findings and clinical significance. AJR Am J Roentgenol 1994;163(6):1375–9.

[13] Smerud MJ, Johnson CD, Stephens DH. Diagnosis of bowel infarction: a comparison of plain films and CT scans in 23 cases. AJR Am J Roentgenol 1990;154(1):99–103.

[14] Wiesner W, Mortele KJ, Glickman JN, et al. Pneumatosis intestinalis and portomesenteric venous gas in intestinal ischemia: correlation of CT findings with severity of ischemia and clinical outcome. AJR Am J Roentgenol 2001;177(6):1319–23.

[15] Balthazar EJ, Birnbaum BA, Megibow AJ, et al. Closed-loop and strangulating intestinal obstruction: CT signs. Radiology 1992;185(3):769–75.

[16] Balthazar EJ, Liebeskind ME, Macari M. Intestinal ischemia in patients in whom small bowel obstruction is suspected: evaluation of accuracy, limitations, and clinical implications of CT in diagnosis. Radiology 1997;205(2):519–22.

[17] Sheedy SP, Earnest Ft, Fletcher JG, et al. CT of small-bowel ischemia associated with obstruction in emergency department patients: diagnostic performance evaluation. Radiology 2006; 241(3):729–36.

[18] Frager D, Baer JW, Medwid SW, et al. Detection of intestinal ischemia in patients with acute small-bowel obstruction due to adhesions or hernia: efficacy of CT. AJR Am J Roentgenol 1996;166(1):67–71.

[19] Cademartiri F, Raaijmakers RH, Kuiper JW, et al. Multi-detector row CT angiography in patients with abdominal angina. Radiographics 2004; 24(4):969–84.

RADIOLOGIC
CLINICS
OF NORTH AMERICA

Radiol Clin N Am 45 (2007) 601–607

Index

Note: Page numbers of article titles are in **boldface** type.

doi:10.1016/S0033-8389(07)00073-5

W

Moving?

Make sure your subscription moves with you!

To notify us of your new address, find your **Clinics Account Number** (located on your mailing label above your name), and contact customer service at:

E-mail: elspcs@elsevier.com

800-654-2452 (subscribers in the U.S. & Canada)
407-345-4000 (subscribers outside of the U.S. & Canada)

Fax number: 407-363-9661

Elsevier Periodicals Customer Service
6277 Sea Harbor Drive
Orlando, FL 32887-4800

*To ensure uninterrupted delivery of your subscription, please notify us at least 4 weeks in advance of move.